Cycling

Editors

ANGELA N. CORTEZ
DANA H. KOTLER

PHYSICAL MEDICINE AND REHABILITATION CLINICS OF NORTH AMERICA

www.pmr.theclinics.com

Consulting Editor
SANTOS F. MARTINEZ

February 2022 • Volume 33 • Number 1

ELSEVIER

1600 John F. Kennedy Boulevard • Suite 1800 • Philadelphia, Pennsylvania, 19103-2899

http://www.theclinics.com

PHYSICAL MEDICINE AND REHABILITATION CLINICS OF NORTH AMERICA Volume 33, Number 1
February 2022 ISSN 1047-9651, 978-0-323-89712-9

Editor: Lauren Boyle
Developmental Editor: Diana Grace Ang

Reprints. For copies of 100 or more of articles in this publication, please contact the Commercial Reprints Department, Elsevier Inc., 360 Park Avenue South, New York, NY 10010-1710. Tel.: 212-633-3874; Fax: 212-633-3820; E-mail: reprints@elsevier.com.

Physical Medicine and Rehabilitation Clinics of North America (ISSN 1047-9651) is published quarterly by Elsevier Inc., 360 Park Avenue South, New York, NY 10010-1710. Months of issue are February, May, August, and November. Business and Editorial Offices: 1600 John F. Kennedy Blvd., Suite 1800, Philadelphia, PA 19103-2899. Customer Service Office: 3251 Riverport Lane, Maryland Heights, MO 63043. Periodicals postage paid at New York, NY and additional mailing offices. Subscription price per year is $332.00 (US individuals), $905.00 (US institutions), $100.00 (US students), $377.00 (Canadian individuals), $932.00 (Canadian institutions), $100.00 (Canadian students), $477.00 (foreign individuals), $932.00 (foreign institutions), and $210.00 (foreign students). Foreign air speed delivery is included in all *Clinics* subscription prices. All prices are subject to change without notice. **POSTMASTER:** Send address changes to *Physical Medicine and Rehabilitation Clinics of North America*, Customer Service Office: Elsevier Health Sciences Division, Subscription Customer Service, 3251 Riverport Lane, Maryland Heights, MO 63043. **Customer Service: 1-800-654-2452 (US). From outside of the United States, call 314-447-8871. Fax: 314-447-8029. E-mail: JournalsCustomer Service-usa@elsevier.com (for print support); JournalsOnlineSupport-usa@elsevier.com (for online support).**

Physical Medicine and Rehabilitation Clinics of North America is indexed in *Excerpta Medica, MEDLINE/ PubMed (Index Medicus), Cinahl, and Cumulative Index to Nursing and Allied Health Literature.*

Contributors

CONSULTING EDITOR

SANTOS F. MARTINEZ, MD, MS
Diplomate, American Academy of Physical Medicine and Rehabilitation; Certificate of Added Qualification Sports Medicine, Assistant Professor, Department of Orthopaedics, Campbell Clinic Orthopaedics, University of Tennessee, Memphis, Tennessee, USA

EDITORS

ANGELA N. CORTEZ, MD
Assistant Professor, H. Ben Taub Department of Physical Medicine and Rehabilitation, Baylor College of Medicine, Houston, Texas, USA

DANA H. KOTLER, MD
Instructor, Physical Medicine and Rehabilitation, Harvard Medical School, Boston, Massachusetts, USA; Director, Cycling Medicine Program, Spaulding Rehabilitation Hospital, Spaulding Outpatient Center – Wellesley, Wellesley, Massachusetts, USA; Newton-Wellesley Hospital, Newton, Massachusetts, USA

AUTHORS

ANNE M. ALTHAUSEN PLANTE, MD
Assistant Professor, Obstetrics and Gynecology, Harvard Medical School, Massachusetts General Hospital, Boston, Massachusetts, USA

ANTJE BARREVELD, MD
Assistant Professor, Anesthesiology, Tufts University School of Medicine, Boston, Massachusetts, USA; Medical Director, Pain Management Services, Newton-Wellesley Hospital, Newton, Massachusetts, USA

DEBORAH BERGFELD, MD
Physical Medicine and Rehabilitation, Department of Neurology, The University of Texas at Austin, Dell Medical School, Austin, Texas, USA

SAURABHA BHATNAGAR, MD
Department of Physical Medicine and Rehabilitation, Harvard Medical School, Spaulding Rehabilitation Hospital, Boston, Massachusetts, USA; US Department of Veterans Affairs, Washington, DC, USA

NAMRITA KUMAR BROOKE, PhD, RD
Adjunct Professor, Department of Movement Sciences and Health, University of West Florida, Pensacola, Florida, USA

ANGELA N. CORTEZ, MD
Assistant Professor, H. Ben Taub Department of Physical Medicine and Rehabilitation, Baylor College of Medicine, Houston, Texas, USA

LUDMILA COSIO-LIMA, PhD
Professor, Exercise Science and Program Coordinator, Department of Movement Sciences and Health, University of West Florida, Pensacola, Florida, USA

DANIEL M. CUSHMAN, MD
Division of Physical Medicine and Rehabilitation, University of Utah, Salt Lake City, Utah, USA

ANDREA CYR, DO
Sports Medicine Fellow, Department of Family Medicine, University of Illinois College of Medicine, UIC Sports Medicine Center, Flames Athletic Center, Chicago, Illinois, USA

NATHAN DOWLING, PT
Department of Physical Therapy, University of Utah, Salt Lake City, Utah, USA

MEREDITH EHN, DO
Division of Physical Medicine and Rehabilitation, University of Utah, Salt Lake City, Utah, USA

CHRISTOPHER GILBERT, AM
Post-Baccalaureate Student, Harvard University Extension, Cambridge, Massachusetts, USA

GABRIELLE T. GOODLIN, MD
Physical Medicine and Rehabilitation, Department of Neurology, The University of Texas at Austin, Dell Medical School, Austin, Texas, USA

ELAINE GREGORY, MD
H. Ben Taub Department of Physical Medicine and Rehabilitation, Baylor College of Medicine, Houston, Texas, USA

MARK GREVE, MD, FACEP
Clinical Assistant Professor, Department of Emergency Medicine, Division of Sports Medicine, Warren Alpert School of Medicine, Brown University, Providence, Rhode Island, USA

ALEXANDRIA HASELHORST, DO
Physical Medicine and Rehabilitation, Department of Neurology, The University of Texas at Austin, Dell Medical School, Austin, Texas, USA

SETH HERMAN, MD
Brain Injury Medical Director, California Rehabilitation Institute, Los Angeles, California, USA

WENDY HOLLIDAY, BSc Physiotherapy, PhD Exercise Science
Department of Human Biology, Division of Exercise Science and Sports Medicine, University of Cape Town, Cape Town, South Africa

MARY ALEXIS IACCARINO, MD
Department of Physical Medicine and Rehabilitation, Harvard Medical School, Spaulding Rehabilitation Hospital, Massachusetts General Hospital, Boston, Massachusetts, USA

STACEY ISIDRO, MD
H. Ben Taub Department of Physical Medicine and Rehabilitation, Baylor College of Medicine, Houston, Texas, USA

TRACEY ISIDRO, MD
H. Ben Taub Department of Physical Medicine and Rehabilitation, Baylor College of Medicine, Houston, Texas, USA

DANA H. KOTLER, MD
Instructor, Physical Medicine and Rehabilitation, Harvard Medical School, Boston, Massachusetts, USA; Director, Cycling Medicine Program, Spaulding Rehabilitation Hospital, Wellesley, Massachusetts, USA; Newton-Wellesley Hospital, Newton, Massachusetts, USA

LAURA LACHMAN, MD
H. Ben Taub Department of Physical Medicine and Rehabilitation, Baylor College of Medicine, Houston, Texas, USA

KOLIE MOORE, BS Biology
Founder and Head Coach, Empirical Cycling, Medford, Massachusetts, USA

ROZANNE M. PULEO, FNP-BC, ONP-C
Sports Medicine, Lynn Community Health Center, Lynn, Massachusetts, USA

SARAH RICE, PhD, DPT
Physical Therapist, Athletico Physical Therapy, Chicago, Illinois, USA

KEVIN RIX, PhD, MPH
Postdoctoral Research Fellow, Penn Injury Science Center, University of Pennsylvania, Philadelphia, Pennsylvania, USA, Dell Seton Medical Center at the University of Texas, Austin, Texas, USA

C. GREG ROBIDOUX, PT
Clinical Specialist, Co-Director, Cycling Medicine Program, Outpatient Physical Therapy, Spaulding Rehabilitation Hospital, Wellesley, Massachusetts, USA

ISABELL SAKAMOTO, MS, CHES
Suicide and Injury Prevention Program Manager, Seattle Children's Hospital, Community Health and Benefit, Seattle, Washington, USA

LINDSEY STEINBECK, MD
Physical Medicine and Rehabilitation, Department of Neurology, The University of Texas at Austin, Dell Medical School, Austin, Texas, USA

JEROEN SWART, MBChB, MPhil (SEM), PhD
Department of Human Biology, Division of Exercise Science and Sports Medicine, University of Cape Town, Cape Town, South Africa

Contents

Cycling biomechanics is a complex analysis of the cyclist and the bicycle. It is important to assess the cyclist dynamically because kinematics and muscle patterns are influenced by their type of riding and fatigue and intensity. Intrinsic factors such as anthropometrics and flexibility should guide the initial bicycle configuration. Static kinematics are a valid and reliable tool in the process of bike fitting, providing an initial fast and cost-effective method of assessing the cyclist. Dynamic assessment methods should then be used to fine tune the bicycle configuration according to the specific needs and workloads of the cyclist.

Cycling has grown in popularity over the past 20 to 30 years, serving as transportation, fitness, and sport. Cycling is unique for several reasons: it is a non–weight-bearing sport, nearly all of the motion is in the sagittal plane, and it is one of the only sports where an individual remains attached to a machine for a long duration. As such, the cycling athlete has unique needs compared with other endurance-based athletes. The complex biomechanical interaction of bicycle and rider requires a systematic process for assessment, which provides the framework for understanding, evaluating, and treating overuse injury in cyclists.

Increased awareness, recognition, and accessibility has led to an increase in the popularity of adaptive cycling. This article aims to provide up-to-date information for clinicians about available adaptations, participation options, and resources. We review the para-cycling classification system and 4 main categories of cycles. There are multiple considerations for fit and customization depending on an individual's disability to improve efficiency and comfort. Virtual platforms that allow riders to train and compete online have grown in popularity among para-cycling communities and offer an alternative to riding outdoors. Many national and local

Para-cycling has high rates of acute injuries. The underlying medical conditions of para-athletes predispose these cyclists to injury patterns and sequelae different from those of their able-bodied counterparts. Such injuries include an increased incidence of upper-extremity and soft tissue injuries, along with predisposition for respiratory, skin, genitourinary, and heat-related illnesses. There are no validated sideline assessment tools or return-to-play protocols for sports-related concussion in wheelchair user para-athletes or those with balance deficits. Para-cyclists may be at increased risk for relative energy deficiency in sport due to competitive pressure to maintain certain weights and increased incidence of low bone mineral density.

Previously a male-dominated activity, female cyclists now make up nearly half of all cyclists in the United States. Although cycling provides a significant number of health benefits, it is an activity that carries risk of injury, both traumatic and nontraumatic. Sex differences are seen in chest trauma and breast injury, as well as pelvic, given the inherent differences in anatomy. Understanding the relationship of the bicycle to the anatomy of the rider can help mitigate risks for injury.

Triathlon is an increasingly popular sport that includes swimming, cycling, followed by running. The triathlete should not be seen merely as a cyclist who also swims and runs. Notable differences are seen in the type of bike used, training patterns, lower extremity demands, and cumulative nature of the sport. Injury prevention and treatment strategies need to take into account the triathlon distance, the type of bike used, athletic experience, prior injuries, risk factors, and a thorough understanding of the demands placed on the body through all 3 disciplines (swim, bike, and run).

Cycling is an important form of exercise, recreation, and transportation. Following traumatic brain injury, the benefits of cycling for health, fitness, and community mobility must be considered alongside potential risk for recurrent injury. In addition to medical concerns and exercise tolerance, key domains include motor function, attention, and visuospatial and executive function, which have previously been explored with regard to driving.

Cycling skill is a combination of cognitive and motor function, and can be trained with appropriate education and intervention. We discuss the relationship of brain injury rehabilitation to specific features of cycling, including case studies.

After cycling crashes, orthopedic and neurologic complaints are often the focus of evaluation and management. However, the trauma sustained may not be limited to physical injury; psychological issues brought on by or co-morbid with the crash also warrant treatment. In this original research, we evaluated the presence of fear or anxiety after cycling crashes and examined factors associated with this mechanism of injury through a survey. Post-crash fear or anxiety was associated with female gender, a history of depression, and greater crash severity. Few cyclists received treatment and most returned to cycling at their previous level, but the timeline varied.

The focus of this article centers on bicycle injury prevention and related infrastructure. The article discusses the current epidemiology of cycling injuries, and known prevention strategies, specifically individual recommended practices related to helmet use in both adult and pediatric populations. The article also discusses different ways in which the environment plays a role in protecting cyclists from injuries, and what environmental changes have been adopted to reduce the likelihood for cycling injuries.

The overall activity of cycling, although profoundly heterogenous, often occurs with mechanisms consistent with motor vehicle collisions. Advanced trauma life support is the standard of care. Traumatic brain injury is the leading cause of death, and concussions are common in cyclists. Road rash is the most common injury, and management should be synonymous with other kinds of burns. A unique aspect of cycling medicine is that it often is done on public roadways in close proximity to the athletes during competition. Clinicians who care for cyclists in the field setting should be prepared to manage a broad spectrum of traumatic injuries.

Cycling is predominantly an endurance sport in which fuel utilization for energy production relies on the availability and delivery of oxygen to exercising muscle. Nutrition and training interventions to improve endurance performance are continually evolving, but ultimately, prescription should aim to generate improvements in cycling power and velocity while prioritizing athlete health and well-being. The wide range of cycling events and the different environments in which events take place pose a variety of nutrition-related challenges for cyclists. This review addresses some of these challenges and highlights recent advancements in nutrition for cycling performance.

Guiding cyclists in their return from illness and injury can be managed in many ways. Understanding how cyclists use power-derived training metrics can give care providers a common language to aid in this return. A general understanding of these metrics may be used to monitor cyclists for signs of nonfunctional overreaching or overtraining. Understanding aspects of training and detraining, particularly hematological, is helpful in communicating fitness expectations. Three populations of cyclists are discussed in terms of their expected knowledge of these metrics, typical training volume and intensity, and relationship with a coach or coaches.

Upper extremity nerve injuries in cyclists include carpal tunnel syndrome and ulnar neuropathy at the wrist. Electromyography and nerve conduction studies aid in the diagnosis of neuropathies. Diagnostic ultrasonography or MRI can also be helpful for evaluation. Overuse injuries in the upper extremity includes biker's elbow, or a tendinopathy of the common flexor or extensor tendons, which is more common in mountain biking. Neck pain is also a common issue for cyclists. Treatment of these conditions varies from conservative management to surgical options, but a bicycle fit assessment is recommended for any ongoing symptoms.

Both lower extremities and lower back are common sources of injury for cyclists. For providers to optimize care within this area of sports medicine, they need to understand the most common sources of injury in this population. Cycling presents a unique challenge: treating both the athlete and the complex relationship between rider and bicycle. Physicians should not replace the role of a professional bike fitter and should view these individuals as integral members of the team to alleviate current and prevent future injury. This article explores common lower extremity and lumbar back overuse injuries in cyclists and their medical management.

PHYSICAL MEDICINE AND REHABILITATION CLINICS OF NORTH AMERICA

SERIES OF RELATED INTEREST

Orthopedic Clinics
https://www.orthopedic.theclinics.com/
Neurologic Clinics
https://www.neurologic.theclinics.com/
Clinics in Sports Medicine
https://www.sportsmed.theclinics.com/

VISIT THE CLINICS ONLINE!
Access your subscription at:
www.theclinics.com

Foreword
Cycling to the Finish

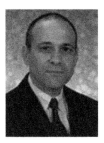

Santos F. Martinez, MD, MS
Consulting Editor

My first memories regarding cycling take me back to when I was about 5 or 6 years old and my older brother (8 years old) was so kind to mentor me. The technique went something like this. You found a hill, and with precision, pushed the unsuspecting novice down it, and of course, the first commandment was to keep pedaling. Naturally, you needed a protective barrier at the bottom, which in our case was the garage. Unfortunately, it was not until my second lesson that I learned about brakes. I do not think this is what they had in mind when using the epigram of "hitting the wall." It is amazing how your proficiency improves after a few scrapes and collisions. Naturally, the incentive in those days was for recreational purposes, as kids were riding bicycles with their friends for hours. Jump ahead 50 years, and my younger brother, George, developed such a passion for cycling that he and a couple of friends bought a bicycle shop (Oconee Outfitters) in our small college town of Milledgeville, Georgia. Yes, cycling has become a boom even in small town America.

There are a number of contributing factors for the increased growth and visibility of cycling globally. It is a cost-effective means of transportation and fitness, not only for able-bodied individuals but also for those who may have certain restrictions and limitations. In some cases, it becomes a family event that can be enjoyed across generations. The dominance of running as the preeminent option for cardiovascular fitness is also making a transition as our aging population looks for joint-conservation options. Cycling certainly provides cardiovascular benefits, and a recent *JAMA* article among others reports reductions in all-cause mortality by greater than 20%. Add to this is a more environmentally conscious culture with growth of dedicated municipality-protected lanes and off-road paths. The growth in sales particularly during the pandemic has been demonstrated by sales across the board from mountain bikes to hybrid e-bikes. Even sales for children's bikes were increased greater than 50%. Because of the various shutdowns, marketing also focused on cycling equipment for home indoor exercise with socially connected exercise classes and training. It is not clear how these sales patterns may revert as society reaches normalization, but our culture and use of

Phys Med Rehabil Clin N Am 33 (2022) xiii–xiv
https://doi.org/10.1016/j.pmr.2021.10.001
1047-9651/22/© 2021 Published by Elsevier Inc.

cycling probably will never reach the levels found in countries such as Denmark and the Netherlands.

Cycling also provides an outlet for those who want to challenge their competitive spirit, with a number of clubs and racing options. This certainly brings in a number of sports-specific medical and training considerations, which is the subject of this issue. The issue certainly is not an all-inclusive text on cycling medicine but attempts to give an across-the-board glimpse of factors of interest for the Physiatrist assisting with providing care from the casual cyclist to the more involved medical coverage of events. No matter your proclivity, there is a race for you, whether against yourself or for the enjoyment of other competitors. Be careful with the wall.

I would like to thank Dr Cortez, Dr Kotler, and their respective authors for making this issue possible.

Santos F. Martinez, MD, MS
Physical Medicine and Rehabilitation
Department of Orthopaedic Surgery and
Biomedical Engineering
University of Tennessee College of Medicine
Campbell Clinic
Memphis, TN 38104, USA

E-mail address:
smartinez@campbellclinic.com

Preface

Cycling Medicine

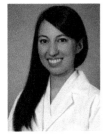 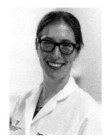

Angela N. Cortez, MD   Dana H. Kotler, MD
Editors

It is our honor to present the first issue of Cycling Medicine for the *Physical Medicine and Rehabilitation Clinics of North America*. We are cycling medicine physicians and dedicated cyclists; as such, we are invested in the enrichment of this growing field. Our contributing authors have a wide range of expertise, and all share a commitment to improving athlete performance, improving safety, and facilitating return from injury.

Cycling commands unique attention within sports medicine. It takes various forms, including recreation, sport, and transportation for a diverse population of athletes and commuters. The physician must consider both the cyclist and the bicycle and the respective demands across various disciplines and over various terrain, from city streets to mountain trails. To capture this complexity, review articles in this issue focus on cycling biomechanics and performance, specific populations, and emerging research in the field. This includes several articles discussing common cycling injuries, both acute and chronic, as well as articles on biomechanics and performance. Highlighted populations include the female cyclist, the adaptive cyclist, and the triathlete.

The assembled issue attempts to combine best practices for cycling injury rehabilitation and prevention with forward-thinking research focused on gaps in current cycling medicine knowledge. We hope this issue can serve as a valuable resource for clinicians, cyclists, and medical staff. We would like to thank all the outstanding

Phys Med Rehabil Clin N Am 33 (2022) xv–xvi
https://doi.org/10.1016/j.pmr.2021.09.001
1047-9651/22/© 2021 Published by Elsevier Inc.

authors for their efforts on this issue and their important ongoing contributions to the field of cycling medicine.

Angela N. Cortez, MD
Baylor Medicine
7200 Cambridge Street, #A10.264
MS: BCM635
Houston, TX 77030, USA

Dana H. Kotler, MD
Spaulding Outpatient Center – Wellesley
65 Walnut Street, Suite 250
Wellesley, MA 02481, USA

E-mail addresses:
angela.cortez@bcm.edu (A.N. Cortez)
dkotler@mgh.harvard.edu (D.H. Kotler)

A Dynamic Approach to Cycling Biomechanics

Wendy Holliday, BSc Physiotherapy, PhD Exercise Science*, Jeroen Swart, MBChB, MPhil (SEM), PhD

KEYWORDS

- Bicycle • Biomechanics • Kinetics • Kinematics • EMG • Static • Dynamic
- Posture

KEY POINTS

- With increasing cycling intensity and fatigue, joint kinematics and muscle patterns alter.
- Increased hamstring flexibility is associated with a more aerodynamic position and an increased power output.
- The comfort and individual anthropometrics of cyclists need to be taken into account.
- Dynamic assessment of the cyclist is recommended to fine tune the optimal position.

INTRODUCTION

Cycling is a dynamic sport that has become increasingly popular over the years. Cycling biomechanics is a complex analysis of both the cyclist and the bicycle. It is important to consider both aspects to fully understand the science of bike fitting. To date there are many static methods used to configure the bicycle optimally; however, with the advancement of technology, 2-dimensional (2D) and 3-dimensional (3D) dynamic methods are now being used more routinely.[1] Likewise, there is a growing body of literature pertaining to how the cyclists' kinematics and muscle patterns are influenced by fatigue, speed, and intensity.

Bike fitting methods should be developed with an evidence-based approach. An emerging body of research is now available to guide such methods. A cyclist usually seeks a bike fitting consultation for 2 primary reasons: to improve their performance or their comfort.[2–4] Bike fitting can be grouped into 2 categories: the optimal range fit and the accommodated fit.[5] The optimal range fit is defined as a set of variables that the fitter is able to accomplish whereby the cyclist is positioned within optimal ranges for the type of cycling they are partaking in, that is, the ideal individualized position that meets the goals of the cyclist is met. Whereas the accommodated fit is considered when there are limitations, either owing to the cyclist's own limitations (eg, flexibility)

Department of Human Biology, Division of Exercise Science and Sports Medicine, University of Boundary Rd, Newlands, Cape Town 7700, South Africa
* Corresponding author.
E-mail address: hllwen005@myuct.ac.za

Phys Med Rehabil Clin N Am 33 (2022) 1–13
https://doi.org/10.1016/j.pmr.2021.08.001
1047-9651/22/© 2021 Elsevier Inc. All rights reserved.

or to components of the bicycle that are not ideally sized (eg, the frame or integrated stem and handlebars). An unsurpassed position is when the bicycle is optimally configured to the cyclist and the cyclist is considered to be in an ideal, comfortable, and sustainable position on the bicycle. To achieve this unsurpassed position, the individual anthropometrics, flexibility, training history, type of cycling, and comfort of the cyclist needs to be taken into account. Previous methods used for configuring the bicycle have not always considered comfort, and thus cyclists may have experienced a degree of discomfort to perform optimally.[2] Nor did the previous methods take into consideration individual characteristics such as leg length, flexibility, and pedaling technique.[6] These factors should be considered during the customizing of the configuration for comfort. The other common goal of most sports participants is to improve their performance. Similarly, the recommended ranges for performance do not always consider individual variations of technique or type of training and racing.

This review explores the current existing literature pertaining to the influence of intrinsic factors on individual bicycle configuration, the different methods of bicycle configuration (namely, static and dynamic kinematics), and the change in the cyclist's kinematics and muscle magnitudes during both steady state cycling and increasing workloads.

The keywords used in the search of literature were bicycle, biomechanics, kinetics, kinematics, EMG, static, dynamic, comfort, and posture.

FULL BODY KINEMATICS

Bicycle configuration guidelines should consider the body position adopted during training or racing.[7] Bini and colleagues[7] investigated the different body positions of cyclists and triathletes on the bicycle. A large difference in bicycle configuration and body position between competitive cyclists and competitive triathletes was demonstrated, specifically with regard to the frontal area and trunk and pelvic angles. Competitive triathletes demonstrated significantly lower frontal areas compared with competitive cyclists, with greater anterior knee projections and greater trunk and pelvic angles. This aggressive position is adopted by triathletes to decrease their frontal surface area and the resultant aerodynamic drag.[8] Only a moderate difference was demonstrated between competitive and recreational cyclists' trunk angles.[7] A limitation of this study was the use of static poses, which may differ during dynamic cycling analysis, and it was suggested that further research should compare joint kinematics during a dynamic assessment.[7] Similarly, dynamic bike fitting should be conducted at the intensity that a cyclist will perform the majority of their training or racing in.[9]

Peveler and colleagues[9] compared the alterations to ankle and knee angles when transitioning from a static position to active pedaling. This work demonstrated differences in both ankle and knee angles, as well as demonstrating a difference in joint kinematics with increasing cycling intensities. The ankle plantarflexion and knee flexion angle were significantly lower at higher intensities. The increase into ankle dorsiflexion at higher intensities may be due to the cyclists compensating to overcome the ergometer saddle height setting of 25° knee flexion angle, not at the cyclist's own freely chosen configuration.

Those results were similar to another study that did configure the test subjects' bicycles to match their own preferred setup.[10] Their results also indicated an increase in ankle dorsiflexion with an increase in workload. It was proposed that this increase was caused by the greater forces being applied on the pedal at higher intensities. The ankle joint functions to transfer force from the legs to the crank.[11] The changes in ankle mean angles into dorsiflexion with increased intensity may be attributable to cyclists adapting their pedaling technique to overcome fatigue and the higher workload, as well as trying to maintain a controlled pedaling cadence.[9,12,13]

An increase in knee and hip extension was also demonstrated at maximal workloads[11,12] and could be linked to a shift in forward position on the bicycle.[13] Cyclists, using their own bicycles at their preferred bicycle configuration, may intuitively move forward on the saddle to enhance the contribution of knee joint extensor muscles to deliver power on the pedal.[14] However, when the cyclist's saddle height was not set according to their freely chosen position, this factor could have resulted in the cyclists changing their ankle and knee angles during the test to pedal within a knee flexion angle that they were accustomed to.[9]

Holliday and colleagues[15] investigated how 3 different cycling intensities affected kinematics and muscle activity during cycling. Cyclists were investigated using an ergometer position matching their own freely chosen bicycle position. There were significant changes in joint angles between 60%, 80%, and 90% intensity. The elbow and thoracic and lumbar spine all adopted a more flexed position with an increase in intensity. As with previous research,[11,12] the ankle moved into greater dorsiflexion, and subsequently the knee adopted a more extended position. They recommend that the use of dynamic measuring methods should consider knee flexion angle in relation to the riding intensity, with the suggestion that optimal dynamic knee flexion angle should range from 33° to 43° at low intensity and 30° to 40° at a higher intensity.[15]

The only other study to date that has assessed the relationship between workload intensity and 3D kinematics demonstrated no workload effects on any of the variables.[16] However, only hip adduction, thigh rotation, shank rotation, pelvis inclination, and spine inclination and rotation were analyzed. The main findings were small to moderate difference in lateral spine inclination and spine rotation between recreational and competitive cyclists.[16]

MUSCLE ACTIVITY

Cyclists train and compete at different intensities, yet it remains unclear how muscle activity is affected by cycling at different intensities. The typical muscle activation pattern displayed during cycling has been studied in more depth owing to the recent advances in technology.[17] For simplification, the pedal revolution can be divided into 4 quadrants, starting with the crank at the top dead center position (0°/TDC). Quadrant 1 corresponds with 0° to 90°, quadrant 2 corresponds with 90° to 180°, quadrant 3 corresponds with 180° to 270°, and quadrant 4 corresponds with 270° to 360°. Quadrants 1 and 2 are variably described as the active, push phase, or knee extension phase, with the foot pushing down on the pedal. Quadrants 3 and 4 are described as the passive, pull phase, or knee flexion phase, where the pedal returns to the TDC position. The gluteus maximus (GMax) is a powerful hip extender and is active during the push phase; from TDC to approximately 130° of the crank rotation cycle. The vastus lateralis oblique and vastus medialis oblique extend the knee and are activated from just before the TDC position and terminate activation at just beyond 90°. The rectus femoris (RF) is a biarticular muscle and works to flex the hip, as well as extend the knee. It is active from approximately 270° to 90°. The tibialis anterior (TA) functions to dorsiflex the ankle, activating from 270° to lift the foot over the TDC and terminates shortly afterward. The gastrocnemius muscles are also biarticular muscles and plantarflex the foot and flex the knee. They activate just after the termination of TA at ±30° and work until 270° in plantarflexing the ankle and therefore acting as the final lever applying force from the foot to the pedal, until the start of the knee flexion phase.

The hamstring muscles have shown greater variability in research studies, with some demonstrating activation from just after TDC through to the bottom dead center position of the crank, or variably until 270°.[18,19] The hamstrings are biarticular muscles, which are active in the transfer of energy at specific times in the pedaling cycle, and in the control of force direction on the pedal, whereas the uniarticular muscles have been linked to being the primary power producers.[17]

Uniarticular muscles are classified as muscles that have their origin and insertion only crossing 1 joint, for example, the TA muscle, which originates from the tibial condyle and crosses the ankle joint to insert into the medial cuneiform and first metatarsal. Biarticular muscles will thus cross 2 joints between origin and insertion, such as the RF which originates from the anterior superior iliac spine and crosses the hip and knee joint to insert into the patella via the quadriceps tendon. Biarticular muscles are complex to understand; however, they are thought to transfer force between the joints and control the direction of the movement.[20] Prilutsky and Gregor[21] suggested that fatigue and rating of perceived exertion may be decreased by preferential activation of biarticular muscles during certain phases of the cycling movement, as well as coactivation of uniarticular muscles with their biarticular antagonists. More recently, the muscle coordination during an all-out sprint cycling task was investigated.[22] Fifteen well-trained cyclists performed 2 submaximal exercises, followed by an all-out seated sprint at 80% of their optimal pedaling rate. The relative contribution of all of the lower limb muscles tested displayed a significant change between the submaximal and maximal cycling exercises. The increase in the duration of all muscle activity during the sprint is suggestive of a strategy to enhance the work generated by each of the muscle groups. During the all-out sprint, there was a large increase in hip flexor activity, a lesser extent to the knee flexor activity, whereas the plantarflexors and knee extensors displayed an even smaller increase. The large increase in activity of the RF muscle during an all-out sprint is possibly explained by its biarticular function, and the authors suggested that it functions largely as a hip flexor during the sprint.[22] During a 60-minute self-paced cycling time trial, participants were asked to perform a 1 minute all-out sprint every 10 minutes.[23] There was a decrease in RF electromyography (EMG) activity during the cycling sprints, which may be indicative of an alteration in the coordination pattern of the cycling movement with the development of fatigue and it is possible that alternative muscles are recruited as fatigue accumulates in working muscles. All of these studies were investigated at maximal power or to exhaustion, and it is difficult to distinguish the change in EMG activity levels with regard to the effects of power output increases or the onset of muscle fatigue.

Blake and colleagues[24] and Holliday and colleagues[15] demonstrated similar results, indicating that there was a general increase in muscle activation as intensity increased. Both studies demonstrated an increase in EMG activity of TA and RF across the top of the pedal stroke. The GMax demonstrated the largest significant change from a low to a high workload, whereas the vastus medialis oblique, vastus lateralis oblique, and biceps femoris all demonstrated significant changes in activity in the quadrant they are most active in.[15] The medial and lateral gastrocnemius demonstrated an early plateau in activity when transitioning from low to high workloads, suggesting that these muscles are already recruited at relatively low workloads as they transfer force from the relatively larger GM, vastus medialis oblique, and vastus lateralis oblique to the pedal. As such their relatively smaller muscle mass may require greater recruitment throughout cycling intensities.[15] Racing at a workload of 55% to 60%, the Vo_{2max} has been suggested as a strategic way to maximize power output while minimizing the risk of early fatigue.[24] Dingwell and colleagues[14] established that, as fatigue occurs, cyclists may change their muscle activation patterns to maintain performance, and this change subsequently may lead to maladaptive joint loading caused by changes in kinematics with fatigue. Thus, strengthening muscles at their specific ranges in the pedal revolution could be beneficial to optimizing riding position and muscle activity (**Table 1**).

ANTHROPOMETRICS AND BICYCLE CONFIGURATION

There are several methods based on anthropometric characteristics that have been described in attempts to optimally configure the bicycle.[28,29] These recommendations are based on existing biomechanical research outside of the field of cycling as well as personal opinion based on experience.

Optimal saddle height, which is the most discussed aspect of bicycle configuration, is determined by leg length measurements and knee flexion angle.[30,31] It has been recommended that the optimal saddle height should take into account individual femur and tibial leg length variations.[32] Similarly, the crank length is commonly determined by the individual leg length, with a ratio of approximately 20% of the in-seam length being recommended.[33] More recently, Holliday and Swart[34] demonstrated similar results to previous studies, and that the optimal saddle height can be determined by leg length measurement.

It has been recommended that the length of an individual's foot and femur should also be taken into consideration when determining the cleat position and saddle setback, respectively.[28] The handlebar reach and handlebar drop position have been described more subjectively, with full arm and upper body length described as being important considerations in optimal frame size, stem length and handlebar height.[29]

FLEXIBILITY AND BICYCLE CONFIGURATION

An assessment of the cyclist's lower back and hamstring flexibility plays an important role in bike fitting.[35] Lumbosacral and hamstring flexibility has been correlated with an increased saddle height.[34] Burke[8] demonstrated similar results where a lower saddle height was selected by cyclists with decreased flexibility of the hamstring muscles; however, this outcome was contradicted by the results of the study by Hynd and associates,[36] who determined that hamstring flexibility did not have an effect on preselected saddle height.

It was hypothesized that a cyclist's spinal flexibility may have an influence on handlebar reach and handlebar drop34, however, there were nonsignificant results. Despite this finding, there was a significant association between hamstring flexibility and a lower handlebar drop position.[34] They concluded that the greater hamstring flexibility allows greater anterior rotation of the pelvis, which allows the cyclist to reach further and lower thereby adopting a more aerodynamic position. This finding is also relevant to the cycling discipline in triathlon, which is often performed as a time trial, and therefore may require a greater upper body flexion to decrease the frontal area for optimal aerodynamics.[8]

Fewer than 50% of experienced cyclists met the recommended standards for flexibility and strength in a study conducted to assess intrinsic and extrinsic factors related to injury of club-level cyclists.[37] Only 22% to 25% of the participants met the required definition of good or okay for the active knee extension test, indicating that fewer than one-quarter of the participants had acceptable hamstring flexibility. Additionally, cyclists who had undergone bike fitting for optimal performance and aerodynamics still reported some degree of discomfort.[37]

Table 1
Workload effects on lower limb muscle recruitment pattern

Study	Muscles Used for EMG Analysis	Aims of Study	Testing Method	No. of Subjects	Main Results and Notes
Ericson et al,[25] 1985	GMax, VLO, RF, VMO, BF, ST, GM	EMG activity during different workloads	Power output increased from 120 W to 240 W	11 healthy subjects	An increase in workload significantly increased the mean maximum activity in all the muscles investigated.
Hautier et al,[26] 2000	GMax, RF, VLO, LG, BF	EMG changes during fatigue produced by repeated maximal sprints	15 repeated 5-s sprints, with a 25-s rest period between each sprint.	8 male subjects 2 female subjects All trained for 9 wk and detrained for 7 wk	GMax and VL remained unchanged after maximal cycling sprints, however the force and power required was reduced. After fatigue, BF and LG were less activated. There is an adaptation of the muscular coordination pattern to transfer force and power to the pedal.
Laplaud et al,[27] 2006	VLO, RF, VMO, SM, BF, LG, MG, TA	Investigate the reproducibility of 8 lower limb muscles activity levels during a pedaling exercise performed to exhaustion	2 × incremental test until exhaustion	8 healthy male subjects	Good reproducibility of activity level of muscles during a progressive pedaling exercise performed until exhaustion. Subnote: All muscles demonstrated an increase in RMS values throughout the incremental exercise.

Dingwell et al,[14] 2008	VLO, BF, LG, TA	Changes in movement kinematics and muscle activity as fatigue progresses.	Cycled at 100% VO_{2max} until exhaustion	7 highly trained male cyclists	Significant muscle fatigue in BF and LG across all subjects. Muscle fatigue preceded changes in trunk angle.
Blake et al,[24] 2012	TA, MG, LG, Sol, VMO, RF, VLO, ST, BF, GMax	To determine muscle timing and coordination, pedal force application and total muscle activity the maximizes cycling efficiency.	3-min intervals at 25%, 40%, 55%, 60%, 75%, and 90% VO_{2max}	9 experienced competitive male cyclists.	Muscle coordination patterns vary with workload. GMax increased activity from low to high resistance. RF and TA demonstrated increased intensity across the TDC with increasing resistance. To maximize the muscle coordination patterns used in competition, it was suggested that cyclists' train in similar conditions.
Holliday et al,[15] 2019	GMax, VMO, VLO, TA, RF, MG, BF	To assess how muscle recruitment patterns are influenced by different workloads	3 intensities: 60%, 80% and 90% of maximum heart rate	17 well-trained male cyclists.	Muscle recruitment patterns vary with workload, there were significant increases in EMG signal for all muscles at higher intensities.

Abbreviations: BF, biceps femoris; GMax, gluteus maximus; LG, lateral gastrocnemius; MG, medial gastrocnemius; RF, rectus femoris; RMS, root mean square; ST, semitendinosus; SM, semimembranosus; Sol, soleus muscles; TA, tibialis anterior; TDC, top dead center; VMO, vastus medialis oblique; VLO, vastus lateralis oblique.

PERFORMANCE GOALS

One of the main goals of bike fitting is to improve performance.[5,29,38] Optimal saddle height for performance has been well-researched; however, other variables related to bicycle configuration and power are largely based on empirical suggestions[8,28,29,38] and limited scientific studies. A recent study demonstrated a greater handlebar drop was associated with an increased relative peak power output.[39] A greater saddle setback was also associated with an increased absolute peak power output.[39] The saddle fore–aft position alters the effective seat tube angle and determines the relative muscle contributions to the pedal force.[40,41] For example, a forward saddle position was associated with a greater peak of the quadriceps muscles during the first one-half of the crank rotation, whereas a greater peak of the GMax, plantarflexors, and hamstring muscles was demonstrated at a further rearwards saddle position.[40] Further research demonstrated that a steeper effective seat tube angle resulted in a significant increase of the RF muscle activity, particularly during the downstroke, which is an important phase for power production.[42]

Another variable that has not been studied in detail is the relationship between flexibility and cycling performance. No significant differences were demonstrated between successful and less successful cyclists' hamstring, iliopsoas, and quadriceps flexibility characteristics.[43] Holliday and Swart[39] investigated 50 well-trained cyclists and demonstrated that increased hamstring flexibility was associated with a significantly greater relative Vo_{2max} and relative peak power output.[39] A review of running-related literature concluded that there are mixed results with regard to flexibility and greater running economy; however, the overall opinion was that increased flexibility improved performance.[44] This finding should be explored further with regard to cycling and optimal performance.

COMFORT AND INDIVIDUAL RIDING STYLE

Cyclists' perceptions of comfort should be considered as they are related to improvements in performance and injury prevention.[3] An online survey identifying factors contributing to bicycle comfort was conducted and, of the 244 respondents, 90% of the cyclists agreed that comfort is a concern when riding a bicycle, whereas 46% of enthusiastic cyclists agree that comfort is reached at the expense of performance.[2] A recreational cyclist will generally prefer to sit more upright, whereas a competitive cyclist will want to be positioned in a more aerodynamic position, adopting a greater trunk flexion angle.[3] There are further differences between cyclists, with novice cyclists demonstrating greater variability in the pedaling technique than a more experienced cyclist[9] and these should be considered during bike fitting.

DYNAMIC BIKE FITTING

To date, there are many static methods used to configure the bicycle optimally.[1] With the advancement of technology, 2D and 3D dynamic kinematic methods are increasingly being used, but there is a paucity of scientific evidence with respect to reference points recommended for the optimal fit. The ability to capture data during real-time cycling enables the bike fitter to assess the body position dynamically, yet the recommended joint angle ranges from static bike fitting cannot be interchanged with dynamic methods.[45,46]

The kinematic comparison of alterations to knee and ankle angles from resting measures to active pedaling during a graded exercise protocol has been investigated, and it was established that knee and ankle angles changed significantly from a stationary position to a dynamic pedaling action measured using 2D video analysis.[9]

Comparing static (Holmes method) with dynamic (photogrammetry of reflective markers for 3D analysis) measures of the lower limb joint angles during cycling demonstrated significant changes for both the ankle and knee joint when transitioning from static to dynamic.[47] Ankle plantarflexion and knee flexion angle increased by approximately 8° from static to dynamic measures.

In another study, dynamic knee flexion angles measured with an electrogoniometer and a high-speed camera (2D kinematics) were significantly underestimated when compared with 3D kinematics.[48] The knee flexion angle as measured with a goniometer was also underestimated compared with 3D and 2D kinematics. The authors suggested that goniometer use should be discouraged for bike fitting, and that precise 2D video analysis can only be reached by adding a 2.2° correction factor to the knee angle assessment.[48]

Holliday and colleagues[45] compared 2 static methods (goniometer and inclinometer) with 3D motion capture and, although all 3 measurement methods were reliable, the typical error of measurement between sessions was higher for 3D motion capture then the static methods. It was concluded that static methods are not interchangeable with 3D motion capture, and new dynamic joint angle recommendations should be established, taking into consideration workload.[45,46]

Kinematics measured in 3D are considered more accurate compared with 2D systems, because the 2D systems cannot measure movement in the transverse plane[49] and, despite the small sample size, there were frontal plane differences in the ankle joint ranges between 2D and 3D assessments.[50]

Using a 3D motion analysis system, the implications for iliotibial band friction syndrome during force and repetition in cycling were investigated.[51] The saddle height for each participant was set with the knee at 25° to 30° flexion at bottom dead center by using a goniometer before the start of the trial. During the cycling tests, the knee flexion angle, as measured with a 3D motion analysis system, reached 30° to 35°, and upon further investigation it was determined that lateral pelvic rocking contributed 5° to 6° to this knee flexion angle increase. The authors thus recommended a dynamic knee flexion angle of 30° to 40° as the optimal range when measured dynamically. Holliday and colleagues[15] recommend that this range take relative workload into account, with a dynamic knee flexion angle of 33° to 43° for low intensity and 30° to 40° for a higher intensity.[15]

Based on these findings, Bini and colleagues,[47] Fonda and colleagues,[48] and Farrell and colleagues[51] have all suggested that kinematic rather than static analysis should be used to assess the lower limb cycling motion and to optimize bike fit. Practically, it has been suggested that a high speed 2D video system with the correction factor would be suitable for commercial bike fitting centers, but that scientific studies should use 3D motion analysis for knee angle assessment during cycling, because it had the most valid results.[48]

SUMMARY AND FUTURE DIRECTIONS

The bike fitting industry, both bike fitting and bike fitting technology, has seen an exceptional growth in the past few years. With the advancement of technology and measuring systems, bicycle configuration has become a science rather than the art form it was back in the formative years of cycling. Furthermore, intrinsic factors that may affect bicycle configuration are now being taken into account to achieve that unsurpassed position where the bicycle is configured optimally to the cyclist and the cyclist is considered to be in an optimal position on the bicycle.

The previous methods of using static measurements for bike fitting cannot be translated to dynamic methods. Static bike fitting may be advantageous because it is a simple, less costly method and highly reliable[45,52]; however, a dynamic method is a more accurate representation of the cyclist's position and movement, especially during increases in workload.[9,15] Dynamic kinematic measurements differ depending on the cyclists' relative power output and should be assessed at relative power outputs according to the cyclists racing needs.[15]

Dynamic bike fitting is recommended for high quality assessment and correction of bike fit; however, owing to the time-consuming process of measuring and analyzing dynamic methods, it has been suggested that a progressive approach that commences with a static fit to correct gross abnormalities and progresses to dynamic assessment to improve final outcomes.[1] The use of static methods to measure joint angles can be used to guide the initial position for saddle height, saddle setback, handlebar reach, and handlebar drop because these methods are easy to perform, reliable, time efficient, and inexpensive.[45] Bike fitting should also be viewed as an ongoing process, because a cyclists' performance parameters, strength, and flexibility may adapt as they train for specific races. The individual variables such as riding style, stature, arm and leg length, flexibility and performance of cyclists should be considered when configuring their bicycle into an optimal position.

CLINICS CARE POINTS

- With increasing cycling intensity and fatigue, joint kinematics and muscle patterns alter.
- Increased hamstring flexibility is associated with a more aerodynamic position and an increased power output.
- Comfort and individual anthropometrics of cyclists need to be taken into account.
- Dynamic assessment of the cyclist is recommended to fine tune the optimal position.

DISCLOSURE

The authors have nothing to disclose.

REFERENCES

1. Swart J, Holliday W. Cycling biomechanics optimization—the (R) evolution of bicycle fitting. Curr Sports Med Rep 2019;18(12):490–6.
2. Ayachi F, Dorey J, Guastavino C. Identifying factors of bicycle comfort: an online survey with enthusiast cyclists. Appl Ergon 2015;46(Part A):124–36.
3. Priego Quesada I, Pérez-soriano P, Lucas-Cuevos A, et al. Effect of bike-fit in the perception of comfort, fatigue and pain. J Sports Sci 2017;35(14):1459–65.
4. Priego Quesada J, Kerr Z, Bertucci W, et al. The association of bike fitting with injury, comfort and pain during cycling: an international retrospective survey. Eur J Sport Sci 2018;1391:1–8.
5. Medicine of Cycling. Medicine of cycling bike fit task force consensus statement. Bike Fitting Consensus Statements Summary Document 2013.
6. Peveler W, Green J. Effects of saddle height on economy and anaerobic power in well-trained cyclists. J Strength Cond Res 2011;25(3):629–33.
7. Bini R, Hume P, Croft J. Cyclists and triathletes have different body positions on the bicycle. Eur J Sport Sci 2014;14(S1):109–15.
8. Burke E. High-tech cycling. Second. Human Kinetics; 2003.

9. Peveler W, Shew B, Johnson S, et al. A kinematic comparison of alterations to knee and ankle angles from resting measures to active pedaling during a graded exercise protocol. J Strength Cond Res 2012;26(11):3004–9.
10. Kautz S, Feltner M, Coyle E, et al. The pedaling technique of elite endurance cyclists: changes with increasing workload at constant cadence. Int J Sports Biomech 1991;7:29–53.
11. Bini R, Diefenthaeler F. Kinetics and kinematics analysis of incremental cycling to exhaustion. Sports Biomech 2010;9(4):223–35.
12. Bini R, Diefenthaeler F, Mota C. Fatigue effects on the coordinative pattern during cycling: kinetics and kinematics evaluation. J Electromyogr Kinesiol 2010;20(1): 102–7.
13. Bini R, Senger D, Lanferdini F, et al. Joint kinematics assessment during cycling incremental test to exhaustion. Isokinet Exerc Sci 2012;20(2):99–105.
14. Dingwell J, Joubert J, Diefenthaeler F, et al. Changes in muscle activity and kinematics of highly trained cyclists during fatigue. IEEE Trans Biomed Eng 2008; 55(11):2666–74.
15. Holliday W, Theo R, Fisher J, et al. Cycling: joint kinematics and muscle activity during differing intensities. Sports Biomech 2019. https://doi.org/10.1080/ 14763141.2019.1640279.
16. Bini R, Dagnese F, Rocha E, et al. Three-dimensional kinematics of competitive and recreational cyclists across different workloads during cycling. Eur J Sport Sci 2016;16(5):553–9.
17. Hug F, Dorel S. Electromyographic analysis of pedaling: a review. J Electromyogr Kinesiol 2009;19(2):182–98.
18. Jorge M, Hull M. Analysis of EMG measurements during bicycle pedalling. J Biomech 1986;19(9):683–94.
19. Dorel S, Couturier A, Hug F. Intra-session repeatability of lower limb muscles activation pattern during pedaling. J Electromyogr Kinesiol 2008;18(5):857–65.
20. Von Tscharner V. Time-frequency and principal-component methods for the analysis of EMGs recorded during a mildly fatiguing exercise on a cycle ergometer. J Electromyogr Kinesiol 2002;12(6):479–92.
21. Prilutsky B, Gregor R. Analysis of muscle coordination strategies in cycling. IEEE Trans Rehabil Eng 2000;8(3):362–70.
22. Dorel S, Guilhem G, Couturier A, et al. Adjustment of muscle coordination during an all-out sprint cycling task. Med Sci Sports Exerc 2012;44(11):2154–64.
23. Kay D, Marino F, Cannon J, et al. Evidence for neuromuscular fatigue during high-intensity cycling in warm, humid conditions. Eur J Appl Physiol 2001;84(1–2): 115–21.
24. Blake O, Champoux Y, Wakeling J. Muscle coordination patterns for efficient cycling. Med Sci Sports Exerc 2012;44(5):926–38.
25. Ericson M, Nisell R, Arborelius U, et al. Muscular activity during ergometer cycling. Scand J Rehabil Med 1985;17(2):53–61.
26. Hautier CA, Arsac LM, Deghdegh K, et al. Influence of fatigue on EMG/force ratio and cocontraction in cycling. Med Sci Sports Exerc 2000;32(4):839–43.
27. Laplaud D, Hug F, Grélot L. Reproducibility of eight lower limb muscles activity level in the course of an incremental pedaling exercise. J Electromyogr Kinesiol 2006;16(2):158–66.
28. de Vey Mestdagh K. Personal perspective: in search of an optimum cycling posture. Appl Ergon 1998;29(5):325–34.
29. Silberman M, Webner D, Collina S, et al. Road bicycle fit. Clin J Sport Med 2005; 15(4):271–6.

30. Hamley E, Thomas V. Physiological and postural factors in the calibration of the bicycle ergometer. J Physiol 1967;191(2):55–6.
31. Peveler W, Bishop P, Smith J, et al. Comparing methods for setting saddle height in trained cyclists. J Exerc Physiol Online 2005;8(1):51–5.
32. Peveler W. Effects of saddle height on economy in cycling. J Strength Cond Res 2008;22(4):1355–9.
33. Gross V, Bennett C. Bicycle crank length. Proc Hum Factors Ergon Soc Annu Meet 1976;20(18):415–21.
34. Holliday W, Swart J. Anthropometrics, flexibility and training history as determinants for bicycle configuration. Sports Med Health Sci 2021. https://doi.org/10.1016/j.smhs.2021.02.007.
35. Kotler D, Babu A, Robidoux G. Prevention, evaluation, and rehabilitation of cycling-related injury. Am Coll Sports Med 2016;15(3):199–206.
36. Hynd J, Crowle D, Stephenson C. The influence of hamstring extensibility on pre-selected saddle height within experienced competitive cyclists. J Sci Cycl 2014; 3(2):22.
37. Dahlquist M, Leisz M, Finkelstein M. The club-level road cyclist. Clin J Sport Med 2015;25(2):88–94.
38. Burt P. Bike fit: optimise your bike position for high performance and injury avoidance. London: Bloomsbury Publishing Plc; 2014. p. 37–67.
39. Holliday W, Swart J. Performance variables associated with bicycle configuration and flexibility. J Sci Med Sport 2020;24(3):312–7.
40. Hayot C, Domalain M, Bernard J, et al. Muscle force strategies in relation to saddle setback management in cycling. Comput Methods Biomech Biomed Engin 2013;16(sup1):106–8.
41. Chye T, Swart J. The effect of alterations in effective seat tube angle on cycling performance, economy and muscle recruitment. University of Cape Town: Master thesis; 2017.
42. Duggan W, Donne B, Fleming N. Effect of seat tube angle and exercise intensity on muscle activity patterns in cyclists. Int J Exerc Sci 2017;10(8):1145–56.
43. Coetzee B, Malan D. Laboratory-based physical and physiological test results that serve as predictors of male, amateur road cyclists' performance levels. J Strength Cond Res 2018;32(10):2897–906.
44. Barnes K, Kilding A. Strategies to improve running economy. Sports Med 2014; 45(1):37–56.
45. Holliday W, Fisher J, Theo R, et al. Static versus dynamic kinematics in cyclists: a comparison of goniometer, inclinometer and 3D motion capture. Eur J Sport Sci 2017;17(9):1129–42.
46. Ferrer-Roca V, Roig A, Galilea P, et al. Influence of saddle height on lower limb kinematics in well-trained cyclists: static versus dynamic evaluation in bike fitting. J Strength Cond Res 2012;26(11):3025–9.
47. Bini R, Hume P, Croft J, et al. Effects of saddle position on pedalling technique and methods to assess pedalling kinetics and kinematics of cyclists and triathletes. Auckland University of Technology: PhD thesis; 2011.
48. Fonda B, Sarabon N, Li F. Validity and reliability of different kinematics methods used for bike fitting. J Sports Sci 2014;32(10):940–6.
49. Couto P, Filipe V, Magalhães L, et al. A comparison of two-dimensional and three-dimensional techniques for the determination of hindlimb kinematics during treadmill locomotion in rats following spinal cord injury. J Neurosci Methods 2008;173(2):193–200.

50. Umberger B, Martin P. Testing the planar assumption during ergometer cycling. J Appl Biomech 2001;17:55–62.
51. Farrell K, Reisinger K, Tillman M. Force and repetition in cycling: possible implications for iliotibial band friction syndrome. Knee 2003;10(1):103–9.
52. Visentini P, Clarsen B. Overuse injuries in cycling: the wheel is turning towards evidence-based practice. Aspetar Sports Med J 2016;5:486–92.

A Practical Approach to the Evaluation of a Cyclist with Overuse Injury

C. Greg Robidoux, PT*

KEYWORDS

- Cycling assessment • Bike fit • Overuse injury • Chronic injury • Cyclist • Bicycle

KEY POINTS

- It is Important to have an understanding of the unique nature of a cycling athlete compared with other endurance athletes.
- The sport of cycling and bike riding in general has significantly grown in popularity in the last 20 years.
- The cyclist-bicycle interaction is a unique relationship in endurance sports requiring an understanding of the bicycle as a whole as well as all of it's component parts.
- It is imperative to employ a consistent and cohesive methodology for evaluating the cyclist with an overuse injury.

INTRODUCTION

Although cycling has been gaining popularity as both fitness activity and transportation, the needs of a cyclist have not been well understood by the medical community at large. Several aspects of the sport of cycling make it a unique human biomechanical endeavor, specifically the amount of time connected to a machine performing a relatively small and repetitive movement. The bio-mechanics of human locomotion on a bicycle are distinctly different from sports where the athletes propel their body through space on their feet. The interaction of human and bicycle requires a different perspective and paradigm of evaluation when assessing for both human performance and potential injury. Cyclists can develop injury due to imbalance in their body, poor biomechanics with the bicycle, or a combination of the 2. Therefore, evaluation and treatment of the cyclist must address both the on-the-bicycle and off-the-bicycle needs. This article aims to lay out a methodology for evaluating a cycling athlete; first, understanding the bicycle and its component parts is needed, followed by the human-bicycle interaction and lastly the potential problem areas if that interaction is not ideal.

Cycling Medicine Program, Outpatient Physical Therapy, Spaulding Rehabilitation Hospital, Wellesley, MA, USA
* 65 Walnut street, suite 260, Wellesley MA 02481.
E-mail addresses: crobidoux@partners.org; SIClgetfit@gmail.com

Phys Med Rehabil Clin N Am 33 (2022) 15–29
https://doi.org/10.1016/j.pmr.2021.08.002
1047-9651/22/© 2021 Elsevier Inc. All rights reserved.

The goal is to provide a construct that assist the clinicians in deciphering overuse injuries that are rooted in the biomechanical interaction between bicycle and rider.

HISTORY

What is thought of as the modern bicycle first appeared in the late 1800s. It proved to be an innovative and efficient form of transportation.[1] This bicycle was dubbed the "safety bicycle," due to the perception that it was much safer than its predecessors, the penny-farthing, or the high wheel, bicycle. The term, *breakneck speed*, came from the potential for going over the front wheel of a penny-farthing at a speed that would catapult the rider forward and onto their head with potential catastrophic effect. Although this illustrates some of the more spectacular ways of injuring oneself on a bicycle, it is far more common to develop chronic or overuse injury due to the repetitive nature and limited range of motion of the pedal stroke.[2] To better illustrate this point, suppose an athlete has a 5-Inch deviation of the knee in the frontal plane from the top of the pedal stroke to the bottom. If this athlete were to complete a 100-mile ride at an average cadence of 95 revolutions per minute and average speed of 14 miles per hour, the knee would travel 3.87 miles laterally over the distance of that single ride. Unsurprisingly, the most common area affected by overuse injury on the bicycle is the knee. One cross-sectional study of more than 20,000 cyclists found that the knee (26.3%), shoulder (13%), and lower back (11.5%) were most affected.[3] Specifically, anterior knee pain was the most common of all overuse injuries evaluated. Many cyclists reported symptoms lasting more than a year, and more than one-third of the subjects had overuse injuries that were severe enough to reduce or prevent cycling.[3] Muscular imbalances, faulty mechanics, and improper gear setup may be tolerated for some time prior to symptom onset (particularly because cyclists often are able to continue to ride in spite of pain), which may lead to an increased prevalence or likelihood of cycling related overuse injury.

Modern cycling comprises many forms and disciplines. It can be undertaken as pure recreation, fitness, competition, or transportation. The most common form of bicycle riding is road cycling, which includes commuting, touring, recreational riding, and competitive road racing, time trial, and triathlon. Mountain biking takes place entirely off-road and includes cross-country riding and downhill or gravity riding. A hybrid of road and mountain biking exists in subsets of the sport like cyclocross and gravel riding, which utilize bicycles that look similar to road bikes but are designed for multiple types of terrain. Additional competitive disciplines include track riding, which takes place on a velodrome and was tremendously popular in the 1920s through the 1940s,[1] and bicycle motocross (BMX), which is derived from motocross racing and takes place on a purpose-built off-road race track. Although now sequestered to a handful of venues around the United States, track racing was one of the most popular sports. Madison Square Garden played host to many feats of endurance and bravery in its storied 6-day bicycle races and even lends its name to a style of track racing that still exists today, the Madison. Although the popularity of cycling has ebbed and flowed since its inception, the past 20 years to 30 years have demonstrated steady growth. Bicycle sales in the past year have increased by more than 50% compared with previous years. People seeking alternate forms of physical fitness and transportation have flocked to purchasing bicycles, bringing a huge influx of new riders into the sport. It has been reported that nearly 1 in every 10 American's note that they have returned to cycling after a year or more in 2020.[4] This influx further increases the need for medical professionals who are versed in understanding the sport of cycling to help treat or prevent cycling-related chronic injury.

WHAT MEDICAL PROFESSIONALS NEED TO KNOW ABOUT THE BICYCLE

Medical professionals excel at understanding and assessment of the human body, but there often is a knowledge gap in terminology, assessment, and documentation of the bicycle configuration (**Fig. 1**). The area used most commonly for a point of reference on the bicycle is the bottom bracket, a fixed point in the frame that is the center of rotation of the crank. It is used for many measures of bike position, including position of both handlebars and saddle (**Table 1**). The core measurements that provide the most useful information are saddle height, saddle setback, nose of saddle to the center of the handlebar, and drop or differential of saddle to handlebar height (see **Table 1**). It also is important to understand the compounding factors associated with adjusting aspects of the bicycle. For instance, because of the angle of the seat tube, raising the seat post in order to raise the saddle height also moves the saddle backwards, away from the bottom bracket. Similarly, moving the saddle forward on the rails effectively lowers the saddle height by bringing the rider closer to the bottom bracket. On the front end of the bicycle, positioning the handlebars includes adjusting both height and fore-aft position, either along the axis of the steerer tube or by changing the angle and length of the stem. When considering a steeper angle for the stem (higher position for the handlebars), note that the handlebars travel in an arc; this means that a stem of the same length with a steeper angle effectively is shorter.

Understanding how bicycle sizing is measured is critical when documenting a bicycle and the position of all of its component parts. Historically, the size of an adult bike was determined by measuring from the center of the bottom bracket to the center of the top tube along the seat tube. The compact geometry of many modern bikes does not allow this measurement; rather, the measurement is taken to a point along the seat tube measured parallel to the ground (see **Table 1**). This measurement typically is listed in centimeters on road bikes and in inches on most mountain bikes. It is best practice to record all position measurements on the bicycle in centimeters or millimeters.

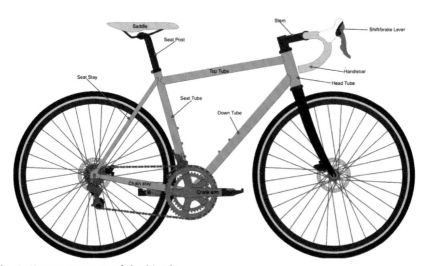

Fig. 1. Key components of the bicycle.

Table 1
Measurements of the bicycle

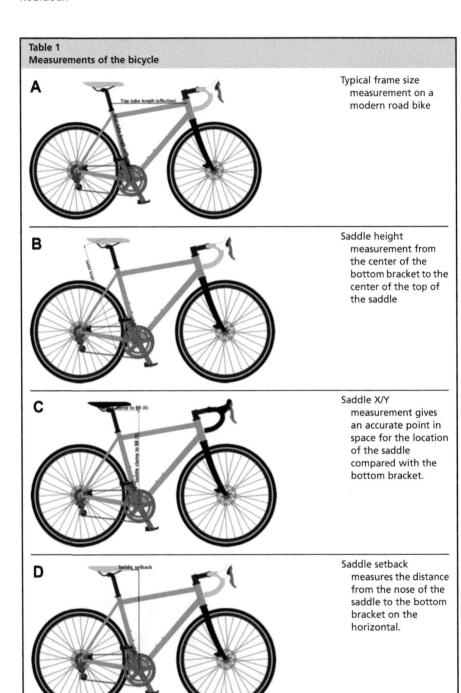

A	Typical frame size measurement on a modern road bike
B	Saddle height measurement from the center of the bottom bracket to the center of the top of the saddle
C	Saddle X/Y measurement gives an accurate point in space for the location of the saddle compared with the bottom bracket.
D	Saddle setback measures the distance from the nose of the saddle to the bottom bracket on the horizontal.

(continued on next page)

Table 1 (continued)	
E 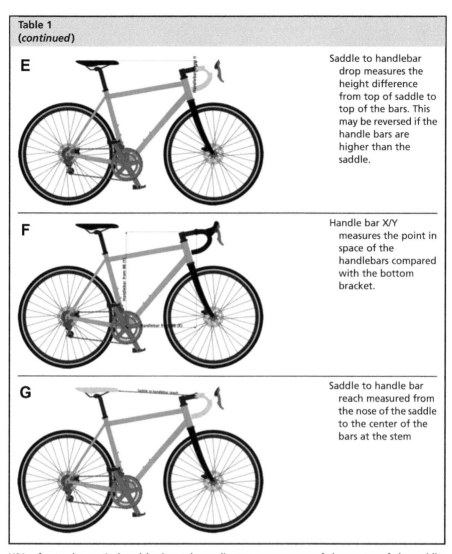	Saddle to handlebar drop measures the height difference from top of saddle to top of the bars. This may be reversed if the handle bars are higher than the saddle.
F	Handle bar X/Y measures the point in space of the handlebars compared with the bottom bracket.
G	Saddle to handle bar reach measured from the nose of the saddle to the center of the bars at the stem

X/Y refer to the vertical and horizontal coordinates or measures of the center of the saddle, measured from the center of the bottom bracket.

EVALUATION

In the pre-assessment, a significant amount of data can be captured in the evaluation and assessment of the cycling athlete, including demographic information and typical medical history as well as bicycle-specific information. These data help to better define the cycling athlete and often expose many of the potential causes for chronic injury on the bike as well as preparing the examiner to have all equipment necessary to accommodate the type of bicycle being evaluated (**Table 2**). A self-administered history tool describing disciplines and training volume may allow the provider to streamline and tailor an in-person visit while still maintaining accuracy.[5] An example of this information is included in **Fig. 1**.

Table 2
Cyclist preassessment

Cycling history

What type of bicycle will be evaluated? Please check all features that apply to your bicycle.	Quick release skewer, thru-axle (rear), road bike, cyclocross bike, gravel bike, mountain bike, triathlon bike or time trail bike, hybrid bike, tandem bike, recumbent bike, modified or adaptive bike, track bike or fixed gear, e-bike
In which disciplines of cycling do you participate?	Road, track, cyclocross, mountain bike, triathlon/time trial, BMX, touring, commuting, gravel, paracycling or handcycling
For how many years have you been riding a bicycle on a regular basis?	<1 y, 1–5 y, 5–10 y, 10–20 y, >20 y
Estimate your total cycling mileage/wk.	< 25 miles, 25–50 miles, 51–75 miles, 76–100 miles, 101–125 miles, 126–150 miles, >150
Estimate your average length of ROAD training ride.	< 5 miles, 5–10 miles, 11–20 miles, 21–30 miles, 31–40 miles, 41–50 miles, 51–60 miles, 61–70 miles 71–80 miles, >80 miles
What is your average speed for a road training ride?	< 10 mph, 10–12 mph, 13–15 mph, 16–18 mph, >19 mph, I do not know my average speed
Estimate the length of average mountain bike ride.	< 5 miles, 5–10 miles, 11–20 miles, 21–30 miles, 31–40 miles, 41–50 miles, 51–60 miles, 61–70 miles 71–80 miles, >80 miles
Estimate your average length of commute by bicycle (1-way).	<5 miles, 5–10 miles, 11–20 miles, >21 miles
Do you typically ride alone or with others?	Alone, with 1 other person, in a group
Do you wear an approved cycling helmet on the majority of your rides?	Yes, no
Is the helmet that you wear <3 y old and/or still under warranty?	Yes, no
Do you train with a power meter (on bike or smart trainer)?	Yes, no

(continued on next page)

Table 2
(continued)

What is your 20-min power/FTP in watts if known?	_____watts
Bicycle racing	
Do you compete in bicycle racing?	Yes, no
In what disciplines of competitive bicycle racing do you participate?	Road, track, cyclocross, mountain bike, triathlon/time trial, BMX, touring, commuting, gravel, paracycling or handcycling
For how many years have you been racing bicycles?	<1 y, 1–5 y, 5–10 y, 10–20 y, >20 y
Do you train with a coach?	Yes, no
What is your ROAD racing category?	Men pro/1, men 2, men 3, men 4, men 5, woman pro/1, women 2, women 3, women 4, women 5 junior boy/girl
What is your MOUNTAIN BIKING race category?	Men pro/1, men 2, men 3, woman pro/1, women 2, women 3, junior boy/girl
Exercise history	
What other types of exercise do you regularly participate in?	Running, swimming, cardio (ie, elliptical, stair climbing), strength/weight lifting, core training/Pilates, yoga, other (check all that apply)
How many times per wk do you run?	1, 2, 3, 7, 5, 6, 7
How many times per wk do you strength/weight train?	1, 2, 3, 7, 5, 6, 7
How many times per wk do you do yoga or flexibility training?	1, 2, 3, 7, 5, 6, 7
Bicycle crash history	
Have you been in 1 or more serious cycling crashes in the last 2 y?	Yes, no
Have you been diagnosed with a concussion or traumatic brain injury?	Yes, no
Nontraumatic/chronic/overuse injury	
Do you have any chronic (>3 mo) areas of discomfort that affect your ability to ride a bicycle?	Yes, no
Which of the following best describes the	Musculoskeletal (ie, joint pain, muscle pain, sprain, fracture),

(continued on next page)

Table 2 (continued)	
problems you had/currently have related to cycling?	spine (ie, neck or low back pain), neurologic (ie, concussion, migraine, numbness, tingling, weakness), cardiopulmonary (ie, palpitations, shortness of breath, wheezing), gastrointestinal, dermatologic (ie, skin breakdown, sores, rashes)
Where do you have the most significant discomfort?	Lower back, neck, hip, knee, foot/ankle, shoulder, elbow, wrist, hand, groin/perineum/genitalia, other
When do you experience this discomfort?	On the bike only, off the bike only, both on and off the bike
Have you sought prior medical care or opinion for the areas of discomfort?	Yes, no

EVALUATION OF THE CYCLING ATHLETE

It is essential to start with a robust history as well as an understanding of goals, expectations, and the psyche of a cyclist. As a population, athletes tend to have a higher pain threshold than nonathletes; endurance athletes, such as cyclists, have been shown to have improved pain inhibition over other types of athletes.[6] This inhibition of pain likely is due to the prolonged duration of exercise but also to the fact that tolerance of pain is coveted and revered in the sport. The very definition of a "good" cyclist is one who can endure more pain than the others around them. It is not unexpected then that these athletes can become desensitized not only to the pain of endurance sport but also to the warning signs that pain is the precursor to injury. One of the most difficult aspects of understanding a history given by a cycling athlete is that an overuse injury often has an undetectable cause (to the athlete) or a perceived catalyst that does not seem to align with the amount of discomfort in their presentation. This is due, in part, not only to the aforementioned tendency to ignore or inhibit pain but also due to the fact that, biomechanically, cycling is a non–weight-bearing sport. The lack of ground reaction force coupled with the repetitive motion of the pedal stroke, which almost exclusively is in the sagittal plane, can prolong the amount of time that it takes for an abnormal movement to become pathologic. When abnormal biomechanics are at play, it often is difficult for an athlete to understand and report on the mechanism of injury. Similar to a patient who suffers an acute flare of significant lower back pain from simply bending over to pick up a sock, it is not the action of picking up the sock that created the injury, rather the months or years of dysfunction prior to that moment. The result is that special care and attention should be paid while conducting the interview to consider what the athlete reports though the lens of the cyclist archetype. Other key factors that should be considered from the history are the use of nonsteroidal anti-inflammatory drugs or analgesics prior to or during sport, the presence of chronic disease, and significant increase in training volume or intensity (>10% per week) as well as the cyclist's age.[7] A cross-sectional study of 21,824 cyclist from New Zealand in 2020 indicated a significant increase in risk of gradual-onset injury based on the risk factors of increased training volume, chronic disease, age greater than 50 years, and use of analgesic/anti-inflammatory medication.[3] Furthermore, it is important to inquire about the specific aspects of cycling that initiate or perpetuate pain, such as time in the saddle, terrain, cadence, and intensity. In addition to potentially revealing biomechanical causes of pain or injury, a history provides the first filter through which what to look at on the bicycle is narrowed down.

PHYSICAL EXAMINATION OF THE CYCLING ATHLETE: OFF THE BIKE

The movement pattern and typical duration and intensity of the cycling, coupled with tendencies to avoid other types of strength or flexibility training, may lead to significant imbalance in length-tension relationships throughout a cyclist's body. When approaching the physical examination of the cyclist, as with any patient with overuse injury, the evaluator should tailor the examination to the primary complaint.[8] There are assessment techniques, however, that are valuable to the evaluation of any cyclist, because they illuminate the outcomes of abnormal biomechanics on the bike. These assessment techniques and typical findings are discussed; some have been modified to better evaluate the cycling athlete.

Hamstring Flexibility

Hamstring flexibility is measured with the patient in supine on the treatment table with both legs out straight. One leg should be elevated to the point where the slack is taken out of the hamstring and the pelvis starts to rotate posteriorly.[9] This can be visualized by posterior rotation at the sacroiliac joint, or posterior superior iliac spine (PSIS), or by movement of the opposite leg. This is not a measure of maximum flexibility; the range beyond the point where the pelvis starts to rotate is not clinically relevant to cycling position. With substantial hamstring inflexibility, however, there is potential that even in normal riding position, the cyclist could elicit a stretch reflex on the bike when rapidly extending the knee through the bottom portion of the pedal stroke, potentially causing reciprocal inhibition of the quadriceps[10,11] and potentially reducing power and/or exposing the rider to greater risk of overuse injury.

Hip Range of Motion

Maximal hip flexion is the measure most pertinent to the cycling athlete. With the patient supine, the hip should be flexed toward the chest in a straight line. If the leg has a tendency to move laterally or externally rotate at the top of the range of motion, then the measure should be taken prior to the point of lateral deviation. On the bike, the occurrence of maximal hip flexion depends on the torso angle maintained by the rider when the foot reaches top dead center of the pedal stroke.[9] Decreased range of motion due to femoroacetabular impingement or hip arthritis can alter the pedal stroke, causing the knee to deviate laterally at the top of the pedal stroke.

Gluteus Medius Manual Muscle Test

The gluteus medius manual muscle test, as described by Florence Kendall,[12] suggests that the patient be in a side-lying position with the hips stacked 1 over the other, the top leg positioned in slight abduction, slight hip extension, and slight external rotation. The examiner may need to stabilize the hips to prevent rolling backwards or forwards.

It goes on to suggest that pressure should be applied to the leg at the lateral calf in the direction of adduction and slight flexion.[12] Because the cycling athlete completes the pedaling motion almost exclusively in the sagittal plane, muscle recruitment of the gluteus medius can prove difficult (especially if the patient is exclusively a cyclist). This creates a tendency to over-recruit the hip flexors and tensor fasciae latae when trying to complete this test, causing the athlete to translate the leg forward away from the tester instead of in an abduction.[9,13] As a result of this tendency, the gluteus medius strength test can be modified to roll the pelvis slightly forward and maintain slight extension of the rotate the lower extremity slightly internally, reducing the potential for recruitment of tensor fasciae latae, iliopsoas, and rectus femoris. Functional testing, such as a single-leg squat (described later), can be used to determine if the athlete is able to use the gluteus medius to stabilize the pelvis in standing. In cycling, because the pelvis is stabilized by the saddle, the result of gluteus medius weakness may be medial knee tracking through the power phase of the pedal stroke.

Modified Thomas Test

Both hip flexor and iliotibial band (ITB) tightness can be evaluated effectively by employing the modified Thomas test.[14,15] The athlete starts supine with knees to chest at the end of the treatment table. The evaluator holds 1 knee close to the chest while the other hip is allowed to extend while keeping the knee at 90°. The inability to achieve extension parallel to the ground indicates limitation in the iliopsoas, rectus femoris, and possibly the ITB as well as potential joint or capsular restriction. Lateral thigh deviation primarily indicates ITB tightness. Similar to the limitation in flexibility of the hamstrings, limiting the quadriceps through reciprocal inhibition, tight hip flexors may limit the gluteus maximus in the power phase of the pedal stroke.[10,11,16]

Single-leg Mini-squat

Although the gluteus medius strength test is employed to understand isolated hip abduction strength, the single-leg squat test allows an examiner to better understand the movement strategies and functional use of the athlete's available strength. This test may result in several movement patterns, each indicating a different pattern of weakness. Ideally, the athlete should be able to balance on 1 foot and squat to a knee angle of approximately 45° from vertical, while maintaining a level pelvis, mostly vertical torso, and without marked medial/lateral knee deviation. Contralateral hip drop indicates weakness or inability to effectively stabilize with the gluteus medius[17]; excessive torso lean to 1 side may indicate weak core muscles; and medial knee drive can indicate poor foot stability or weak hip stabilizers. In the cycling population, it is common to see both medial knee drive as well as contralateral hip drop.[9,17]

Craig's Test

Craig's test can be utilized to shed additional light on poor frontal plane mechanics throughout the pedal stroke. In the presence of femoral anteversion, the knees may track in toward the top tube while pedaling, even while the feet are well supported and the hip is strong and stable.[18]

Pelvic Alignment

Checking the sacroiliac joint and the 2 halves of the pelvis at the anterior superior iliac spine and PSIS for symmetry give insight into how the pelvis may interact with the saddle.[19] Ideally, on a road bike, the saddle should support the anterior aspect of the ischial tuberosities and pubic rami. Sacroiliac dysfunction or pelvic obliquity can affect a rider's ability to feel as though they are sitting square in the saddle significantly. In more extreme cases, this may cause the rider to appear windswept, with 1 knee deviating medially toward the top tube and the other deviating laterally. This phenomenon can happen when 1 ischial tuberosity is ahead of the other and the pelvis must rotate on the saddle for those bones to be square.

Foot Measurement

The role of the foot in cycling differs from its role in walking or running. The foot has 2 phases for walking or running and has only 1 for cycling. In the initial stance phase of gait, the foot should remain rigid until the tibia translates forward, unlocking the navicular, which then translates medially, allowing the foot to pronate; at this point, the foot loses rigidity and becomes flexible, allowing the person to propel forward into the next step. In cycling, the foot should remain a rigid lever to deliver force to the pedal, and, as such, supportive inserts in a cycling shoe post from the midfoot forward rather than the midfoot rearward, as is seen in walking or running orthotics.[20]

The Brannock device is the gold standard for basic foot measurement.[21] It is able to capture overall length and width of the foot as well as medial longitudinal arch, which are important for correct shoe sizing. Cycling shoes typically are measured in European sizes, so the corresponding Brannock device should be used. For the cyclist, measures of overall and arch length as well as width should be taken both in full weight bearing and in a seated or non–weight-bearing position. The suggested cycling shoe size is based on the longest recorded measurement. The longest measure may not be the overall length, as seen when an individual has a long arch and short toes. Although this foot would fit into the corresponding shoe size based on the overall length, the entirety of the arch would not be supported, allowing for greater arch collapse. If there is a difference of a full shoe size or more between weighted and nonweighted length measures, then a cycling specific insole or orthotic should be considered. The amount of support and its effect on overall pedaling biomechanics is individualized but has been shown to effectively reduce internal tibial torsion, which translates to reduced medial knee movement in the power phase of the pedal stroke and thereby reduces reduced potential overuse injury at the knee.[21]

Navicular Drop

The navicular drop measurement refers to the displacement of the navicular from a talonavicular neutral (talus congruent with the navicular) position to its position in unsupported stance.[22] This measurement helps to further define the type of support the foot requires in the cycling shoe. If the relative drop is greater than 1 cm, then additional forefoot support, in the form of a forefoot wedge inserted under the insole may be considered.

ON-THE-BIKE EVALUATION

Although optimizing bike fit may be a part of injury management in the cyclist, it is a separate process from the initial clinical evaluation (and typically is not covered by insurance). Assessment by a clinician is not intended to take the place of an independent bike fitting session but rather to better understand the biomechanical contributors to injury and plan effective treatment. This is important particularly because treatment of the cyclist usually involves a combination of both on-the-bike and off-the-bike strategies to improve core strength, stability, efficiency, and biomechanics.[23]

A systematic assessment of cycling position starts with evaluation of the foot; then, knee angle, fore and aft positions (knee over pedal spindle), saddle support, and pelvic posture; and, finaly, the position of the torso and upper extremity. This approach allows a clinician to synthesize the information from the history and physical evaluation to make educated decisions on how each joint will be affected by adjustment at each position. On-the-bike assessment should be performed using the bike that the athlete uses the most[9] or the bike where the pain or dysfunction is present. The bike should be stabilized on a stationary trainer that has the appropriate attachment points for the type of axle present on the bike, and the front axle should be leveled to the rear axle. Riders should warm up at a comfortable cadence and power, typical of the way they would start an outdoor ride, which allows for observation of any abnormalities in pedal stroke, posture, or body movement. The clinician should consider any deficits seen in the physical assessment, viewing from both the sagittal and frontal planes. In addition to general assessment of posture and pedal stroke, special attention should be paid to the contact points, pedal, saddle, and handlebars.

The pedal contact point includes the pedals, the cleats, and the shoes as a system. A properly placed cleat should be located between the first and fifth metatarsal heads, in line with the second toe, and should allow for a few degrees of float in both internal and external rotation (float). With the foot supported in the correct size and width shoe and with correct cleat placement, the knee should track straight up and down throughout the pedal stroke (if there are no limitations at the knee or hip).[24] Cleat position should be set to accommodate normal rotation in stance and should not be used to drive the foot or the knee in a specific direction, because this causes increased torque at either the hip or the knee. For example, if the heel is rubbing the crank arm or chain stay throughout the pedal stroke, stance width should be increased instead of forcing the heal away by rotating the cleat.

With the foot properly positioned, focus can shift to the knee. With an appropriate saddle height, at the point of greatest knee extension (crank arm in line with the seat tube), the knee angle should measure somewhere between 25° and 35° from full (180°) extension.[25] Within this range, when the crank arm is at the 90° position, the tibial tuberosity should be located within 2 cm in front of or behind the pedal spindle. These ranges of knee extension and fore/aft placement allow for optimal firing of the quadraceps and gluteal muscles with minimal shear forces at the anterior and posterior knee.[25]

Saddle comfort is achieved through careful selection of the correct saddle and clothing combination as well as an understanding of how to sit on the saddle. Saddle adjustment is one of the most challenging and complex areas of bike fit, due to the variability of pelvic shape, soft tissue anatomy, and postural stability. The combination of width, shape, and support provides the structure and foundation for proper pelvic alignment, with support distributed over the ischial tuberosities and slightly onto the pubic rami,[26] and the rider's torso positioned at approximately 45° without excessive posterior rotation of the pelvis. This allows core and gluteal activation as well as positioning the rider's center of mass over the bottom bracket. Simply choosing a softer saddle to alleviate discomfort can cause more problems because the extra padding can protrude up into more sensitive soft tissue structures in the pelvis, potentially causing pain, numbness, or friction in the genital region. An additional challenge is the difficulty many cyclists have in describing and localizing sensations in this region. Use of anatomic models, self-palpation, and cueing may help a cyclist understand and sense the appropriate contact point of the pelvis to the saddle. Saddle pressure mapping technology can be employed to provide better objective data for this contact point.

The torso and arm should form an approximately 90° angle. The hands and wrists should be positioned neutrally on the hoods or grips to allow for easy access to the brakes and shifters and the elbows bent between 15° and 30°. This relationship should allow the rider to describe an approximate perceived 60:40 weight distribution from saddle to hands and allow for optimal control of the bicycle.

When a bike is fit by a fitter, adjustments typically are made sequentially at the contact point (described previously), starting in the sagittal plane. Each small adjustment typically has an effect along the kinetic chain: adjustments at the foot can affect the knee; adjustments at the knee can affect the hip; adjustments at the hip and pelvis can affect the torso; and so on. Small changes at each segment typically are tolerated better by a cyclist than a single large adjustment at 1 segment and allow for a larger overall effect.[27] Often, careful adjustment in the sagittal plane corrects most abnormalities in the frontal plane; however, if some medial or lateral knee deviation persists, it can be corrected with small changes to stance width or wedging of the shoe/cleat.

The inclusion of the on-the-bike assessment as part of the overall evaluation of the cyclist helps ensure that a treatment plan addresses all potential causes of current injury as well as prevention of future injury. The injured cyclist may require periodic physical and biomechanical assessment as their strength mobility, pain, and training demands change with time. Likewise, the uninjured cyclist can benefit from this as well, secondary to the dynamic nature of the human body interacting with the relatively fixed position on a bicycle.

SUMMARY

When an individual chooses to use cycling as transportation, fitness, or competition, the repetitive nature of the pedal stroke in a confined range of motion presents a high likelihood of overuse injury if not performed with ideal biomechanics. The needs of the cycling athlete have not been well understood by the medical community at large. Cycling has been described as the interaction of an adaptable athlete with an adjustable machine.[28] This interaction creates a wide variety of possible issues for the medical provider to consider. The evaluation of the cycling athlete should be based on a basic understanding of bicycle geometry and components; an understanding the athlete's goals, motivations, and tendencies; and a systematic methodology for evaluating the kinetic chain of a cyclist on a bicycle. These 3 concepts, when applied in concert, allow the provider to successfully navigate a cycling evaluation and construct a robust treatment plan. Just as the assessment requires a multimodal approach, the treatment plan most likely needs to address the cyclist both on and off the bike. Optimizing the position on a bicycle by reducing movements outside of the ideal track of the pedal stroke, especially in the frontal plane, reduces risk of cycling-related overuse injury. Off the bike, treatment of cyclists should be thought of like truing a bicycle wheel. A bicycle wheel is said to be true when each opposing spoke is balanced in equal tension. Cyclists are prone to significant areas of tightness as well as typically demonstrating significant strength through the sagittal plane and potential weakness in the frontal plane (specifically the hip stabilizers). Efforts to true the cyclist by improving length-tension relationships and better balancing strength, stability, and flexibility will help most cyclists avoid overuse or chronic cycling injury.

CLINICS CARE POINTS

- It is important to understand the cyclist as a unique endurance athlete. When taking a comprehensive history, it is important to keep in mind that the typical recreational to competitive cyclist has trained to be more pain tolerant than other types of athletes and, therefore, may be less likely to recognize a transition from discomfort to injury.

- Cycling is a non–weight-bearing sport and, as a result, overuse injury caused by poor biomechanics on the bike may take a long time (1–2 seasons of riding) to present.
- A key aspect of both evaluation and treatment of a cycling athlete is to be able to assess biomechanics both on and off the bike. Treatment typically requires changes to both the bicycle and the athlete in tandem.
- Bicycle fitting is specific to the type of bicycle and discipline of riding. Adjustments that are made to a road bike, for instance, typically are not the same as a mountain bike ridden by the same rider.
- When evaluating a cyclist on the bicycle, the evaluator should start at the foot and work up the kinetic chain identifying any biomechanical abnormality or pathology at each joint and contact point (pedals, saddle, and handlebar) that is encountered along the way.
- When adjusting a bicycle for a rider, small adjustments at each point in the kinetic chain often add up to larger overall improvement in biomechanics as well as decreased likelihood of chronic or overuse injury.

DISCLOSURE

The author is the owner and executive director of the Serotta International Cycling Institute.

REFERENCES

1. Nathalie Lagerfeld. America's Short, Violent Love Affair With Indoor Track Cycling.
2. Perrin AE. Cycling-related injury. Conn Med 2012;76(8):461–6.
3. du Toit F, Schwellnus M, Wood P, et al. Epidemiology, clinical characteristics and severity of gradual onset injuries in recreational road cyclists: A cross-sectional study in 21,824 cyclists - SAFER XIII. Phys Ther Sport 2020;46:113–9.
4. Bernhard A. The Great bicycle Boom of 2020. BBC.
5. Boissonnault WG, Badke MB. Collecting health history information: the accuracy of a patient self-administered questionnaire in an orthopedic outpatient setting. Phys Ther 2005;85(6):531–43.
6. Assa T, Geva N, Zarkh Y, et al. The type of sport matters: pain perception of endurance athletes versus strength athletes. Eur J Pain (United Kingdom) 2019;23(4):686–96.
7. Rivara FP, Thompson DC, Thompson RS. Epidemiology of bicycle injuries and risk factors for serious injury. 1997. Inj Prev J Int Soc Child Adolesc Inj Prev 2015;21(1):47–51.
8. Kotler DH, Babu AN, Robidoux G. Prevention, evaluation, and rehabilitation of cycling-related injury. Curr Sports Med Rep 2016;15(3):199–206.
9. Wadsworth DJS, Weinrauch P. The role of a bike fit in cyclists with hip pain. A clinical commentary. Int J Sports Phys Ther 2019;14(3):468–86.
10. Mills M, Frank B, Goto S, et al. Effect of restricted hip flexor muscle length on hip extensor muscle activity and lower extremity biomechanics in college-aged female soccer players. Int J Sports Phys Ther 2015;10(7):946–54.
11. Stokes M, Young A. The contribution of reflex inhibition to arthrogenous muscle weakness. Clin Sci 1984;67(1):7–14.
12. Kendall F, McCreary E. Muscles testing and function. third. Williams & Wilkins; 1983.
13. Frese E, Brown M, Norton BJ. Clinical reliability of manual muscle testing: middle trapezius and gluteus medius muscles. Phys Ther 1987;67(7):1072–6.

14. Vigotsky AD, Lehman GJ, Beardsley C, et al. The modified Thomas test is not a valid measure of hip extension unless pelvic tilt is controlled. PeerJ 2016; 2016(8):1–12.
15. Kim GM, Ha SM. Reliability of the modified Thomas test using a lumbo-plevic stabilization. J Phys Ther Sci 2015;27(2):447.
16. Tashiro Y, Hasegawa S, Nishiguchi S, et al. Body characteristics of professional Japanese keirin cyclists: flexibility, pelvic tilt, and muscle strength. J Sport Sci 2016;4(6):341–5.
17. Ressman J, Grooten WJA, Rasmussen Barr E. Visual assessment of movement quality in the single leg squat test: A review and meta-analysis of inter-rater and intrarater reliability. BMJ Open Sport Exerc Med 2019;5(1):1–10.
18. Choi BR, Kang SY. Intra-and inter-examiner reliability of goniometer and inclinometer use in Craig's test. J Phys Ther Sci 2015;27(4):1141–4.
19. Al-Subahi M, Alayat M, Alshehri MA, et al. The effectiveness of physiotherapy interventions for sacroiliac joint dysfunction: A systematic review. J Phys Ther Sci 2017;29(9):1689–94.
20. O'Neill BC, Graham K, Moresi M, et al. Custom formed orthoses in cycling. J Sci Med Sport 2011;14(6):529–34.
21. Blazer MM, Jamrog LB, Schnack LL. Does the Shoe fit? Considerations for proper shoe fitting. Orthop Nurs 2018;37(3):169–74.
22. Zuil-Escobar JC, Martínez-Cepa CB, Martín-Urrialde JA, et al. Medial longitudinal arch: accuracy, reliability, and correlation between navicular drop test and footprint parameters. J Manipulative Physiol Ther 2018;41(8):672–9.
23. Piotrowska SE, Majchrzycki M, Rogala P, et al. Lower extremity and spine pain in cyclists. Ann Agric Environ Med 2017;24(4):654–8.
24. Bini R, Flores-Bini A. Potential factors associated with knee pain in cyclists: a systematic review. Open Access J Sport Med 2018;9:99–106. https://doi.org/10.2147/oajsm.s136653.
25. Millour G, Duc S, Puel F, et al. Comparison of static and dynamic methods based on knee kinematics to determine optimal saddle height in cycling. Acta Bioeng Biomech 2019;21(4):93–9.
26. Salai M, Brosh T, Blankstein A, et al. Effect of changing the saddle angle on the incidence of low back pain in recreational bicyclists. Br J Sports Med 1999;33(6):398–400.
27. Priego Quesada JI, Pérez-Soriano P, Lucas-Cuevas AG, et al. Effect of bike-fit in the perception of comfort, fatigue and pain. J Sports Sci 2017;35(14):1459–65.
28. Burke ER. High-tech cycling. In: McNeely E, MacEntire C, editors. Second Edition. Human Kinetics; 2003.

Adaptive Cycling
Classification, Adaptations, and Biomechanics

Gabrielle T. Goodlin, MD, Lindsey Steinbeck, MD,
Deborah Bergfeld, MD, Alexandria Haselhorst, DO*

KEYWORDS

- Para-cycling • Adaptive sports • Handcycle • Tricycle • Tandem cycling

KEY POINTS

- Para-cycling is now the third largest Paralympic sport after swimming and track and field; there are 8 impairment categories for participation in sanctioned events including limb deficiency, leg length difference, impaired muscle power, impaired passive range of movement, hypertonia, athetosis, ataxia, and visual impairment.
- The major adaptive cycling categories include tandem cycling, handcycling, tricycle, and standard bicycle.
- Special care should be taken regarding the fit and configuration of adapted bikes because this para-athlete population can have altered physiology and mechanics.
- Virtual platforms that allow riders to train and complete online have grown in popularity among para-cycling communities and offer an alternative to riding outdoors.
- There are many organizations that offer grants and assistance to para-cyclists, because the cost of equipment can be a barrier to entry and participation.

INTRODUCTION

The world of amateur and competitive adaptive cycling has grown in the last few decades. This expansion is attributed to increased awareness, innovation, and adaptation in the worlds of medicine, engineering, prosthetics, and orthotics. These changes in adaptive cycling have allowed more athletes with physical and cognitive impairments to experience the benefit of exercise, leading to improved physical, mental, and social health outcomes. Numerous national and international organizations have helped foster this inclusive growth in adaptive sports including: the International Paralympic Committee, the Union Cycliste Internationale (UCI), US Adaptive, Move United, Challenged Athletes, and One Chair at a Time, just to name a few.

Physical Medicine & Rehabilitation, Department of Neurology, The University of Texas at Austin, Dell Medical School, 1400 North IH-35, Suite 2.230, Austin, TX 78701, USA
* Corresponding author.
E-mail address: ajhaselhorst@ascension.org
Twitter: @gabi_goodlin (G.T.G.); @AliHaselhorstDO (A.H.)

Phys Med Rehabil Clin N Am 33 (2022) 31–43
https://doi.org/10.1016/j.pmr.2021.08.003

HISTORY AND GROWTH OF ADAPTIVE CYCLING

The sport of adaptive cycling has blossomed from the days of the premiere of road para-cycling at the Paralympic games in 1984 to the now 50 cycling events that were offered in the 2016 Rio Paralympic Games.[1] Para-cycling is now the third largest Paralympic sport after track and field and swimming. There were 269 participants in the 2016 Paralympic games, with the largest pool of athletes from the United States.[2] Key international competitions include Paralympic Games, the World Championships, and the World Cup. Qualifying events are broken into 2 domains: road cycling and track cycling. Adaptive handcycling was initially designed as a mobility tool for World War I veterans. It has progressed to be recognized as a sport by the International Paralympic Committee first in 1999 and now has its own governing body.[3] Since 2007, the UCI has overseen the expansion of the organization's classification system for para-cycling based on athlete impairment. At the 2016 Paralympic Games, handcycling contributed to 39% of the events in the road cycling schedule and was incorporated within the wheelchair class of the paratriathlon.[4] Despite this headway, there is still some ground to cover because there are no mountain biking circuits for individuals with disabilities. These riders must compete alongside able-bodied riders.[5]

CLASSIFICATION SYSTEM IN ADAPTIVE CYCLING

There are 8 impairment categories that qualify Paralympic athletes for inclusion in para-cycling established by the UCI. These include limb deficiency, leg length difference, impaired muscle power, impaired passive range of movement, hypertonia, athetosis, ataxia, and visual impairment. Impairments outside of those that are commonly encountered in recreational adaptive cycling include cognitive impairment, hypotonia, hearing impairment, impaired metabolic function, joint instability, and hypermobility. The UCI uses a functional system classification based on the type and extent of disability consisting of 4 main adaptive categories: tandem cycling, handcycling, tricycle, and standard bicycle.

Handcycles are used by adaptive athletes with lower limb amputations and those with para- or tetraplegia. Hand cyclists are classified into 5 groups (H1–H5) based on impairment level, with 1 being the most impaired (**Table 1**).[3] H1 to H4 athletes compete in a recumbent lying position, whereas H5 athletes compete in a kneeling position. Tricyclists are athletes with balance deficits preventing the use of a standard bicycle, such as those with dystonia, ataxia, or athetosis. They are classified into 2 groups, T1 and T2 (see **Table 1**).[3] Those capable of riding a standard bicycle with adaptations are classified into 5 groups, C1 to C5 (see **Table 1**).[3] Athletes in this category include those with neurologic conditions resulting in dystonia, spasticity, impaired muscle power, movement disorders, and those with limb deficiency or amputation. The final classification category is for those with vision impairment or blindness using tandem cycles with a "sighted" pilot (see **Table 1**).[3] Despite there only being 1 class, visually impaired athletes are designated B1 to B3 based on their degree of vision impairment. B1 athletes have no sight, B2 athletes can see a diameter up to 10°, and B3 athletes can see a diameter up to 40°.[3]

Currently, there is no equal classification system for competition in off-road para-cycling or adaptive mountain biking (aMTB).[6] There is an Adaptive Trail Rating system that was developed for trail makers and event managers to provide guidelines and resources to promote aMTB. The Adaptive Trail Rating system includes aMTB trail ratings, directional mobility, and access signs that can be placed along trails. The aMTB trail ratings are on a 0 to 5 scale, with 0 being not accessible and 5 being fully accessible.[6] This is just one example of ways to make all types of cycling more accessible.

Table 1	
UCI event classification system for adaptive cyclists	
Handcycle	
H1	Tetraplegia, with impairment of majority of upper limb (C6 and above) and inability to use trunk or legs
H2	Tetraplegia, typically with impairment of ≤50% of upper limb function (C7 or C8); often with significant dystonia or movement disorder
H3	Paraplegia, with thoracic impairment (T1–T10), limited truncal stability
H4	Impairment T11 and below, unable to sustain kneeling position
H5	Impairment T11 and below (typically paraplegia or limb deficiency), compete in kneeling position using bilateral upper limbs and trunk
Tricycle	
T1	Severe dystonia/spasticity, ataxia, athetosis
T2	Moderate dystonia/spasticity, ataxia, athetosis
Bicycle	
C1	Single or double limb deficiency, significant limb and/or truncal weakness and/or significant limb dystonia/spasticity
C2	Moderate dystonia/spasticity involving upper and lower limbs, typically predominant lower limb, with possible athetosis, ataxia, limb deficiency
C3	Mild upper limb dystonia/spasticity with mild to moderate lower limb dystonia/spasticity, with less athetosis or ataxia, possible limb deficiency
C4	Mild lower limb dystonia/spasticity with possible athetosis or ataxia, possible limb deficiency/amputation
C5	Single limb amputation, spastic or dystonic monoplegia, mild locomotion impairment
Tandem	
B1	Blind
B2	Visually impaired: Able to see a diameter up to 10°
B3	Visually impaired: Able to see a diameter up to 40°

TYPES OF CYCLING ADAPTATIONS

There are a variety of adaptations to standard bicycles and unique para-cycling configurations of bikes to accommodate the disability of the para-cyclist.

Handcycles

Handcycles have a variety of configurations and are typically used by para-athletes with spinal cord injury, spina bifida, or proximal bilateral lower extremity amputations and/or limb deficiencies.[7] The simplest form is a wheel connected to a crank system that can be attached to a standard wheelchair.[7] This system is ideal for individuals who do not have access to an adapted cycle or prefer not to transfer from their wheelchair. Although wheelchairs are well-suited for low-level activity or activities of daily living, it can be more cumbersome for high-speed recreational activities.

Rigid frame handcycles are more commonly used for recreational activities and elite competition. Typically, the front wheel is propelled synchronously with a conventional cycle drivetrain propelled by handgrips instead of pedals.[8] Handcycles allow para-cyclists to adopt a more upright (**Fig. 1**), touring backrest position (**Fig. 2**), or a horizontal recumbent position (**Fig. 3**).[7] Alternatively, there are also handcycles available in kneeling/prone positions in which the crank is positioned below the shoulder level

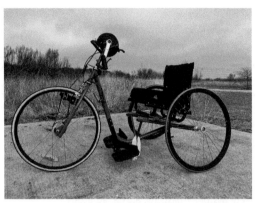

Fig. 1. Upright handcycle. This is an example of a handcycle with an upright seating config-uration. The drivetrain and brake act solely on the front wheel, whereas the back 2 wheels provide stability. The seating can be customized with interchangeable cushions and the de-gree of back support provided. These are usually entry-level bikes for para-athletes who are new to the sport. The upright position can be beneficial for individuals with poor truncal control; however, the para-athlete will experience increased air resistance and drag compared with more recumbent configurations. Owing to the high center of gravity, up-right handcycles are not suitable for speeds of more than 15 miles per hour. Upright hand-cycles can be easier for individuals to transfer in and out of compared with recumbent handcycles, which are much lower to the ground.

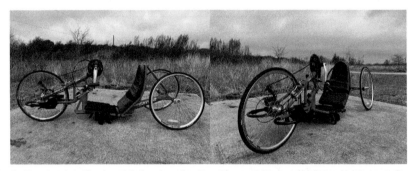

Fig. 2. Touring handcycle. This is a handcycle with a touring recumbent seating configura-tion. Although elite para-cyclists compete in a more horizontal and thus aerodynamic posi-tion, the touring bike pictured is ideal for recreational comfort over longer distances. This position allows the rider to visualize the road more easily compared with the racing hand-cycle position. This bike uses cable gearing, which requires the rider to orient the hand grips with the cables facing up so that they clear the bike and the athlete during the hand crank cycle. Electrical shifting is also available, which minimizes the presence of cables and does not require specific orientation of the hand grips. There are 2 typical steering options: fork steer and lean to steer. Fork steering is more widespread and uses a traditional frame where the fork turns independently. This steer option works well for individuals with low-level and high-level disabilities. The handcycle pictured here uses fork steering. Lean to steering requires a 2-piece frame where the top swivels over the bottom frame and the front wheel turns along with the seat. The rider initiates a turn by leaning the whole body, similar to monoskiing.

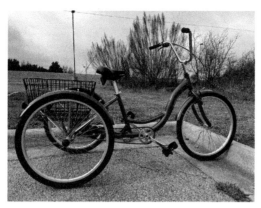

Fig. 3. Tricycle. The tricycle provides stability for athletes who struggle to maintain balance on a standard bicycle. Although the 3-wheel configuration is very similar to upright hand-cycles, the drivetrain uses pedals and acts on the back axle, which powers the 2 back wheels. The handcycle drivetrain instead powers the front wheel. Tricycles can be fitted with standard bicycle seats as pictured here, or with backrest options that offer varying degrees of truncal support.

of the para-cyclist.[7] Kneeling handcycles have the theoretic potential for increased power owing to the advantage of the body weight placed over the crank set; however, studies show slower velocities when compared with recumbent cycles owing to increased drag from the athletes' frontal surface area.[9] The kneeling position may be favored for off-road recreation because the individual has a more advantageous position from which to see the upcoming terrain.[10] This better vantage point may allow the athlete to avoid upcoming obstacles and prevent injury. Prone hand cycles may benefit athletes with conditions such as cerebral palsy with high extensor tone and poor head and trunk control.[11] Similar to tricycles, handcycles also have 3 wheels, but are uniquely powered by the upper extremities. The placement of the wheels depends on the activity and where the desired center of gravity of the athlete should be placed.[12]

Tandem Bicycles

Tandem bicycles are ideal for para-athletes with visual impairments participating in road cycles or mountain biking events. The blind or visually impaired rider, referred to as the stoker, rides behind a sighted rider, who is referred to as the pilot.[13] The stoker focuses on providing power, and the pilot is responsible for navigation, gearing, braking, and additional power.[14] Safety consideration for balance must be taken into account because the 2 riders can weight shift independently on the bike. To adapt, turns are taken wider to accommodate for the length of the bike. Mounting and dismounting carry an increased risk of falls.[14] High levels of communication are required between the pilot and the stoker so that the stoker can anticipate turns, stops, and changes in cadence.

Tricycles

Tricycles are typically used by athletes with conditions that impair balance or lead to severe pedaling restrictions.[12] The 3-wheel configuration provides more balance and stability than a standard 2-wheeled cycle (**Fig. 4**).[12] Most athletes use the upright and recumbent cycle styles. Although not as common, some manufacturers offer a prone

A 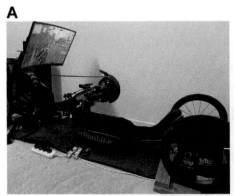 **B**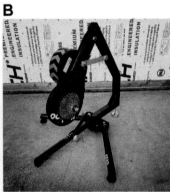

Fig. 4. Stationary handcycle setup for virtual training. (*A*) An example of a handcycle stationary setup using a smart trainer so that the rider can participate in virtual training on Zwift. This product is one of many multiplayer online platforms that allows cyclists to interact, train, and compete in virtual worlds with a global community. (*B*) A modified Kickr smart trainer that has been adapted with a customized bracket that allows the rider to mount a handcycle on the trainer instead of a standard bicycle. Handcycles have drivetrains that act on the front wheel instead of the rear wheel, making it difficult to use some stationary trainers available on the market; however, multiple online communities have published instructions and suggestions on how to modify standard trainers for adapted virtual uses.

recumbent configuration for cyclists with high extensor tone and poor head and/or trunk control.[11] Tricycles can be fitted with standard bicycle seats or seating options with varying degrees of truncal support.[15,16] Additional customizable accessories are available, such as abductor pads to help to align lower extremities to assist with pedal efficiency in patients with spasticity.[16]

Adaptations to Standard Bicycles

Standard bicycles can be adapted to accommodate for certain impairments. Cyclists with upper limb hemiparesis may benefit from modified handlebars or switching brakes to the stronger side.[17] Those with lower limb hemiparesis or dystonia may benefit from toe cages, clips, or Velcro foot straps if deemed safe by the provider.[17] Adult sized training wheels can be considered in those with mild balance impairments or ataxia.

Para-cyclists with an upper extremity amputation often require use of prosthetic limbs to provide support, stability, and aid in steering/gearing of a standard bicycle.[18] Upper extremity amputee individuals can participate in para-cycling by:

1. Using a regular bicycle with modifications,
2. Wearing an upper extremity prosthesis, and
3. Riding one handed.[19]

Upper extremity prostheses can aid athletes in gripping the handlebar, in steering, and in operating the gears and brakes. Prosthetic hands fitted with voluntary opening/closing mechanisms are typically sufficient.[20,21] For above-elbow amputees, elbow units of the prosthesis can be locked at different angles or left unlocked to allow the para-cyclist to assume various positions during a ride or race.[21,22] Most children with congenital amputations choose not to wear prostheses for play activities; however, cup adaptations can be attached to handlebars to place a residual limb to allow for steering and balance.[19]

Athletes with transtibial amputations may elect to wear a lower extremity prosthesis during cycling to help transfer power through the crank interface.[18] Whereas transfemoral amputees may choose not to ride with a prosthesis owing to poor power production and discomfort.[23] To limit friction issues caused by ischial containment sockets, transfemoral amputee para-athletes will often choose to lower the height of the medial wall of the socket for increased comfort.[23] These sockets may be used because the stability of the hip musculature is not as important during cycling as it is during ambulation or running. Many para-cyclists prefer stirrups over toe clips for ease and speed of mounting and dismounting their bike; however, some transtibial para-cyclists directly attach their prosthesis to the pedal or the crank. This process requires a socket design that allows the rider to don the limb quickly as they mount or sit on the saddle.[23] In the event of a flat tire, it would take more time for a para-cyclist to dismount and detach their prosthesis to walk to an aid station. This factor may add unwanted additional time to an elite competitive para-cyclist.

Bike Accessories

There are recumbent foot cycles that can be used by individuals who may benefit from a lower center of gravity for more stability, including those with traumatic brain injuries, cerebral palsy, stroke, or other neurologic injuries. Custom foot plates with ratcheted straps can be made to fit around shoes and braces.[11] Custom foot plates can be placed in the optimal position for athletes with spasticity to allow for leg alignment, promote neutral hip/knee positioning, and decrease heel flexion.[11] Proper foot pedal placement can allow riders to propel downwards to achieve reciprocal patterning. Four-point chest harnesses can be added to seat backs to keep the rider in the upright position.[11] These harnesses may be useful in athletes with truncal weakness and spinal deformities. Some custom bikes come with an adjustable tilt fork that can be increased to up to 6 inches of tilt without changing the position of the seat or crank.[11] The ability to change the tilt can allow for more rider comfortability. Options are available to add rear steering to bikes so that a caregiver or therapist can gear and brake.[11] Rear steering improves rider safety and awareness when learning to use the bike. The gears can be adjusted to where the rider has more control of steering and gearing as their skills improve.

BIOMECHANICAL AND PHYSIOLOGIC CONSIDERATIONS FOR ADAPTIVE CYCLING

As the popularity of para-cycling has grown over the last several decades, new understandings in biomechanics have improved comfort and efficiency for para-athletes when selecting specific prosthetic and bike models.

Physiology

Any degree of lower limb amputation will decrease the total propulsive torque on the amputated side, requiring compensatory strategies from the para-athlete to account for asymmetry between the lower extremities.[24] Transtibial amputated limbs display lower magnitudes of hip extensor, knee flexor, and extensor moments that contribute to work asymmetry.[24] Studies have demonstrated notable differences in the timing of muscle activation between an individual's dominant and amputated limb during the pedal cycle. This difference is seen specifically with a delayed peak activation of the rectus femoris and gastrocnemius on the residual limb.[24,25] These asymmetries not only lead to decreased power, but may set up the para-athlete for overuse injuries as well.

Handcycling Considerations

Handcycling is a closed-chain motion, so the configuration of the handbike affects the technique and efficiency of the handcyclist. Studies have investigated the optimal placement of cranks and hand grips. With able-bodied cycling, saddle height adjustments offer the ideal placement of the athlete for the optimal crank power and ergonomic positions to decrease injuries. Saddle height is determined using a percentage of the inseam length and knee angle.[26,27] The equivalent in handcycling would be a combination of arm length percentage and elbow angle; however, this metric fails to consider the position and orientation of the wrists, humerus, and shoulder girdle.[28] Standard horizontal crank positions between 97% and 100% of an athlete's total arm length have been found to be the most efficient configuration for handcyling.[28] In those with spinal cord injury with paraplegia, evidence supports a decreased load on the shoulder, without significantly compromising efficiency, with more upright backrest positioning and distant crank placement.[29]

Transfemoral Amputations

For individuals with transfemoral amputations who desire to ride an upright or recumbent bike, some publications recommend a prosthesis with a Barlett tendon knee, with the possible addition of a flexion stop to the knee joint.[30] Brian Bartlett, who was a prior member of the US Ski team before his above-the-knee amputation, helped to design this prosthesis to allow him compete in elite level downhill mountain bike racing and road cycling competitions alongside able-bodied athletes.[31] The added benefit of the Barlett tendon knee is that it allows for stability in stance phase for para-cyclists who prefer to stand out of the saddle.[5] Many athletes require greater knee flexion for cycling than is typically used for a running prosthesis.[23] The use of locking liners, 1-way suction valves, or seal-in liner systems eliminates the need for an external sleeve suspension system that can limit knee range of motion during the pedal stroke.[23]

Socket and Liner Considerations

Residual limb volumes can fluctuate, which can present a challenge to athletes' prosthetic suspension, especially for those new to the sport. Training can decrease body fat and change muscle composition, which may reshape the residual limb. Loss of body fluids during long rides can contribute to the decrease in residual limb volume and create excessive movement within the socket.[23] Modifications with leather or pelite pads within the socket surface or using socks can accommodate for minor fluctuations.[23] The use of silicone or gel suspension sleeves will assist in the reduction of shear forces, compression, and peak pressures against the residual limb.[32] Excessive knee flexion at the top of the pedal stroke can apply pressure from the proximal posterior and anterior distal walls of the socket against the transtibial residual limb, leading to skin breakdown.[33] Either a silicone or urethane liner system with the knee preflexed to 5° to 10° can help to decrease the material bunching and skin pressure in the posterior aspect of the knee.[23] Suspension sleeves with wave or undulated features can be designed to allow for increased knee flexion without gathering excess material.[23] Para-cyclists with transtibial amputations and short residual limbs can use a supracondylar cuff strap or elastic 2-inch waist belt with inverted Y strap that will help to augment suspension.[23]

Competitive para-cyclists typically require specialized foot and ankle cycling prosthetic devices to allow for aerodynamic designs and stiffness that contribute to performance.[33] Energy-storing prosthetic feet will cause a loss of propulsive pedaling power, which is more noticeable with increased cycling frequency and longer distances.[33] For elite cyclists, a standard J-shaped carbon fiber prosthetic foot affords ankle rigidity, whereas other custom-made foot attachments with rigid ankles are constructed for the sole purpose of cycling.[33,34] Some racing para-cyclists remove the foot altogether and connect the pedal directly to the prosthetic pylon using a toe cleat.[33]

VIRTUAL RIDING OPTIONS

Stationary cycling has been a viable training option for some time. The coronavirus disease 2019 pandemic, however, triggered an exponential growth in virtual training platforms that allow athletes to train and compete from the safety of their own homes. In 2020, the inaugural Virtual Tour de France took place on the virtual platform Zwift after sanctioned in-person competitions were canceled.[35] This event included 92 men and 68 women from 40 different teams.[35] Individuals can use their regular road bike, tricycle, or handcycle to participate with the addition of a bike trainer. Bike trainers are used to hold the regular cycle of choice in place and to provide resistance either through friction resistance or by attaching the cassette directly to the trainer (see **Fig. 3**). Wheel-on trainers are those in which the rear wheel attaches to a roller, which provides resistance. In contrast, direct drive trainers involve connecting the bike to the trainer's cassette after removing the rear wheel. Direct- drive models are more costly but provide more realistic resistance, less noise, and prevent wear on the rear wheel.[36] Riders can participate in group rides or structured workouts in a virtual environment with other riders from all over the world. There is a growing para-cycling community on these platforms. For example, the para-cycling coach of the Norwegian Cycling Federation started hosting a virtual group ride on Zwift during the pandemic.[37] Zwift does not yet include avatars representative of adaptive cyclists, but there is active discussion about this as a future direction on its online community forum.[38] Popular platforms used for training and competition include:

- Zwift[39]
- Bkool[40]
- Rouvy[41]
- RGT Cycling[42]
- The Sufferfest[43]
- Trainer Road[44]

These virtual options allow for para-cyclists to connect with each other in online communities. Some individuals may also prefer stationary indoor para-cycling for increased safety compared with riding outside on roads that are shared with cars. This may allow for injury prevention while athletes can continue to prosper from the health benefits of para-cycling. Furthermore, virtual riding options decrease the need for transportation to and from organized in-person programs, which is a known barrier to participation in adaptive sports.[45,46]

ORGANIZATIONS AND FUNDING ASSISTANCE

The cost of a handcycle or adapting a bicycle can be a barrier for many people with disabilities who are interested in getting involved in adaptive cycling. There are multiple groups and organizations that provide para-athletes with financial resources, scholarships or grants to lower the financial barrier of getting adaptive equipment. These organizations also provide community support by loaning adaptive equipment and offer recreational and training opportunities for adaptive sports. Prominent national organizations include the following.

- *Challenged Athletes Foundation (CAF)*: The CAF offers Access for Athletes grants for adaptive sports equipment in addition to providing resources for training and competition expenses[47]
- *Move United* provides national leadership and opportunities for individuals with disabilities in more than 60 different adaptive sports. Move United has a national network of more than 180 local member organizations and maintains fund programs specifically for youth para-athletes, victims of gun violence or acts of terrorism, and those disabled during active military service.[48]
- *High Fives Non-Profit Foundation*: The Empowerment Fund provides resources and inspiration to individuals who have suffered a life-altering injury, such as spinal cord injuries, traumatic brain injuries, amputation, or other mobility-limiting injuries that occurred while participating in outdoor sports.[49]
- *IM Able Foundation*: Grants are awarded to disabled individuals, specifically to provide handcycles and other adaptive athletic gear in addition to instructional training programs.[50]
- *Kelly Brush Foundation*: The Active Fund, through the Kelly Brush Foundation, provides grants to individuals with spinal cord injuries to purchase adaptive sports equipment.[51]
- *The Semper Fi Fund* provides support in a variety of ways for injured veterans, including assistance with specialized and adaptive equipment.[52]
- *Travis Roy Foundation* gives financial assistance for adaptive sports equipment and assistive technology to individuals with spinal cord injuries.[53]
- *US Department of Veterans Affairs (VA)*: The VA Adaptive Sports Grant program provides opportunities for Veterans to improve their independence, well-being, and quality of life through adaptive sports and therapeutic arts programs.[54]
- *Achilles International*: Global organization in 25 countries, including the United States, that provides athletic programs for people with disabilities. This includes a dedicated handcycle program.[55]

Local spinal cord injury nonprofit organizations also often offer small grants specifically for adaptive sports equipment within the communities that they serve. One example is the Lone Star Paralysis Foundation based in Austin, Texas, that offers free adaptive sporting events and loans adaptive equipment to local citizens with disabilities.

SUMMARY

The world of amateur and competitive adaptive cycling has grown in both scope and popularity over the last few decades. Increased recreational, therapeutic, and competitive participation makes it increasingly important for clinicians to become familiar with the field. The 8 impairment categories defined by the UCI for para-cycling classification include limb deficiency, leg length difference, impaired muscle power, impaired passive range of movement, hypertonia, athetosis, ataxia, and visual impairment. The 4 main adaptive categories include tandem cycling, handcycling, tricycle, and standard bicycle. There are multiple considerations for fit and customization depending on the individual's disability and adapted bike to improve efficiency and comfort. Virtual platforms that allow riders to train and compete online have grown in popularity among para-cycling communities and offer an alternative to riding outdoors. Many national and local organizations offer grants and programs to assist with adaptive cycling equipment and offer opportunities for training and competition.

CLINICS CARE POINTS

- Para-cycling is now the third largest Paralympic sport after track and field and swimming; there are 8 impairment categories for participation in sanctioned events including limb deficiency, leg length difference, impaired muscle power, impaired passive range of movement, hypertonia, athetosis, ataxia, and visual impairment.
- The major adaptive cycling categories include tandem cycling, handcycling, tricycle, and standard bicycle.
- Special care should be taken regarding the fit and configuration of adapted bikes because this para-athlete population can have altered physiology and mechanics.
- Virtual platforms that allow riders to train and complete online have grown in popularity among para-cycling communities and offer an alternative to riding outdoors.
- There are many organizations that offer grants and assistance to para-cyclists, because the cost of equipment can be a barrier to entry and participation.

DISCLOSURE

The authors have nothing to disclose.

REFERENCES

1. Rio 2016 results archive - cycling | international Paralympic committee. International Paralympic Committee. 2021. Available at: https://www.paralympic.org/rio-2016/results/cycling. Accessed March 1, 2021.
2. About paracylcing. Union Cycliste Internationale. 2021. Available at: https://www.uci.org/para-cycling/about-paracycling. Accessed March 1, 2021.
3. Para-cycling: UCI cycling regulations. Union Cycliste Internationale. 2021. Available at: https://www.uci.org/docs/default-source/rules-and-regulations/16-par-20210101-e.pdf. Accessed March 1, 2021.
4. Rio 2016 - results | international Paralympic committee. 2021. Available at: https://www.paralympic.org/rio-2016/results. Accessed March 1, 2021.
5. Eveleth R. The man who built himself an 'impossible' knee. Mosaic: BBC Future; 2015.
6. Boundary BT. What is adaptive MTB?. Available at: https://breaktheboundary.com.au/resources/what-is-adaptive-mountain-biking/. Accessed May 26, 2021.
7. Stephenson BT, Stone B, Mason BS, et al. Physiology of handcycling: a current sports perspective. Scand J Med Sci Sports 2021;31(1):4–20.
8. Zipfel E, Olson J, Puhlman J, et al. Design of a custom racing hand-cycle: review and analysis. Disabil Rehabil Assist Technol 2009;4(2):119–28.
9. Groen WG, Van Der Woude LHV, De Koning JJ. A power balance model for hand-cycling. Disabil Rehabil 2010;32(26):2165–71.
10. ReActive adaptations | offroad handcycles - bomber offroad handcycle. Reactive adaptations. 2021. Available at: https://reactiveadaptations.com/bomber-rs-offroad-handcycle/. Accessed March 2, 2021.
11. Adaptive bikes. Freedom Concepts Inc. Available at: https://www.freedomconcepts.com/product-lines/adaptive-bikes/. Accessed March 2, 2021.
12. Para cycling | Canadian Paralympic committee. Available at: https://paralympic.ca/paralympic-sports/para-cycling. Accessed March 2, 2021.
13. About para-cycling. British cycling. 2021. Available at: https://www.britishcycling.org.uk/aboutpara-cycling?c=EN. Accessed March 2, 2021.

14. Cycling - United States association of blind athletes. USABA. 2021. Available at: https://www.usaba.org/sports/cycling/. Accessed March 2, 2021.

15. Adaptive bicycles. Cerebral palsy foundation. 2021. Available at: https://www.yourcpf.org/cpproduct/adaptive-bicycles/. Accessed March 2, 2021.

16. Adaptive tricycles: exercise with all the fun of riding. Rifton Equipment. 2021. Available at: https://www.rifton.com/products/special-needs-tricycles/adaptive-tricycles. Accessed March 2, 2021.

17. Bikes and trikes - CHASA. Children's hemiplegia and stroke association. Available at: https://chasa.org/disability-sports/bikes-and-trikes/. Accessed May 26, 2021.

18. Dyer B. The importance of aerodynamics for prosthetic limb design used by competitive cyclists with an amputation: an introduction. Prosthet Orthot Int 2015;39(3):232–7.

19. Baker SA, Calhoun VD. A custom bicycle handlebar adaptation for children with below elbow amputations. J Hand Ther 2014;27(3):258–60.

20. Radocy B. Upper-limb prosthetic adaptations for sports and recreation. In: Bowker H, Michael J, Smith D, editors. Atlas of amputations and limb deficiencies: surgical, prosthetic, and rehabilitation principles. 3rd edition. American Academy of Orthopedic Surgeons; 2004. p. 327–38.

21. Bragaru M, Dekker R, Geertzen JH. Sport prostheses and prosthetic adaptations for the upper and lower limb amputees: an overview of peer reviewed literature. Prosthet Orthot Int 2012;36(3):290–6.

22. Riel L-P, Adam-Côté J, Daviault S, et al. Design and development of a new right arm prosthetic kit for a racing cyclist. Prosthet Orthot Int 2009;33(3):284–91.

23. Gailey R, Harsch P. Introduction to triathlon for the lower limb amputee triathlete. Prosthet Orthot Int 2009;33(3):242–55.

24. Lee Childers W, Prilutsky BI, Gregor RJ. Motor adaptation to prosthetic cycling in people with trans-tibial amputation. J Biomech 2014;47(10):2306–13.

25. Childers LW, Hodson-Tole EF, Gregor RJ. Activation changes in the gastrocnemius muscle: adaptation to a new functional role following amputation. Med Sci Sports Exerc 2009;45(5):S168.

26. Ferrer-Roca V, Roig A, Galilea P, et al. Influence of saddle height on lower limb kinematics in well-trained cyclists: statis vs. dynamic evaluation in bike fitting. J Strength Cond Res 2012;26(11):3025–9.

27. Bini R, Hume PA, Croft JL. Effects of bicycle saddle height on knee injury risk and cycling performance. Sports Med 2011;41(6):463–76.

28. Stone B, Mason BS, Warner MB, et al. Horizontal crank position affects economy and upper limb kinematics of recumbent handcyclists. Med Sci Sports Exerc 2019;51(11):2265–73.

29. Arnet U, Van Drongelen S, Schlüssel M, et al. The effect of crank position and backrest inclination on shoulder load and mechanical efficiency during handcycling. Scand J Med Sci Sports 2014;24(2):386–94.

30. Harvey ZT, Loomis GA, Mitsch S, et al. Advanced rehabilitation techniques for the multi-limb amputee. J Surg Orthop Adv 2012;21(1):50–7.

31. Eveleth R. Going out on a limb: skier Brian Bartlett needed a new knee, so he invented one. 2015. Available at: https://www.newsweek.com/going-out-limb-skier-brian-bartlett-needed-new-knee-so-he-invented-one-334060.

32. Sanders JE, Nicholoson BS, Zachariah SG, et al. Testing of elastomeric liners used in limb prosthetics: classification of 15 products by mechanical performance. J Rehabil Res Dev 2004;41(2):175–86.

33. Childers WL, Kistenberg RS, Gregor RJ. The biomechanics of cycling with a transtibial amputation: recommendations for prosthetic design and direction for future research. Prosthet Orthot Int 2009;33(3):256–71.

34. Childers WL, Kistenberg RS, Gregor RJ. Pedaling asymmetries in cyclists with unilateral transtibial amputation: effect of prosthetic foot stiffness. J Appl Biomech 2011;27(4):314–21.

35. Petri J. Get ready for a virtual Tour de France. Bloomberg. 2020. Available at: https://www.bloomberg.com/news/articles/2020-06-29/tour-de-france-zwift-ready-an-unprecedented-virtual-cycling-race. Accessed March 14, 2021.

36. Johnson A. The difference between a wheel on and wheel off bike trainer. Indoor cycling tips. Available at: https://indoorcyclingtips.com/the-difference-between-wheel-on-and-wheel-off-trainers/. Accessed May 26, 2021.

37. Paracycling group ride hosted by NCF. Zwift. Available at: https://www.zwift.com/events/view/622702?. Accessed March 14, 2021.

38. Paracyclist: custom avatar request. Zwift | Forums. Available at: https://forums.zwift.com/t/paracyclist-custom-avatar-request/238072. Accessed May 26, 2021.

39. The at home cycling & running virtual training app - Zwift. Available at: https://www.zwift.com/. Accessed March 15, 2021.

40. BKOOL. The most realistic indoor cycling simulator. Available at: https://www.bkool.com/en. Accessed March 15, 2021.

41. Rouvy | #1 indoor cycling workout app. Available at: https://rouvy.com/en/. Accessed March 15, 2021.

42. Indoor cycling & virtual bike training app - RGT cycling. Available at: https://www.rgtcycling.com/. Accessed March 15, 2021.

43. The Sufferfest: complete training app for cyclists and triathletes. Available at: https://thesufferfest.com/. Accessed March 15, 2021.

44. Trainer road | get faster with trainerroad. Available at: https://www.trainerroad.com/. Accessed March 15, 2021.

45. Bezyak JL, Sabella SA, Gattis RH. Public transportation: an investigation of barriers for people with disabilities. J Disabil Policy Stud 2017;28(1):52–60.

46. Rimmer JH. Barriers associated with exercise and community access for individuals with stroke. J Rehabil Res Dev 2008;45(2):315–22.

47. Grant program | challenged athletes foundation. Available at: https://www.challengedathletes.org/programs/grants/. Accessed March 15, 2021.

48. Move United. Available at: https://www.moveunitedsport.org/. Accessed March 15, 2021.

49. High fives foundation | an adaptive sports foundation with heart. Available at: https://highfivesfoundation.org/. Accessed March 15, 2021.

50. IM Able Foundation | Programs. 2014. Available at: https://imablefoundation.org/programs/. Accessed March 15, 2021.

51. The active fund - Kelly Brush Foundation. Available at: https://kellybrushfoundation.org/theactivefund/. Accessed March 15, 2021.

52. Semper Fi & America's Fund. Available at: https://semperfifund.org/. Accessed March 15, 2021.

53. Travis Roy Foundation | spinal cord injury grants & research. Available at: https://www.travisroyfoundation.org/. Accessed March 15, 2021.

54. VA adaptive sports grant program. https://www.blogs.va.gov/nvspse/grant-program/. Accessed March 15, 2021.

55. Handcycle program — Achilles international. Available at: https://www.achillesinternational.org/handcycle-program. Accessed March 15, 2021.

Adaptive Cycling
Injuries and Health Concerns

Gabrielle T. Goodlin, MD, Lindsey Steinbeck, MD,
Deborah Bergfeld, MD, Alexandria Haselhorst, DO*

KEYWORDS

- Para-cycling • Paralympics • Injury • Sports-related concussion

KEY POINTS

- Para-cycling is one of 5 Paralympic sports with the highest rates of acute injuries, which account for 71% to 75% of injuries reported at the Paralympic Games
- Limited injury data exist specifically for para-cyclists; however, general para-athlete trends can be applied to this population, including increased incidence of upper extremity injuries and predisposition for injury and illness depending on the para-athlete's underlying condition
- It is unclear how standard concussion assessment tools and return-to-play protocols can be applied to wheelchair user para-cyclists or those with baseline balance or vestibulo-ocular deficits because no validated alternatives exist
- Para-cyclists with spinal cord injury or increased metabolic rates are at increased risk for heat-related illness during training and competition
- Para-cyclists may be at increased risk for RED-S among para-athletes because their health conditions typically predispose many athletes to low bone mineral density and more than 50% of para-cyclists report pressure to maintain specific weights for competition and performance

INTRODUCTION

All sports carry an inherent risk of injury, and para-cycling is not exempt. The underlying medical conditions that define para-athletes' classifications predispose this unique population of cyclists to certain injury patterns and sequelae that are different from those of their able-bodied counterparts. The popularity of amateur and competitive para-cycling has exponentially increased over the past several decades, and providers should understand the unique injury and illness characteristics of these para-athletes when providing care to support continued participation in such a beneficial

Physical Medicine & Rehabilitation, Department of Neurology, The University of Texas at Austin, Dell Medical School, 1400 North IH-35, Suite 2.230, Austin, TX 78701, USA
* Corresponding author.
E-mail address: ajhaselhorst@ascension.org
Twitter: @gabi_goodlin (G.T.G.); @AliHaselhorstDO (A.H.)

Phys Med Rehabil Clin N Am 33 (2022) 45–60
https://doi.org/10.1016/j.pmr.2021.08.004
1047-9651/22/© 2021 Elsevier Inc. All rights reserved.

physical activity. Although data for this population remain scarce, we seek to lay out what is known in this field and identify areas for further research and investigation.

INJURIES IN PARA-CYCLING

Epidemiologic data for injury rates among para-cycling athletes at the pediatric, recreational, and elite levels are limited. There has been a concerted effort over the past decade to increase data surveillance at elite levels of competition. Systemic injury surveillance was widely implemented for summer Paralympic sports starting with the 2012 London Paralympic Games. The overall injury incidence rate among the 274 participating para-cyclists during the 2012 London Paralympics was 6.7 per 1000 athlete-days (9.3%) in road cycling and 9.3 per 1000 athlete-days (13%) in track cycling.[1] In comparison, the percentage of able-bodied cyclists injured at the 2012 London Olympics was 9% of road cyclists and 3% of track cyclists (**Fig. 1**).[2] In the 2016 Rio Paralympics, road para-cycling and track para-cycling data were presented together. Among the 204 participating para-cyclists, the injury incidence rate was 7.0 per 1000 athlete-days (9.8%), compared with 5.6% of able-bodied road cyclists and 5.3% of able-bodied track cyclists (see **Fig. 1**).[3,4] In the Paralympic Games, both road cycling and track cycling were among the top 5 sports with the highest rates of acute injuries, accounting for 71% to 75% of recorded cycling injuries.[1] Athletes in the class category C1 (single or double limb deficiency, severe limb and/or truncal weakness, and/or severe limb dystonia/spasticity on a standard bicycle) suffered the most frequent injuries.[5] Unfortunately, the injury data available do not further differentiate between anatomic locations of traumatic and nontraumatic injuries among para-cyclists and para-athletes to compare with the injury patterns observed among

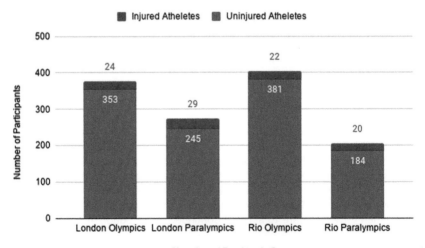

Fig. 1. Comparison of Olympic cycling injuries to Paralympic cycling Injuries in 2012 and 2016. Widespread injury monitoring was implemented at the 2012 London Paralympic Games, allowing for direct comparison with injury data from corresponding Olympic Games during the same year and the subsequent events in Rio during 2016. The overall percentage of cycling (road and track) athletes who were injured at the 2012 London Olympics was 6.4% compared with 10.5% at the London Paralympic Games. The overall percentage of cycling athletes injured at the 2016 Rio Olympics was 5.4% compared with 9.8% at the Rio Paralympics. (*Data from* Refs.[1–4])

able-bodied cyclists. Increased injury surveillance at recreational and elite competitions will help to further our understanding of specific injury patterns among this population beyond the generalities described earlier.

Although the data available specifically for para-cyclists remain limited, there are general inferences that can be made using the pooled Paralympic data and para-sport surveillance. During the 2016 Rio Paralympics, athletes with limb deficiency constituted the group with the highest number of injuries, encompassing 32% of all injured athletes.[3] This injury rate was followed by athletes with visual impairment at 20%, spinal cord injury (SCI) at 18.4%, and central neurologic impairment at 17% of all injured athletes.[3] The injury incidence rates between male and female Paralympic athletes are similar.[1] The incidence rate of upper-limb injuries was higher than that of lower-limb injuries at the 2012 and 2016 Paralympic Games.[1,3] Shoulders were injured at the highest rate, followed by wrist/hand, and then elbow.[1,3] This injury pattern is unique to the para-sport community because lower limb injuries predominate in the able-bodied Olympic athlete population.[2,4] Among lower extremity injuries in para-athletes, the knee is the most commonly injured and is typically seen in athletes with visual impairments, cerebral palsy, and amputations.[1,6] Participants with SCIs have a higher prevalence of fractures that other athletes because of the high prevalence of low bone mineral density (BMD) and osteopenia.[6] Athletes with cerebral palsy have the highest percentages of soft tissue injuries, which is thought to be due to limited range of motion, spasticity, and discoordination that may cause additional stress to muscles, joints, and tendons.[7]

Overuse injuries on average affect 13% of athletes from all adaptive sports.[8] Data available for small cohorts of adaptive cyclists report chronic injuries in a range of 23% to 94.7% over the course of a season, suggesting that this population experiences higher-than-average levels of chronic injuries.[1,5,9] The anatomic distribution of overuse injuries in adaptive cyclists is similar to those of able-bodied cycling, although the incidences of injuries in the low-back, neck, and shoulder are slightly higher for para-cyclists.[9]

ILLNESS IN PARA-CYCLING

Predisposition to illness and health problems are higher in adaptive sports populations when compared with their able-bodied counterparts. Respiratory illnesses account for the most illnesses in the para-athlete population.[3,10] Other common ailments include skin, gastrointestinal, and genitourinary (GU) illnesses.[10,11] Athletes with the highest proportion of illness include those with SCIs (30.8%), limb deficiencies (24.2%), and central neurologic injury (14.8%).[11] Females and para-athletes aged 35 to 75 years have higher rates of illness when compared with male para-athletes and younger age groups.[8,11] Skin illnesses can be attributed to prosthesis use with limb deficiencies or athletes with sensory deficits who spend long periods in a sitting position in wheelchairs or adaptive equipment.[12,13] Respiratory and GU illnesses are reported most frequently in athletes with SCI due to frequent GU instrumentation and impaired respiratory muscle function in tetraplegic athletes.[12,13] Predisposition to illness in athletes with SCIs is likely due to several factors such as decreased immune function leading to immunodeficient states, wheelchair use leading to skin breakdown, and sensory deficits that may lead to imprecise early symptom reporting.[11,14–16]

At the 2016 Rio Paralympic Games, the illness incidence was 10.5% and 13.2% in track and road para-cyclists, respectively.[11] This rate seems to be similar to the overall illness rates for athletes across all Paralympic sports.[10,11] Limited long-term surveillance of elite Paralympic teams showed that at any given time, 28% of athletes reported health problems, with 12% to 14% reporting substantial health problems due to illness that resulted in severe reduction in training volume or complete inability to participate in sport.[8,17] Familiarity with the common medical conditions and disabilities present in para-cycling will help clinicians quickly identify and effectively treat illness in this population so that para-cyclists can return to training and competition.

SPECIAL CONSIDERATIONS ON SAFETY AND INJURY PREVENTION
Sport-Related Concussion and Traumatic Brain Injury

Head injuries and sport-related concussion (SRC) are a recognized risk in adaptive cycling given the high speeds at which athletes compete and the risk for collisions. The Centers of Disease Control and Prevention has reported that of the 207,830 people treated annually for traumatic brain injuries (TBIs) related to sports and recreational activities, cycling accounts for 40,424 cases (19.45%), the highest number in any reported sport.[18] Epidemiologic studies estimate that SRC accounts for 1.3% to 9.1% of all injuries during cycling events, including approximately 2% of injuries at the Tour de France.[19–21] Large-scale epidemiologic data are unavailable for para-cycling; however, Paralympic sports with visually impaired athletes and sports performed at high speeds show particularly high incidences of concussions.[1,12] Unfortunately, the Rio 2016 Paralympic Games saw the death of a para-cycling athlete following head trauma during competition in men's road cycling.[3] Little is known about how the sequelae of SRC may affect athletes with central neurologic injuries, such as cerebral palsy, stroke, or TBI.[22] Baseline screening and prompt diagnosis is the standard of care of SRC treatment; however, large portions of tools used to diagnose SRC such as the Sport Concussion Assessment Tool 5th edition (SCAT5) are not useful for wheelchair athletes or those with baseline balance deficits.[22,23] Athletes with disability have been found to have a greater number of baseline symptoms, including poor immediate memory and balance deficits, resulting in higher total severity scores compared with able-bodied athletes.[24] The Wheelchair Error Scoring System is a proposed modified sideline concussion assessment to replace the standard Balance Error Scoring System used for able-bodied athletes; however, validation is still needed.[23] Participants with visual impairments are unable to use ImPACT, King-Devick, or other concussion screening tools that rely on vision.[23] Consensus recommendations for return to participation may pose additional challenges because of the inability to administer standardized balance assessments and lack of wheelchair-specific return-to-play protocols.

Boosting and Autonomic Dysreflexia

Athletes with SCIs at the T6 level or higher are susceptible to episodes of autonomic dysreflexia (AD), which is an excessive output of the sympathetic nervous system (SNS) in response to noxious stimuli such as an overdistended bladder or restrictive clothing. AD can lead to life-threatening hypertension, tachycardia, diaphoresis, muscle spasms, and skin color changes. Boosting is the deliberate act of inducing an episode of AD to improve performance by drastically increasing blood pressure just before competition.[25] When boosting, the sympathetic reflex triggers peripheral vasoconstriction resulting in hypertension and adrenaline responses, which can overcome the limitations of cardiovascular blunting, increase blood flow to muscles, and reduce rate of perceived exertion.[26,27] Boosting is banned by the International Paralympic Committee (IPC) because of hazardous side effects and potentially life-threatening health risks including dizziness, blurred vision, impaired cognition, intracranial hemorrhage, retinal detachments, seizures, and cardiac arrhythmias.[27] In a survey of

Paralympians with SCI, 54.5% of athletes were aware of AD and 16.7% of all males admitted to boosting.[28] These athletes reported benefit of boosting with marathon-, middle-, and long-distance events.[28] Screening is conducted by the IPC in athletes with SCI immediately before competition by measuring systolic blood pressure. Readings of 160 mm Hg or greater are considered consistent with boosting.[22] The IPC recently decreased the cutoff from 180 mm Hg because it was not sensitive enough to capture athletes who were boosting. In addition, athletes must provide any documentation of hypertension at least 14 days before their event. It is important to counsel para-cycling athletes with SCI on how to identify AD and the associated dangerous risks. Despite education on the dangerous consequences, however, para-athletes may still elect to boost before an event and providers should be prepared to manage hazardous outcomes.

Thermoregulation and Heat-Related Illnesses

The adaptive cycling population faces unique challenges with thermoregulation that result in environmental challenges during recreation and competition. Athletes with SCI experience greater thermal strain compared with able-bodied counterparts both at rest and during exercise in hot ambient climates.[29] Sympathetic outflow, including outflow from cardiac accelerator nerves, efferent vasomotor, and sudomotor fibers, typically occurs between the T1-L2/L3 spinal levels and is therefore affected in most athletes with SCI, although to varying degrees depending on the level of injury.[30] Control of the skin vasculature and sweat glands in the face is mediated from T1-T4, the upper extremities from T3-T7, the trunk from T4-T12, and the lower extremities from T10-L2, whereas sensory innervation of the skin in the upper extremities is mediated from C4-T1, the trunk from T2-T12, and the lower extremities from L1-S4.[31,32] Tetraplegic individuals with cervical injuries effectively lose their SNS. Individuals with SCI with complete tetraplegia lack evaporative cooling capacity through the sympathetic reflex during passive heat stress, and individuals with paraplegia sweat, on average, only 1 dermatomal level below their neurologic level of injury.[33] Owing to the absence of evaporative cooling below the level of the SCI and inability to dissipate heat from insensate skin, athletes with SCI experience an earlier increase in mean skin temperature.[34] Consequently, this increase in skin temperature is not directly detected because of loss of afferent information from skin below the level of injury, resulting in an increased core temperature before appropriate effector mechanisms are initiated.[34] Cardiac blunting occurs when SCI interrupts the cardiac sympathetic outflow from T1-T5, which prevents heat dissipation through elevated heart rate.[31] Peak core temperatures up to 40.4°C (104.72°F) have been recorded in para-athletes with SCI, even in temperate conditions.[35]

Handcycling athletes are at increased risk for elevated core temperatures because of low surface area and air density for convective heat loss in recumbent positions in addition to a closer proximity to the road surface for radiant heat gain (**Fig. 2**).[35] Athletes with tetraplegia already experience greater thermal strain because of the loss of the SNS and are more likely to use handcycles compared with those with paraplegia.[29] Athletes with cerebral palsy may display impaired muscle efficiency due to athetosis, hypertonia, or ataxia resulting in greater metabolic cost and heat production.[36] In addition, many para-athletes with neurologic conditions may use botulinum toxin injections to address limited range of motion due to muscle spasticity. Botulinum toxin temporary blocks the release of acetylcholine, which reduces muscle spasticity, as well as sweat production at the site. This side effect on local sweat production may result in a lower evaporative heat loss capacity and reduced adaptive potential during heat acclimation.[37] Para-cycling athletes with SCI or cerebral palsy who train and

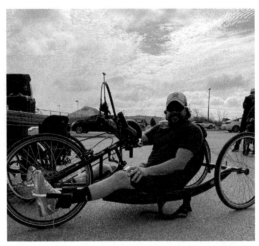

Fig. 2. Orientation of a typical handcycle to road and pavement. Handcyclists are at increased risk for elevated core temperatures because of low surface area and air density for convective heat loss in recumbent positions and a closer proximity to the road surface for radiant heat gain.

compete in warm or humid environments should be educated on their predisposition to develop heat-related illnesses.

STRATEGIES FOR ADAPTIVE CYCLING ATHLETES AND ORGANIZED EVENTS TO PREVENT HEAT-RELATED ILLNESSES
Hydration and Fluid Replacement

- Determine the sweat rate of the athlete to develop an individualized strategy to replete fluid losses.[38,39]
- Additional water and first aid stations may be necessary for prolonged events in warm environments.[38,39]
- Consider acclimation strategies for para-cyclists who compete outdoors

Education

- Signs and symptoms of heat illness should be provided to coaches and support staff.
- Recognize when an athlete needs to stop, be removed from the environment, and/or actively cooled.
- Athletes with intellectual impairments may require additional supervision and guidance regarding hydration advice.[38,39]

Environmental Exposure

- Check anatomic regions that are prone to skin breakdown due to contact with adaptive cycling equipment and/or the accumulation of sweat frequently to avoid skin breakdown.[38,39]
- Avoid sun exposure where possible.
- Use sunscreen to lessen the risk of sunburn and detrimental effects on local sweating ability.

Active Cooling Strategies

- Ice vests can be used during intermittent exercise to reduce thermal strain in athletes with SCI.[38,39]
- Water sprays, cooling garments, extremity cooling, cold water immersion, ice slurries, and mixed method cooling have been previously studied; there are not enough data to recommend one method over the others.[38,39]
- Appropriate cooling methods should be selected to avoid areas of sensory deficits to prevent cold injuries.

Relative Energy Deficiency in Sport and Osteopenia

Relative energy deficiency in sport (RED-S), formally known as the Female Athlete Triad, was first described in 1993 as the triad of disordered eating, amenorrhea, and osteoporosis in females. The definition was broadened in 2014 by the IPC to include the physiologic and performance consequences of low energy availability in both males and females.[40] The condition is characterized by insufficient caloric intake and/or excessive energy expenditure that can alter many physiologic systems including metabolism, endocrine function, menstrual function, bone health, immunity, protein synthesis, cardiovascular function, and psychological health.[41,42] The hallmark triad components have been redefined to include low energy availability with or without an eating disorder, menstrual dysfunction, and low BMD.[41] The health consequences and prevalence of risk factors for RED-S in the para-athlete population are largely unknown, but are thought to be disability and sport dependent.[43]

- *Central neurologic injury*: athletes with aberrant movement patterns such as dyskinesis or athetosis may have higher energy expenditures.[44]
- *SCI*: these athletes exhibit reduced energy expenditures by 25% to 75% during exercise when compared with able-bodied individuals; the greatest reduction occurs in athletes with tetraplegia.[45] As discussed in the Thermoregulation and Heat-Related Illnesses section, the amount of SNS activation during exercise varies depending on the neurologic level of injury and may result in cardiovascular blunting or reduction in peak heart rate, blood pressure, and maximal oxygen uptake during exercise, all of which contribute to decreased energy expenditure.[45,46]
- *Spina bifida (SB)*: individuals who are primary wheelchair users are thought to have reduced basal metabolic rate and decreased daily energy requirements. Alternately, ambulatory individuals with SB have higher energy requirements compared with the general population due to inefficiency of gait.[47,48]
- *Amputations and limb deficiencies*: higher energy expenditures in the setting of prosthetic use and resultant pedal cycle asymmetry. Athletes with bilateral amputations and/or more proximal lower-extremity amputations result in higher energy expenditures during ambulation.[49,50]
- *Short stature:* limited research is available in athletic populations. However, studies suggest elevated resting metabolic rate in individuals with achondroplasia, thought to be due to alteration in organ mass or mitochondrial differences.[51] The prevalence of obesity in individuals with achondroplasia, however, is almost twice as high as that of peers of normal stature, likely due to reduced caloric needs in a smaller body habitus.[52]

Both male and female para-athletes may monitor or restrict weight for sports performance purposes, which can increase risk for nutritional deficiencies. In fact, multiple studies have cited concern for relative energy availability in athletes with SCI, indicating insufficient dietary energy and macronutrient intakes.[53–56] One study found that more than 25% of female athletes with SCI had a daily dietary intake that did not meet the estimated average requirement for nutrients, including calcium, magnesium, folate, and vitamin D.[53] Surveys of elite male and female adaptive cyclists have shown that more than 50% were concerned about their weight.[53,57] In a survey conducted by Brook and colleagues,[57] 72% of male para-cyclist respondents felt pressure to maintain a specific body weight, 72% attempted to change their body weight or body composition to improve sport performance, and 66.7% considered themselves overweight.[57] Data were limited for female para-cyclists, but 50% felt pressure to maintain a specific body weight and 62.5% considered themselves overweight. In the same survey, 33% of male para-cyclists exhibited dietary restraint behavior and 38.8% exhibited pathologic eating behaviors, compared with 25% and 12.5%, respectively, in female para-cyclists.[57] These findings seem to be consistent with prior reports of increased levels of dietary restraint among male compared with female elite athletes with SCI.[53] Dietary restraint scores among female athletes with SCI are similar to those of able-bodied populations, whereas male scores were higher than population norms in able-bodied athletes.[53] Epidemiologic data from able-bodied athletes suggests that the prevalence of disordered eating in elite male athletes is between 1.3% and 32.5% and between 6% and 45% among elite female athletes.[58,59] Although further research is needed in mental health and disordered eating at all levels of competition, the available data suggest that there is an above-average prevalence of disordered eating among para-cyclists and that they may be particularly at risk for developing eating disorders due to both the nature of the sport of cycling to maintain competitive weights and underlying changes in metabolism secondary to medical conditions.

Predisposition to changes in bone health is also well documented for in many conditions affecting para-athletes. One survey found that 8.5% of combined male and female para-athletes had a history of low BMD diagnosed by a dual-energy x-ray absorptiometry scan.[57] A much higher prevalence of low BMD was found among para-cyclists, specifically 22.2% of male and 25% of female para-cyclists, although it should be noted that the number of female respondents was low (n = 8).[57] Bone health among the para-athlete population partially depends on unique risk factors associated with disability. It has been well documented that athletes with SCI have disuse osteopenia/osteoporosis affecting the lower extremities.[60] Research in the general population of individuals with SCI has established that osteoporosis is due to reduced skeletal loading over time.[60] The effects of declining bone health have been shown to be greater in females with SCI when compared with the typical bone health decline associated with estrogen loss in able-bodied women.[61] Individuals with SB also frequently have significantly lower BMD than their able-bodied counterparts.[62–64] Females with SB show lower BMD than males.[62] Children with cerebral palsy display a wide range of BMD that averages 1 SD less than the average for age-matched peers.[97] There is a positive correlation between low weight and reduced BMD, suggesting that poor nutritional intake leads to alterations in bone health in cerebral palsy.[65] The severity and subtype of cerebral palsy are important factors affecting BMD. For example, adults with spastic cerebral palsy had lower BMD Z-scores than adults with dyskinetic cerebral palsy.[66] In addition, individuals with central neurologic injuries requiring prolonged use of anticonvulsants have been found to have lower BMD and unilateral amputees may exhibit reduced BMD in their residual limb.[67–70]

The predisposition for low BMD among this population can lead to bone fractures from minor injuries; this should be taken into consideration during injury assessments in para-sport competitions of what may have been deemed as minimal trauma during a similar able-bodied athletic competition.[57,71] Athletes and the general population with SCI are well documented to have disuse osteopenia/osteoporosis affecting the lower extremities.[60] Individuals with complete SCI who remain non-weight-bearing have demonstrated significant loss of BMD in the proximal femur within 1 year following their injury, and reaching fracture threshold within 1 to 5 years.[72] Among individuals with SCI, osteoporotic fractures most commonly occur in the distal femur and proximal tibia, whereas fractures among able-bodied cyclists most commonly occur in the upper extremities with the clavicle being the predominant location.[73–77] There is some evidence to suggest that positive adaptive changes in BMD can occur in the upper extremities among para-athletes who use their upper extremities for wheelchairs in their sport, which may also apply to handcycling.[78] A preliminary investigation on the effects of sports activity on BMD in athletes with SCI suggests that timely return to sport following SCI correlates with higher BMD and may help to attenuate bone loss.[79] Fractures can also occur as the result of reduced coordination, loss of proprioception, or unforeseen obstacles in visually impaired athletes.[71] Many para-athletes may lack sensation accompanying an acute fracture, particularly SCI athletes below their level of injury. In such cases, evidence of abnormal body position, swelling, erythema, bruising, or grinding sensations should be addressed with precautionary stabilization and diagnostic imaging.[71] It should also be noted that acute fractures may cause AD in para-athletes with SCI as a form of noxious stimuli. Management of pain signals and elevated blood pressure may be required to prevent sequelae of AD.

There is a paucity of data on RED-S and menstrual dysfunction patterns in female para-athlete populations. A prior survey on female para-athletes found that 13.4% had a history of delayed menarche and almost half of participants met the criteria for oligomenorrhea or amenorrhea over the course of 1 year.[57] Specific to SCI, 1 in 3 met criteria for oligomenorrhea or amenorrhea.[57] It has been well established that a transient absence of menses can occur in females for an average of 5 months following initial SCI, but this occurs without long-term impact on menstruation or reproductive health.[80] TBI studies have reported that almost 50% of females experience menstrual dysfunction, including amenorrhea, lasting up to 5 years following initial injury.[81,82] Although data on menstruation in individuals with cerebral palsy is scant, one study reported that 29.4% of adolescents with cerebral palsy experienced menstrual dysfunction.[83] Clinical providers should be aware that menstrual dysfunction may be present among female para-athletes as a sequalae of their injury or medical condition and can be difficult to distinguish from menstrual dysfunction in the setting of RED-S.

Athletes participating in adaptive cycling should be screened for low energy availability to reduce complications of RED-S. Unfortunately there are no current screening tools for disordered eating designed for para-athletes that are validated by the *Diagnostic and Statistical Manual of Mental Disorders* (Fifth Edition) criteria.[41] The Periodic Health Examination and the Preparticipation Physical Evaluation include relevant questions that may assist with early detection.[40,41,84] Additionally, the RED-S Clinical Assessment Tool (RED-S CAT) can assist clinicians in screening for RED-S and management for return-to-play decisions, although validation is still needed.[41] The RED-S CAT tool stratifies athletes into low-, moderate-, and high-risk categories and uses a red light, yellow light, green light system in its return-to-play program that could be adapted to guide clinical decision making for para-athletes (**Table 1**).[41] Prevention efforts should include increased awareness among athletes, coaches, and support staffs. A survey by Brook and colleagues[57] showed that only 8.1% of participating elite para-athletes were aware of the Female Athlete Triad/RED-S, including 13.6% of

| Table 1 | | |
| Relative energy deficiency in sport return-to-play model | | |
High Risk Red Light	Moderate Risk Yellow Light	Low Risk Green Light
No clearance for sport	Training allowed within the scope of a treatment plan	Full sport participation
Sport participation may pose a serious health risk to the athlete Use of written contract recommended	Cleared for sport participation under supervision Reevaluation of the athlete's risk is recommended at regular intervals of 1–3 mo	Cleared for full training and competition

Adapted from Mountjoy et al. RED-S CAT. Relative energy deficiency in sport (RED-S) clinical assessment tool (CAT). Br J Sports Med 2015;49:421–3.

female para-athletes and 4.0% of male para-athletes. The International Olympic Committee consensus statement supports educational programs and peer-based disordered eating prevention programs that are gender specific.[85] These programs target athlete's significant others and coaches in addition to promoting changes to sport regulations, policy measures, and the health care system.[85,86]

HEALTH BENEFITS OF ADAPTIVE SPORTS

Medical providers often espouse the benefits of physical activity to their patients as a mainstay of preventive medicine. Mounting evidence has shown that exercise may also alleviate deficits associated with neurologic disorders.[87] Studies have shown improvement across several domains including cardiopulmonary function, physical endurance, body composition, cognition, and mental performance through engagement in adaptive sports.[88] Adaptive cycling programs have been shown to significantly improve balance in the poststroke period and gross motor function in children with cerebral palsy.[89,90] Furthermore, an 8-week structured cycling program helped to improve social coping skills, fine motor skills, and externalization of maladaptive behaviors in adolescents with Down syndrome.[91] Despite this knowledge, less than 20% of those with an acquired neurologic disorder in the United States meet the World Health Organization's recommended minimum of 150 minutes of physical activity per week.[92] With this breadth of benefits, health care providers should promote engagement in adaptive sports among their patient population whenever it is deemed safe and feasible. Adaptations in cycling have evolved so significantly that the degree of disability is rarely a barrier to participation.

SUMMARY

The recent growth in handcycling and other forms of adaptive cycling has encouraged more people with disabilities to participate over the past several decades; however, much remains unknown regarding the injury profile and risk factors of this subpopulation of para-athletes. Further injury and illness monitoring is needed at organized paracycling events to elucidate trends and differences between para-cyclists and able-bodied cyclists. To date data are available only from 2 Summer Paralympics in 2012 and 2016. Unique characteristics of common conditions exist within the para-athlete community that may predispose this population to certain injuries, such as heat-related injuries. Additional focus should also be applied to the development of concussion and RED-S assessment tools for para-athletes and return-to-play protocols for these conditions.

CLINICS CARE POINTS

- Para-cycling is one of 5 Paralympic sports with the highest rates of acute injuries, which account for 71% to 75% of injuries reported at the Paralympic Games

- Limited injury data exist specifically for para-cyclists; however, general para-athlete trends can be applied to this population, including increased incidence of upper-extremity injuries and predisposition for injury and illness depending on the para-athlete's underlying condition

- It is unclear how standard concussion assessment tools and return-to-play protocols can be applied to wheelchair user para-cyclists or those with baseline balance or vestibulo-ocular deficits because no validated alternatives exist

- Para-cyclists with SCI or increased metabolic rates are at increased risk for heat-related illness during training and competition

- Para-cyclists may be at increased risk for RED-S among para-athletes because their health conditions typically predispose many athletes to low BMD and more than 50% of para-cyclists report pressure to maintain specific weights for competition and performance

DISCLOSURE

The authors have nothing to disclose.

REFERENCES

1. Willick SE, Webborn N, Emery C, et al. The epidemiology of injuries at the London 2012 Paralympic Games. Br J Sports Med 2013;47:426–32. https://doi.org/10.1136/bjsports-2013-092374.
2. Engebretsen L, Soligard T, Steffen K, et al. Sports injuries and illnesses during the London Summer Olympic Games 2012. Br J Sports Med 2013;47(7):407–14.
3. Derman W, Runciman P, Schwellnus M, et al. High precompetition injury rate dominates the injury profile at the Rio 2016 Summer Paralympic Games: a prospective cohort study of 51 198 athlete days. Br J Sports Med 2018;52(1):24–31. https://doi.org/10.1136/bjsports-2017-098039.
4. Soligard T, Steffen K, Palmer D, et al. Sports injury and illness incidence in the Rio de Janeiro 2016 Olympic Summer Games: a prospective study of 11274 athletes from 207 countries. Br J Sports Med 2017;51(17):1265–71. https://doi.org/10.1136/bjsports-2017-097956.
5. Hanief YN, Umar F. The characteristics of Indonesian para-cycling athletes' injuries. Adv Rehabil 2020;34(3):37–46.
6. Athanasopoulos S, Dimitris M, Tsakoniti A, et al. The 2004 Paralympic Games: physiotherapy services in the paralympic village polyclinic. Open Sports Med J 2009;3:1–8. https://doi.org/10.2174/1874387000903010001.
7. Patatoukas D, Farmakides A, Aggeli V, et al. Disability-related injuries in athletes with disabilities. Folia Med (Plovdiv) 2011;53(1):40–6.
8. Hirschmüller A, Fassbender K, Kubosch J, et al. Injury and illness surveillance in elite para athletes: an urgent need for suitable illness prevention strategies. Am J Phys Med Rehabil 2021;100(2):173–80.
9. Kromer P, Röcker K, Sommer A, et al. [Acute and overuse injuries in elite paracycling - an epidemiological study]. Sportverletz Sportschaden 2011;25(3):167–72.
10. Derman W, Schwellnus M, Jordaan E, et al. Illness and injury in athletes during the competition period at the London 2012 Paralympic Games: development

and implementation of a web-based surveillance system (WEB-IISS) for team medical staff. Br J Sports Med 2013;47(7):420–5.

11. Derman W, Schwellnus MP, Jordaan E, et al. Sport, sex and age increase risk of illness at the Rio 2016 Summer Paralympic Games: a prospective cohort study of 51 198 athlete days. Br J Sports Med 2018;52(1):17–23.

12. Derman W, Schwellnus MP, Jordaan E, et al. The incidence and patterns of illness at the Sochi 2014 Winter Paralympic Games: a prospective cohort study of 6564 athlete days. Br J Sports Med 2016;50(17):1064–8.

13. Schwellnus M, Derman W, Jordaan E, et al. Factors associated with illness in athletes participating in the London 2012 Paralympic Games: a prospective cohort study involving 49 910 athlete-days - ProQuest. Br J Sports Med 2013;47(7): 433–40.

14. McKibben M, Seed P, Ross S, et al. Urinary tract infection and neurogenic bladder. Urologic Clinics of North America 2015;42(4):527–36.

15. Brommer B, Engel O, Kopp MA, et al. Spinal cord injury-induced immune deficiency syndrome enhances infection susceptibility dependent on lesion level. Brain 2016;139(3):692–707.

16. Derman W, Schwellnus M, Jordaan E. Clinical characteristics of 385 illnesses of athletes with impairment reported on the WEB-IISS system during the london 2012 paralympic games. PM&R. 2014;6(8):S23–30.

17. Fagher K, Dahlström Ö, Jacobsson J, et al. Prevalence of sports-related injuries and illnesses in paralympic athletes. PM&R. 2020;12(3):271–80.

18. Gilchrist J, Thomas KE, Wald M, et al. Nonfatal Traumatic Brain Injuries from Sports and Recreation Activities - United States, 2001-2005 - ProQuest. MMWR Morb Mortal Wkly Rep 2007;56(29):733–7.

19. Roi GS, Tinti R. Requests for medical assistance during an amateur road cycling race. Accid Anal Prev 2014;73:170–3.

20. Emond SD, Tayoun P, Bedolla JP, et al. Injuries in a 1-Day recreational cycling tour: bike new york. Ann Emerg Med 1999;33(1):56–61.

21. Decock M, Wilde LD, Bossche LV, et al. Incidence and aetiology of acute injuries during competitive road cycling. Br J Sports Med 2016;50:669–72. https://doi.org/10.1136/bjsports-2015-095612.

22. Blauwet C, Lexell J, Derman W, et al. The road to rio: medical and scientific perspectives on the 2016 paralympic games. PM&R. 2016;8(8):798–801.

23. Moran RN, Broglio SP, Francioni KK, et al. Exploring baseline concussion-assessment performance in adapted wheelchair sport athletes. J Athl Train 2020;55(8):856–62.

24. Weiler R, Van Mechelen W, Fuller C, et al. Do Neurocognitive SCAT3 baseline test scores differ between footballers (soccer) living with and without disability? a cross-sectional study. Clin J Sport Med 2018;28(1):43–50.

25. Blauwet CA, Benjamin-Laing H, Stomphorst J, et al. Testing for boosting at the Paralympic games: policies, results and future directions. Br J Sports Med 2013;47(13):832–7.

26. West CR, Gee CM, Voss C, et al. Cardiovascular control, autonomic function, and elite endurance performance in spinal cord injury. Scand J Med Sci Sports 2015; 25(4):476–85.

27. Filomena M. "Boosting" in Paralympic athletes with spinal cord injury: doping without drugs. Funct Neurol 2015. https://doi.org/10.11138/fneur/2015.30.2.091.

28. Bhambhani Y, Mactavish J, Warren S, et al. Boosting in athletes with high-level spinal cord injury: knowledge, incidence and attitudes of athletes in paralympic sport. Disabil Rehabil 2010;32(26):2172–90.

29. Price MJ, Campbell IG. Effects of spinal cord lesion level upon thermoregulation during exercise in the heat. Med Sci Sports Exerc 2003;35(7):1100–7.

30. Krassioukov A, Biering-Sørensen F, Donovan W, et al. International standards to document remaining autonomic function after spinal cord injury. J Spinal Cord Med 2012;35(4):201–10.

31. Prévinaire JG, Mathias CJ, El Masri W, et al. The isolated sympathetic spinal cord: cardiovascular and sudomotor assessment in spinal cord injury patients: A literature survey. Ann Phys Rehabil Med 2010;53(8):520–32.

32. Kirshblum SC, Burns SP, Biering-Sorensen F, et al. International standards for neurological classification of spinal cord injury (Revised 2011). The J Spinal Cord Med 2011;34(6):535–46.

33. Trbovich M, Ford A, Wu Y, et al. Correlation of neurological level and sweating level of injury in persons with spinal cord injury. The J Spinal Cord Med 2020;1–8. https://doi.org/10.1080/10790268.2020.1751489.

34. Price MJ, Trbovich M. Thermoregulation following spinal cord injury. Thermoregulation: from basic neuroscience to clinical neurology, Part II. Elsevier; 2018. p. 799–820.

35. Stephenson BT, Hoekstra SP, Tolfrey K, et al. High thermoregulatory strain during competitive paratriathlon racing in the heat. Int J Sports Physiol Perform 2020; 15(2):231–7.

36. Maltais D, Wilk B, Unnithan V, et al. Responses of children with cerebral palsy to treadmill walking exercise in the heat. Med Sci Sports Exerc 2004;36(10): 1674–81.

37. Stephenson BT, Stone B, Mason BS, et al. Physiology of handcycling: a current sports perspective. Scand J Med Sci Sports 2021;31(1):4–20.

38. Griggs KE, Price MJ, Goosey-Tolfrey VL. Cooling athletes with a spinal cord injury. Sports Med 2015;45(1):9–21.

39. Griggs KE, Stephenson BT, Price MJ, et al. Heat-related issues and practical applications for Paralympic athletes at Tokyo 2020. Temperature 2020;7(1):37–57.

40. Ljungqvist A, Jenoure P, Engebretsen L, et al. The International Olympic Committee (IOC) Consensus Statement on periodic health evaluation of elite athletes March 2009. Br J Sports Med 2009;43(9):631–43.

41. Mountjoy M, Sundgot-Borgen J, Burke L, et al. The IOC relative energy deficiency in sport clinical assessment tool (RED-S CAT). Br J Sports Med 2015;49(21): 1354.

42. Statuta SM, Asif IM, Drezner JA. Relative energy deficiency in sport (RED-S). Br J Sports Med 2017;51(21):1570–1.

43. Blauwet CA, Brook EM, Tenforde AS, et al. Low energy availability, menstrual dysfunction, and low bone mineral density in individuals with a disability: implications for the para athlete population. Sports Med 2017;47:1697–708.

44. Crosland J, Boyd C. Cerebral palsy and acquired brain injuries. In: Broad E, editor. Sports nutrition for Paralympic athletes. CRC Press, Taylor & Francis Group; 2021. p. 91–105.

45. Price M. Energy expenditure and metabolism during exercise in persons with a spinal cord injury. Sports Med 2010;40(8):681–96.

46. Krassioukov A, West C. The role of autonomic function on sport performance in athletes with spinal cord injury. PM&R. 2014;6(8):S58–65.

47. Duffy CM, Graham HK, Cosgrove AP. The influence of ankle-foot orthoses on gait and energy…: journal of pediatric orthopaedics. J Pediatr Orthopaedics 2000; 20(3):356–61.

48. Evans EP, Tew B. The energy expenditure of spina bifida children during walking and wheelchair ambulation. Z Kinderchir 1981;34(4):425–7.
49. Gonzalez EG, Corcoran PJ, Reyes RL. Energy expenditure in below-knee amputees: correlation with stump length. Arch Phys Med Rehabil 1974;55(3):111–9.
50. Lee Childers W, Prilutsky BI, Gregor RJ. Motor adaptation to prosthetic cycling in people with trans-tibial amputation. J Biomech 2014;47(10):2306–13.
51. Weaver DS, Owen GM. Nutrition and short stature. Postgrad Med 1977; 62(6):93–9.
52. Hunter AGW, Hecht JT, Scott CI. Standard weight for height curves in achondroplasia. Am J Med Genet 1996;62(3):255–61.
53. Krempien JL, Barr SI. Risk of nutrient inadequacies in elite canadian athletes with spinal cord injury. Int J Sport Nutr Exerc Metab 2011;21(5):417–25.
54. Gerrish HR, Broad E, Lacroix M, et al. Nutrient intake of elite canadian and american athletes with spinal cord injury. Int J Exerc Sci 2017;10(7):1018–28.
55. Goosey-Tolfrey VL, Crosland J. Nutritional practices of competitive british wheelchair games players. Adapt Phys Activ Q 2010;27(1):47–59.
56. Grams L, Garrido G, Villacieros J, et al. Marginal micronutrient intake in high-performance male wheelchair basketball players: a dietary evaluation and the effects of nutritional advice. PLOS ONE 2016;11(7):e0157931.
57. Brook EM, Tenforde AS, Broad EM, et al. Low energy availability, menstrual dysfunction, and impaired bone health: a survey of elite para athletes. Scand J Med Sci Sports 2019;29(5):678–85.
58. Bratland-Sanda S, Sundgot-Borgen J. Eating disorders in athletes: overview of prevalence, risk factors and recommendations for prevention and treatment. Eur J Sport Sci 2013;13(5):499–508.
59. Karrer Y, Halioua R, Mötteli S, et al. Disordered eating and eating disorders in male elite athletes: a scoping review. BMJ Open Sport Exerc Med 2020;6(1): e000801. https://doi.org/10.1136/bmjsem-2020-000801.
60. Jiang S-D, Dai L-Y, Jiang L-S. Osteoporosis after spinal cord injury. Osteoporos Int 2006;17(2):180–92.
61. Slade JM, Bickel CS, Dudley GA. The effect of a repeat bout of exercise on muscle injury in persons with spinal cord injury. Eur J Appl Physiol 2004;92(3). https://doi.org/10.1007/s00421-004-1103-8.
62. Martinelli V, Dell'Atti C, Ausili E, et al. Risk of fracture prevention in spina bifida patients: correlation between bone mineral density, vitamin D, and electrolyte values. Child's Nerv Syst 2015;31(8):1361–5.
63. Marreiros H, Loff C, Calado E. Osteoporosis in paediatric patients with spina bifida. The J Spinal Cord Med 2012;35(1):9–21.
64. Szalay EA, Cheema A. Children with Spina Bifida are at risk for low bone density. Clin Orthop Relat Res 2011;469(5):1253–7.
65. Grossberg R, Blackford MG, Kecskemethy HH, et al. Longitudinal assessment of bone growth and development in a facility-based population of young adults with cerebral palsy. Dev Med Child Neurol 2015;57(11):1064–9.
66. Kim W, Lee SJ, Yoon Y-K, et al. Adults with spastic cerebral palsy have lower bone mass than those with dyskinetic cerebral palsy. Bone 2015;71:89–93. https://doi.org/10.1016/j.bone.2014.10.003.
67. Mergler S, Evenhuis HM, Boot AM, et al. Epidemiology of low bone mineral density and fractures in children with severe cerebral palsy: a systematic review. Dev Med Child Neurol 2009;51(10):773–8.
68. Presedo A, Dabney KW, Miller F. Fractures in patients with cerebral palsy. J Pediatr Orthopaedics 2007;27(2):147–53.

69. Leet A, Mesfin A, Pichard C, et al. Fractures in children with cerebral palsy. J Pediatr Orthopaedics 2006;26(5):624–7.
70. Sherk VD, Bemben MG, Bemben DA. BMD and bone geometry in transtibial and transfemoral amputees. J Bone Miner Res 2008;23(9):1449–57.
71. Webborn N, Van De Vliet P. Paralympic medicine. Lancet 2012;380(9836):65–71.
72. Szollar S, Martin E, Sartoris D, et al. Bone mineral density and indexes of bone metabolism in spinal cord injury. Am J Phys Med Rehabil 1997;77(1):28–35.
73. Vestergaard P, Krogh K, Rejnmark L, et al. Fracture rates and risk factors for fractures in patients with spinal cord injury. Spinal Cord 1998;36(11):790–6.
74. Frotzler A, Cheikh-Sarraf B, Pourtehrani M, et al. Long-bone fractures in persons with spinal cord injury. Spinal Cord 2015;53(9):701–4.
75. Zehnder Y, LüThi M, Michel D, et al. Long-term changes in bone metabolism, bone mineral density, quantitative ultrasound parameters, and fracture incidence after spinal cord injury: a cross-sectional observational study in 100 paraplegic men. Osteoporos Int 2004;15(3):180–9.
76. Grundill WL, Muller R. Bicycle accident injuries. S Afr Med J 1986;70(7):413–4.
77. Tanabe K. Cyclists' fractures in the elderly. Arch Osteoporos 2019;14(1). https://doi.org/10.1007/s11657-019-0627-9.
78. Goktepe AS, Yilmaz B, Alaca R, et al. Bone density loss after spinal cord injury: elite paraplegic. Am J Phys Med Rehabil 2004;83(4):279–83.
79. Miyahara K, Shikata-cho O, Wang DH, et al. Effect of sports activity on bone mineral density in wheelchair athletes. J Bone Miner Metab 2008;26(1):101–6.
80. Huang T-S, Wang Y-H, Lai J-S, et al. The hypothalamus-pituitary-ovary and hypothalamus-pituitary-thyroid axes in spinal cord—injured women. Metabolism 1996;45(6):718–22.
81. Colantonio A, Mar W, Escobar M, et al. Women's health outcomes after traumatic brain injury. J Women's Health 2010;19(6):1109–16.
82. Ripley DL, Harrison-Felix C, Sendroy-Terrill M, et al. The impact of female reproductive function on outcomes after traumatic brain injury. Arch Phys Med Rehabil 2008;89(6):1090–6.
83. Burke LM, Kalpakjian CZ, Smith YR, et al. Gynecologic issues of adolescents with down syndrome, autism, and cerebral palsy. J Pediatr Adolesc Gynecol 2010; 23(1):11–5.
84. Physicians AAoF, Pediatrics AAo, Medicine ACoS, et al. Preparticipation physical Evaluation. 4th Edition. American Academy of Pediatrics; 2010.
85. Mountjoy M, Sundgot-Borgen J, Burke L, et al. International Olympic Committee (IOC) Consensus Statement on Relative Energy Deficiency in Sport (RED-S): 2018 Update. Int J Sport Nutr Exerc Metab 2018;28(4):316–31.
86. De Bruin APK. Athletes with eating disorder symptomatology, a specific population with specific needs. Curr Opin Psychol 2017;16:148–53. https://doi.org/10.1016/j.copsyc.2017.05.009.
87. Woodlee MT, Schallert T. The impact of motor activity and inactivity on the brain. Curr Dir Psychol Sci 2006;15(4):203–6.
88. Declerck L, Kaux J, Vanderthommen M, et al. The effect of adaptive sports on individuals with acquired neurological disabilities and its role in rehabilitation: A systematic review. Curr Sports Med Rep 2019;18(12):458–73.
89. Katz-Leurer M, Sender I, Keren O, et al. The influence of early cycling training on balance in stroke patients at the subacute stage. Results of a preliminary trial. Clin Rehabil 2006;20(5):398–405.

90. Armstrong EL, Boyd RN, Horan SA, et al. Functional electrical stimulation cycling, goal-directed training, and adapted cycling for children with cerebral palsy: a randomized controlled trial. Dev Med Child Neurol 2020;62(12):1406–13.
91. Ringenbach SDR, Holzapfel SD, Arnold NE, et al. Assisted Cycling Therapy (ACT) improves adaptive behaviors in adolescents with down syndrome. J Dev Phys Disabilities 2020;32(3):535–52.
92. Rimmer J, Wolf L, Armour B, et al. Physical activity among adults with a disability-United States, 2005. JAMA 2008;299(11):1255–6.

Unique Concerns of the Woman Cyclist

Rozanne M. Puleo, FNP-BC, ONP-C[a],*, Antje Barreveld, MD[b], Sarah Rice, PhD, DPT[c], Anne M. Althausen Plante, MD[d], Dana H. Kotler, MD[e]

KEYWORDS

- Bike fit • Cycling biomechanics • Female cyclists • Cycling posture • Bicycle saddle
- Pelvic pain • Overuse injury • Traumatic cycling injury

KEY POINTS

- Anatomic differences between female and male individuals in several cycling injury areas (head, breast, hip/knee, upper extremity, and perineal area) may change the incidence, presentation, and treatment of cycling-related injuries.
- Female cyclists with concussion or traumatic brain injury endorse different symptoms than male cyclists, both at baseline and postinjury
- Bicycle design specific for women is controversial; optimizing the bike fit to the rider is of greater value for injury reduction, comfort, and safety.
- Saddle design and choice can influence the overall health of the cyclist.
- Pelvic pain in female cyclists can have many different presentations.

INTRODUCTION

From the origins of cycling in 1817, when women were forbidden from riding,[1] the population of women cyclists has grown to 42.7% of riders in America.[2] In the late nineteenth century, physicians began to recommend cycling as a means for health promotion, but women were discouraged from riding because of concerns about decreased reproductive capacity, uterine displacement, injuries, and notably "Bicycle Face," a condition thought to impact thyroid function.[1,3] Another concern raised by physicians at that time was the impact that cycling would have on sexual health, or more specifically, "sexual purity," and that riding astride on a bicycle saddle was

---

[a] Sports Medicine, Lynn Community Health Center, 269 Union Street, Lynn, MA 01902, USA; [b] Anesthesiology, Tufts University School of Medicine, Pain Management Services, Newton-Wellesley Hospital, 2014 Washington St, Newton, MA 02462, USA; [c] Athletico Physical Therapy, 2143 W Division St, Chicago IL 60622-3006, USA; [d] Obstetrics and Gynecology, Harvard Medical School, Massachusetts General Hospital, 55 Fruit St, Boston, MA 02114, USA; [e] Department of Physical Medicine & Rehabilitation, Harvard Medical School, Spaulding Outpatient Center – Wellesley, 65 Walnut Street, Wellesley, Boston, MA 02481, USA
* Corresponding author.
E-mail address: rozpuleo@yahoo.com

Phys Med Rehabil Clin N Am 33 (2022) 61–79
https://doi.org/10.1016/j.pmr.2021.08.005
1047-9651/22/© 2021 Elsevier Inc. All rights reserved.

not considered feminine and might encourage masturbation.[4] Others were concerned that participating in cycling would cause physiologic sex reversal in women.[1] In spite of the absurdity and sexism of these assertions, it is the earliest recognition of the potential impact of cycling on women's health.[4]

Others in the medical community recognized the potential health benefits that helped grow bicycle adoption among women throughout the century.[1] At the time, progressive physicians claimed that an hour of cycling per day would help with conditions such as insomnia, anemia, and nervousness.[1] More recent research on cycling has provided evidence as a way to promote public health,[5] including benefits such as reduction in the risk of cardiovascular disease, type 2 diabetes, cancer, and obesity mortality.[5] And although women's participation in cycling is no longer considered controversial, cycling remains a male-dominated activity.[6] Data from competitive cycling federations show a significant gender disparity, with more men involved in the sport than women; in the United Kingdom, United States, and Australia, only 15% to 17.5% of athletes competing were registered within the women's cycling fields.[7] The commercial cycling industry is also male dominated, with 89% of all bike shops owned by men.[8]

Cycling-related injuries can range from high-velocity traumatic injuries to nontraumatic injuries that may evolve over an extended period. Overuse injuries predominate but traumatic tend to be more severe.[9,10] The purpose of this article was to provide a broad overview of the current literature on the clinical relevance of gender differences in cycling-related injuries. With respect to gender differences, it is important to note that clinical and research language remains binary, and the words woman/women/female may not encompass all non-cisgender male gender identities. A study on women's and gender-diverse participation in cycling conducted an open-ended demographic questionnaire to accurately define the population of cyclists who do not identify as cisgender male. Although most respondents identified as women, cisgender ("cis") women, or female, 12 additional gender identities were reported.[7] Hormonal changes related to gender transition and hormone replacement have not been thoroughly studied in cycling and are not discussed here. With respect to the cycling-related research that is discussed in this article, please refer to the individual articles cited for details of the study population.

HEAD INJURY

Cycling is a high-speed sport with potential for traumatic injury, particularly to the head. It is the most common sports-related cause of traumatic brain injury (TBI) in female individuals, and second only to football in male individuals.[11] Prior studies have shown an increased risk of head injury/concussion in female compared with male individuals in comparable sports,[12–14] although research on this topic has been historically problematic, as female individuals typically endorse more concussion symptoms at baseline and postconcussion (Kotler DH, Rice S, Iaccarino MA, unpublished data, 2019).[15] As sports-related head injuries are also frequently underreported,[16,17] the question of whether the sex differences in head injury are due to true difference or underreporting is not entirely answered.

Recent research on the expanding set of TBI and concussion surveillance efforts in sport has demonstrated sex differences in performance on both baseline and sideline outcome measures such as the ImPACT and SCAT5. One study showed that female National Collegiate Athletic Association Division 1 athletes demonstrated improved performance on verbal memory, visual motor speed, and reaction time domains of the ImPACT at baseline relative to their male counterparts,[18] whereas others showed that female collegiate athletes endorse more symptoms of sadness, nervousness, and feeling more emotional at baseline than male subjects.[19] These differences may be significant when considering postconcussive symptoms and timing for return to sport.

Helmet use is generally accepted to help prevent TBI and concussion injuries in cycling.[20] Anthropomorphic data on female versus male skull dimensions and cortical bone thickness show that female individuals have straighter foreheads, less pronounced glabellae, and less pronounced orbital rims compared with male individuals.[21] In addition, female individuals undergo more cortical bone resorption during the adult years,[22] and thinner cortical bone offers less protection from skull fracture injuries.[23] There is a lack of sex-specific epidemiologic data, but these factors together suggest that female cyclists may gain substantial protective benefit against TBI by using a well-fitting cycling helmet.

BREAST INJURY

Breast injury includes both traumatic and frictional injury. There is little research investigating breast injuries in sport, and even less regarding support and protection of the breasts. This may be in part because of a lack of reporting of breast injuries.[24] Breast trauma has been previously evaluated in the setting of a motor vehicle accident, but is certainly a risk in contact sports, as well as sports with potential for trauma, including cycling. Most hematomas are mild, with rupture of superficial capillaries secondary to blunt trauma. Fat necrosis can occur following the injury, with cyst formation, palpable nodules, and even calcification. These are not typically symptomatic, but may be evident on imaging and can even be mistaken for malignancy.[25] In the augmented breast, traumatic capsular hematoma can develop, and with more significant trauma, an implant may rupture.[26]

Mondor disease, a superficial thrombophlebitis of the anterior chest wall, may occur spontaneously or can be associated with direct trauma, which is often minimal and potentially not recalled by the athlete. A palpable tender cord may be seen in the location of the superficial vein.[27] This uncommon, benign condition is typically self-limiting but still should be evaluated by a breast specialist to rule out any association with breast carcinoma.

Management of breast trauma includes ice, analgesia, topical or oral anti-inflammatories, and firm support. Aspiration of hematoma may be necessary in some cases. With any abnormal findings on breast examination, mammographic examination should be considered to rule out an underlying malignancy, and abnormal imaging findings may be confirmed with biopsy if needed.

CYCLING AND BONE HEALTH

Cycling is considered nonimpact, which is a favorable quality with regard to wide participation across age groups and levels of fitness. Although cycling requires large muscular effort, there is minimal external loading and ground reaction forces, and as such, it does not promote an increase in bone density.[28] Most of bone mass is developed during adolescence and young adulthood, and is dependent on factors including genetics, weight-bearing/loading exercise, lean body mass, nutrition and energy availability, bone-building nutrients, and reproductive hormone levels.[29]

Prior research has found that decreased bone mineral density (BMD) is prevalent among cyclists, which is concerning for an activity in which there is also a risk of fractures related to crashing.[30–32] Much of the prior research, however, has been limited by a focus on a relatively homogeneous elite male cyclist population, which is not representative of the general cycling population. Male cyclists have frequently demonstrated similar or lower BMD than sedentary controls, and significantly lower BMD than athletes participating in weight-bearing activity.[30] In one study, two-thirds of road cyclists categorized as elite and professional showed low BMD.[31] In a 7-year study of male masters cyclists compared with nonathletes, rates of osteopenia and osteoporosis were more common in the cyclists at baseline, with BMD showing a significantly greater decline in the cyclists throughout the course of the study. Those participating in weight training or impact exercise lost significantly less bone mass than those who did not.[32] Even within the sport of cycling, there are differences between disciplines with respect to bone density. In a comparison of radial bone size and strength between cyclists participating in road versus mountain biking, in which there is more external impact, the mountain bikers' radii showed increased size, density, and strength compared with those of the road cyclists and controls.[33]

Findings in competitive female road cyclists have shown similar decreases in BMD,[34] including when compared with runners. Comparison of the lumbar spine bone density between female cyclists, controls, and runners over 18 months of training showed decreases in the cyclists and controls but not runners, suggesting that the axial load of running may be protective to the lumbar spine bone density.[35] However, more recent research has examined a more diverse group of male and female bike racers to evaluate the contribution of factors including age, USA Cycling category, and racing type on body composition across a road racing season, using dual-energy x-ray absorptiometry and dietary recall. In this case, BMD values did not decrease over time, and in fact the female participants showed higher Z-Scores than male participants. In this study, nearly all female participants met daily calcium and vitamin D intake recommendations, reported calcium and vitamin D supplementation, whereas male participants did not, and female participants also reported weight-bearing physical activity in addition to cycling.[36]

Bone health in endurance sports, particularly cycling, is a challenging topic for research, as many confounding factors are prominent. Cyclists train long hours over many years and may spend little time doing weight-bearing or cross-training activity. In addition, cyclists of lean body type and low body mass index may self-select into their sport, as this phenotype provides an advantage, particularly over hilly terrain where power-to-weight ratio has a major impact on performance.[32] Relative energy deficiency in sport (RED-S) is a syndrome that describes consequences of the low energy availability state, including hormonal dysfunction in both men and women, and is a common issue in endurance athletes, with consequences in both health and performance. Although decreased energy availability is not necessarily a result of disordered eating, risk factors for disordered eating are prevalent in cycling, including the importance of power-to-weight ratio, body-contour-revealing clothing, and difficulty maintaining energy availability during training and competition.[29,37] The nature of cycling, requiring high workloads and caloric expenditure for long periods, poses a challenge for both maintenance of energy availability and calcium homeostasis during a long ride or race. Research has shown that exercise stimulates parathyroid hormone, a marker of bone turnover, including moderate-intensity, long-duration exercise, as seen in endurance cycling.[38] It has also been suggested that dermal calcium loss through sweat may lead to resorption of calcium from bone if not replaced through nutritional intake.[28] Multiple factors in addition to loading contribute to bone regulation, and the lack of a consistent negative correlation of any specific factor is a testament to this complexity.

OVERUSE INJURY AND BIKE FIT

Overuse injury typically results from a combination of muscular imbalances, degenerative change, and suboptimal biomechanics. In a study of Division I college athletes across multiple sports, overuse injury rate was higher among female athletes, although the difference was less between comparable sports.[39] Previously seen alterations in the biomechanics of female individuals include increased knee abduction (valgus), and quadriceps to hamstring ratio during landing in female individuals, which have been associated with anterior cruciate ligament injuries.[40] This has been examined both in a drop and vertical jump, as well as in a single-leg squat, in which women were found to demonstrate increased pelvic rotation, hip internal rotation, hip adduction and rotation range, and knee mediolateral motion compared with men.[41] This lack of pelvic stability appears to also cause downstream effects on the knee, such as patellofemoral pain syndrome, particularly in female individuals.[42] In the cyclist, management of these injuries involves understanding the anatomic and biomechanical factors of the cyclist, the positioning of the rider on the bicycle, and the demands of the discipline of cycling.[10] In considering the fit needs of women cyclists, anatomic differences must be considered, including a wider inter-ischial distance, greater genu and/or coxa valgum, shorter legs, narrower shoulder width, and smaller hands.[43]

A frequent complaint of cyclists is anterior knee pain. Patellofemoral pain syndrome (PFPS) refers to pain in the patella or surrounding soft tissues, and is more common in female individuals.[44,45] Dynamic valgus during functional activity has been associated with PFPS and has been more frequently observed in female athletes compared with male athletes. In cycling, overuse-related knee pain is typically associated with medial deviation of the knee in pedaling and altered activation of the vastus medialis and vastus lateralis muscles.[46] The role of Q-angle in patellofemoral pain syndrome has been debated and is not thoroughly understood.[47] One factor that can contribute to patellofemoral pain is the crank length of the bicycle drive-train. If these are too long for their inherent hip range of motion, cyclists' knees may deviate laterally with some external rotation at the knee joint at the top of the pedal stroke. The larger the Q angle, the greater the deviation between the top and bottom of the pedal stroke. This can result in significant medial-lateral patellar movements that can result in PFPS. Biomechanical imbalances may also contribute to overuse injuries, such as lateral hip pain.[48,49]

Using a shorter crank arm helps to reduce shear force across the knee joint and maximum knee and hip flexion at the top of the pedal stroke, which may be especially beneficial for female riders with shorter legs and increased Q angle.[50] Some biomechanical faults may also be addressed through improved foot support in the shoe, and allowing for slight medial and lateral rotation of the foot, known as pedal float (**Fig. 1**). Saddle position is adjustable, both up and down, as well as fore and aft. Riders with a wider pelvis may require adjustment of stance width (width of the feet) (**Fig. 2**), which can be done through the adjustment of cleat position, the addition of washers to space the pedals, or use of pedal spindle extenders. On the front end of the bike, smaller hands may require repositioning of the shifters and brake levers or use of shims to allow for easier reach (**Fig. 3**). This can be a critical safety issue, as female cyclists' smaller hands may not otherwise easily be able to reach the bicycle brakes from the drop portion of the handlebar. Short-reach or compact geometry handlebars may also improve comfort for some riders.

Upper extremity peripheral nerve injuries, including cervical radiculopathies and ulnar and median entrapment neuropathies, are common in cyclists.[51] The posture of a cyclist on the bike is generally characterized by a forward head, extended neck, and

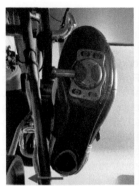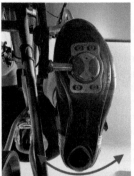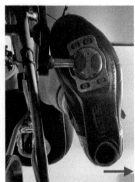

Fig. 1. Having a pedal float allows the foot to rotate while being clipped into the pedal.

significant pressure on the elbows and extended wrists, which can cause entrapment or pressure neuropathies at multiple sites.[52] There are important epidemiologic differences between men and women who experience these injuries. One study showed that women have a twofold lower incidence of ulnar nerve entrapment at the elbow.[53] In contrast, women have twofold to threefold increased incidence of median nerve entrapment at the wrist.[54] For both male and female cyclists, entrapment injuries of the deep branch of the ulnar nerve at the wrist can evade early detection, as lesions of the deep palmar motor branch may present without sensory deficits.[55] A recent study demonstrated that EMG-diagnosed median nerve injuries at the wrist in the absence of ulnar nerve injury may present with pain or reported paresthesias in an apparently ulnar nerve distribution.[56] Together, these lines of evidence support a comprehensive neurologic and electrodiagnostic workup for a female cyclist who is suspected to have the classic "cyclist's palsy" or another upper extremity nerve injury.

Women's specific bicycle design has been the source of some controversy. In the past, the prevalent theme was "Shrink it and pink it," meaning to manufacture smaller sizes and make items that aesthetically appeal to women. This compromised functionality and often resulted in lower-quality equipment. Research and development went into improving bicycle fit for women, primarily based on the assumption that women are shorter and have proportionally shorter torsos than men.[57] However, newer data obtained while a cyclist is in the cycling position, rather than while standing, suggests that the sex differences in bike fit are not nearly as clear as previously thought, and the differences are not dissimilar to the heterogeneity within an all-female or all-male population.[57] A bicycle geometry must work with an individual's proportions, and women have a variety of body types and proportions, some of which may not require a women's-specific bicycle. In addition, variables such as experience level, flexibility, and preferred body position may be more relevant to bike selection than gender. As such, over the past few years, many bicycle manufacturers have reverted to a unisex platform for frame geometry, and now emphasize the importance of bike fitting for the individual rather than gender-specific design.[57,58]

In contrast to frame geometry, saddle design must be more nuanced to accommodate for anatomic differences between individuals. The bicycle saddle is 1 of 3 contact points of the rider with the bicycle and is essential for providing pelvic support to enable efficient pedaling and safe handling of the bicycle.[59] A proper position on the saddle typically involves the cyclist's weight being equally distributed over the ischial tuberosities and the inferior pubic rami, with proportionally less compression over the soft tissues and neurovascular structures.

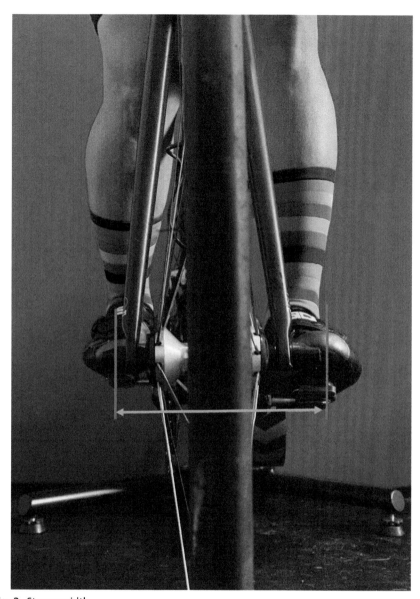

Fig. 2. Stance width.

Saddles can vary widely in shape, width, and other more granular features. Saddle design has evolved to improve comfort, as various ailments can arise from sitting improperly on a saddle, particularly for long durations.[60] Saddle design may include a dome-shaped, flat, or sloping surface, fabricated with different types of material and padding, all of which impact the amount of pelvic movement that occurs while riding and can contribute to adequate support. Some saddles are designed with cut-out centers or channels intended to decompress the neurovascular structures.[61] Modifications to saddle design have included full removal of the nose of the saddle,

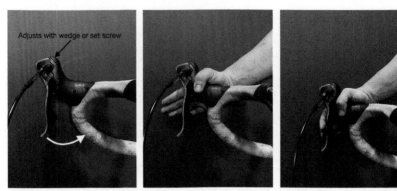

Adjusts with wedge or set screw

Fig. 3. Smaller hands may require repositioning of the shifters and brake levers or use of shims to allow for easier reach.

intended to reduce compression of the perineal area.[61,62] The nose of the saddle itself has been tested at varying widths to assess the impact on pressure distribution and perceived discomfort.[61] Saddle pressure distribution will shift depending on the posture of a rider.[63] A person riding with a fairly upright posture will have their weight distributed differently from a cyclist riding in an aerodynamic posture. Saddles are designed to support the specific weight distribution of the riding discipline. For example, if a rider is going to participate in time-trialing, which requires an aerodynamic position, and will also commute by bike, they will likely benefit from 2 different saddles to support the different postures for each type of riding.

An improper saddle selection or position may contribute to overuse issues elsewhere, such as in the spine, hip, or even the upper extremities.[59] If a saddle is not positioned in a way that optimally supports the rider, excess or imbalanced pelvic motion can occur, and this can translate into dysfunction axially or peripherally.[64] Sauer and colleagues[43] noted sex differences in pelvic motion in seated cycling. Although inherent differences in pelvic anatomy will influence position on the saddle, it was noted that when changing hand positions, female individuals exhibited increased anterior pelvic tilt in the drops position compared with male individuals that was not correlated with lumbar flexibility, but rather the anatomic differences.[43] This highlights the importance of inquiring not only how frequently one rides, but also what type of cycling they participate in, and which positions they prefer.

Although it is important to have a well-positioned saddle that matches the pelvic shape and riding discipline, it is equally important for female cyclists to wear well-fitting bicycle shorts with a chamois (pronounced sham-ee) appropriate for the type of riding. The location of the chamois padding will differ based on the riding discipline and where the pressures are distributed. An overall thicker chamois may increase perineal pressure and is not always recommended.[65] A poorly fitted chamois or one that is too thick can cause pain, even in the presence of an appropriate saddle in the proper position.

It is important to note that there are no data on the effects of the bicycle saddle on transgender women who have undergone gender re-affirming surgery. More research is needed to understand this impact. Many of the studies have been conducted on a binary population, but with the increased acknowledgment of nonbinary populations, future research needs to include these populations in their analyses.

PELVIC PAIN

Causes of pelvic pain specific to cycling can be somatic or neuropathic (**Table 1**),[66–68] and just as an inappropriate saddle can cause dysfunction in other areas of the body, pain, injury, or dysfunction elsewhere in the body can translate into an inability to sit properly on the saddle resulting in pain and dysfunction. Causes of pelvic pain may be related to musculoskeletal pelvic etiologies (eg, postpartum changes in the pelvic floor muscles and joints), cyclist posture/positioning (eg, repetitive muscle or nerve irritation, injury, or compression), or muscle imbalances and overuse/underuse injuries.

Discomfort localized to the saddle region may be attributed to pressure, friction, tissue traction, and shear, sometimes contributing to skin breakdown, and other times causing focal pressure or pain over bony structures, soft tissues, urethra, or neurovascular structures. A basic understanding of the muscles, nerves, skeletal anatomy, and referral patterns can provide clues to the possible causes of pelvic pain in cyclists. Although pelvic pain can be a result of noncycling causes, such as endometriosis or bladder hyperactivity/interstitial cystitis, a thorough pain assessment can provide clues to the cause of pain. For instance, pain in the perineum or genitalia may be a sign of peripheral nerve compression (eg, pudendal nerve entrapment) from an improper bicycle fit, or due to lumbar or hip joint pathology referring to the perineum.

Table 1
Example of somatic versus neuropathic causes of pelvic pain in the cyclist

Somatic	Neuropathic
Hip-related referred pain in the absence of trauma	Pudendal neuralgia • numbness or pain in the rectum, perineum, vagina/penis/scrotum (see *Nantes Criteria*, Labat 2008[102]) • ± sexual dysfunction
Pelvic floor muscle inflammation/tightness (eg, pelvic floor muscle dysfunction leading to dyspareunia, vaginismus, or anorectal pain)	Anterior abdominal cutaneous nerve entrapment syndrome (ACNES) (Scheltinga 2018[101]) • pin-point, localized pain in the abdominal wall • positive Carnet sign • typically relieved by local anesthetic nerve block/trigger point injection in the area of pain
Pubic symphysis instability/inflammation (osteitis pubis)	Ilioinguinal neuralgia (eg, secondary to inguinal hernia or anatomic nerve compression)
Abdominal wall/myofascial inflammation or dysfunction (eg, lumbopelvic pain)	Genitofemoral neuralgia (may lead to clitoral or upper vaginal pain)
Anterior iliopsoas muscle dysfunction	
Labial hypertrophy	
Coccygodynia/coccyx pain	

(*Data from* - Scheltinga M, Roumen R. Anterior cutaneous nerve entrapment syndrome (ACNES). *Hernia.* 2018;22(3):507 to 516; - Labat JJ, Riant T, Robert R, Amarenco G, Lefaucheur JP, Rigaud J. Diagnostic criteria for pudendal neuralgia by pudendal nerve entrapment (Nantes criteria). *Neurourology and Urodynamics: Official Journal of the International Continence Society.* 2008;27(4):306 to 310.)

There are several nerves that innervate the perineum but the pudendal nerve primarily supplies the "undercarriage," including the perineum and genitalia. The pudendal nerve stems from the sacral plexus (S2-3-4) and passes under the sacrospinous ligament through the Alcock canal to innervate the genitalia. In addition, the internal pudendal artery and veins pass through the same canal, which then branches into the various arteries of the genitalia.[69] When seated on a bicycle saddle, there is consistent pressure in the region of these structures, which can lead to dysfunction. Over time, compression can result in chronic fibrotic changes that can reduce blood flow.[69] And although it may be intuitive to use a cut-out saddle to relieve the pressure of these central vessels, one study showed that cut-out saddles have a negative effect on weight distribution, and can increase the pressure on the perineum.[70,71]

PELVIC PAIN ASSESSMENT IN THE CYCLIST

Pain assessment should always begin with the personal pain narrative. This is an opportunity for the cyclist to describe physical symptoms along with the palliating and provocative factors while the provider pays close attention to the important emotional details. This permits the provider to respond empathically to the personal pain narrative.[72] When evaluating a female cyclist, questions should include the volume and type of riding they do, and how aggressive their riding position is. A saddle position that offers a significant drop in height from saddle to handlebars can put increased pressure on the ischiopubic rami, which can lead to painful saddle pathologies and decreased genital sensation.[43,73–75]

Pain assessment also should include an evaluation of functional status, as well as a full medical, sexual, psychosocial, and substance use history. In addition to the impact pelvic pain can have on cycling, acute or chronic pelvic pain can negatively impact day-to-day function and sexual function, as well as overall emotional well-being.

Pain diagrams can aid the physical examination in localizing the pain generators, as the term "pelvic pain" is quite nonspecific. The physical examination should focus on inspection, palpation, hip range of motion or pain, patient guidance to the pain location, and both an external and internal vaginal examination and possibly a rectal examination if indicated based on the patient's symptoms. Often, the pain narrative and diagram can provide the necessary clues to the diagnosis, and an internal examination may not be needed by the general practitioner.

SADDLE SORES

"Saddle sore" is a generic and colloquial term that describes painful skin injuries that occur on the buttocks, perineum, and upper inner thigh.[76] Generally, these occur from saddle pressure and chafing and can lead to ulcerations, folliculitis, nodules, and cysts that interfere with the ability to sit on the saddle.[76–78] Very little empirical evidence exists that describes the prevalence of saddle sores in women cyclists, although anecdotal reports suggest that it is a common occurrence in this population.[76] When these sores are in the form of an abscess, they can be treated conservatively, but if large enough to warrant intervention, they can be treated with incision and drainage, oral antibiotics, and time off the bike for recovery and healing.[79] An unpublished survey of 18 professional female cyclists in the United Kingdom found that all respondents have had painful saddle problems that have interfered with training and competition[80]; however, the specifics of these saddle concerns were not well defined. As a result of this survey, a team of experts was convened to try to address the problem. The team implemented a number of interventions, including antimicrobial wash, paraffin-based moisturizer, and a moratorium on shaving pubic hair.[80] This, combined with subtle adjustments to saddle fit and chamois choice, resulted in an elimination of saddle concerns 6 months postintervention.[80]

More well defined in the literature is the term "cyclist's nodules." These are an underdiagnosed condition of the perineum and have been classified in multiple case studies as perineal nodular induration (PNI).[81–83] These are more extensively reported in male than in female cyclists, which has led these nodules to sometimes be referred to as a "cyclist's third testicle."[81,83–86] Described in case reports as a solid nodule, a painful mass, and a focal area of tenderness with a nodular indurated area in the perineum, PNIs are a type of saddle sore.[81,83,84,87] A histologic analysis reported on vulvar nodules identified in 4 female cyclists with PNI noted that all lesions shared features of ischemic fasciitis, which is a non-neoplastic proliferation of atypical fibroblasts that is thought to result from prolonged pressure on soft tissues.[82]

LABIAL/VULVAR HYPERTROPHY

The vulva is the name of the external female genitalia, and it includes, among other features, the labia majora, often described as the "outer lips" and the labia minora that are often described as the "inner lips." These vary in size and shape from person to person and are rarely symmetric. While cycling, the labia are compressed from the rider being in contact with the saddle and this can result in significant pressure. In addition, there can be repetitive friction and shearing forces from inherent pelvic motion. Over time, both the labia majora and minora can increase in size and interfere with an individual's everyday activities, causing physical and psychological symptoms. Although not common in the general population, a few case reports and observational studies have described female cyclists who have experienced labial hypertrophy.[88–90] A number of factors may contribute to this phenomenon. Chronic inflammation in the vulvoperineal area related to friction and compression of the inguinal lymphatic vessels may contribute to altered lymphatic circulation.[88] Modifying the saddle position to ensure that pressure is well distributed throughout may help mitigate this risk. Saddles with cut-out centers have been designed with the intention of alleviating soft tissue and neurovascular pressure; however, subsequent research on labial hypertrophy discovered that these saddles can worsen hypertrophy in some women because gravity can pull lymphatic fluid into the cut-out portion, and this can exacerbate the swelling.[91]

Hypertrophy can result in irritation, pain, chronic infection, or poor hygiene. Pain and irritation can interfere with daily activities beyond cycling, such as walking, sitting, wearing tightly fitted clothes, and sexual activity. Many patients describe swelling and pain in the labia following activities, which then resolves after the activity is concluded. To mitigate these symptoms, many patients "fold up" their labia or push them into their vagina to decrease their symptoms. There are, however, patients in whom these symptoms do not resolve and continue to progress over time leading them to seek medical consultation for treatment.

Labia majora hypertrophy is characterized by the enlargement of the labia majora, and labia minora hypertrophy is a clinical diagnosis generally described as protuberant labial tissue that projects beyond the labia majora.[92] It is diagnosed by physical examination and based on the presence of physical and/or psychological symptoms that interfere with daily activities. Although there are no standard diagnostic criteria, clinicians describe the labia minora by using labial width. If the labia minora can be stretched greater than 6 cm from the midline to the lateral free edge, they are generally considered hypertrophic. Initially, functional symptoms can be addressed using methods of vulvar care (**Table 2**), reduced time in the saddle, and avoidance of form-fitting clothes.

Table 2 General vulvar care	
Do	**Do Not**
• In everyday situations, wear cotton underwear- or no underwear when possible.	• Wear underwear underneath bike shorts. This will increase friction.
• Wash with lukewarm water.	• Wash the vulva. If you feel like the area needs to be washed, do not scrub.
• Use Vaseline, olive oil or coconut oil on the vulvar skin daily to keep it hydrated. Use nonmedicated chamois creams during cycling activities.	• Use feminine wipes, powders, creams, or other over-the-counter products.
• Avoid scented laundry detergents or fabric softeners for clothes that touch the vulvar skin.	• Douche.
	• Use tea tree oil, witch hazel, Gold Bond powder, Epsom salts or other "cleansing" products, because they irritate the skin.
• Apply ice or cool compress to soothe the area if irritated.	• Use over-the-counter yeast treatments without talking to the provider because they can be irritating to the vulva and may not treat the underlying condition.
• Sleep with gloves or socks on your hands if you scratch in your sleep.	
• Use tampons for menses if possible. Constant contact with a pad causes more irritation.	
• If you use pads, avoid pads with significant latex content (eg, Always brand).	
• Use lubricant to make intercourse more comfortable.	

(*Data from* Mitchell, C MD and Pascal, A DNP General Vulvar Care. [1]Department of Obstetrics and Gynecology, Massachusetts General Hospital, Boston, MA [2]Harvard Medical School, Boston, MA. General Vulvar Care. 12/2015.)

In those with recurrent symptoms who do not respond to conservative care, surgical management can be considered. Labiaplasty describes the surgical procedure that is used to reduce the size or restore symmetry of the labia by resecting the hypertrophic tissue.[93,94] These procedures can be performed using local anesthesia, sedation, or general anesthesia.[95] Careful screening for body dysmorphic disorder should be part of the preoperative evaluation. Alteration of labia in minors that is not deemed medically necessary can be considered female genital mutilation under federal law in the United States,[96] and surgical management in patients younger than 18 should be thoughtfully undertaken. Although labiaplasty is a relatively simple surgical procedure, there are complications, such as infection, bleeding, wound breakdown, and persistent pain.[97] In general, however, most patients experience a high level of satisfaction, and improved self-esteem.[98] Because of the risk of postoperative complications, it is imperative that cyclists remain off the bike for 8 to 12 weeks.

PRACTICAL APPROACHES TO PELVIC CONCERNS IN WOMEN CYCLISTS

Treatment of pelvic concerns is dependent on the most likely etiology, and is most effective using a multimodal and interdisciplinary approach (**Table 3**).There are considerations that should be discussed with the cyclist as part of a plan to promote pelvic health and prevent cycling-related pelvic injury. Bicycle shorts should always be in direct contact with the vulva; underwear should not be worn underneath bike shorts. Chamois creams are commonly used barrier creams that reduce the friction between the cyclists' skin and the chamois of the bicycle shorts to help reduce skin concerns. These should be used for every ride and placed either directly on the skin or directly on

Table 3 Multimodal strategies for the prevention and treatment of pelvic pain in the cyclist	
Treatment Category	**Example Treatment Strategies**
Cycling optimization	• Appropriate saddle/bike fitting • Appropriate clothing, such as bike shorts with properly sized chamois in direct contact with skin • Chamois cream to reduce friction • Avoid pubic hair removal • Cycling pause
Pharmacotherapy	• Topical agents (eg, local anesthetics) • Neuropathic medications (eg, antiepileptics) • Suppositories (eg, muscle relaxants inserted in rectum or vagina)
Physical therapy/exercise	• Pelvic floor vs general musculoskeletal physical therapy • Alternative guided exercise programs, cross-training, and appropriate strengthening vs myofascial relaxation strategies
Interventions	• Injection therapies for diagnostic/therapeutic benefit (eg, nerve blocks, muscle trigger points, or joint injections) • Surgery when indicated (eg, labiaplasty, nerve decompression)
Behavioral strategies	• Mindfulness and cognitive behavioral strategies to promote pain coping techniques and muscle relaxation • Mental health support to address the potential impact chronic pain or inability to cycle can have on psychological well-being
Alternative therapies	• Chiropractic care • Anti-inflammatory dietary strategies • Acupuncture

the chamois. A placebo-controlled study compared 1% hydrocortisone to 10% trolamine salicylate cream to a nonmedicated cream,[99] and showed that the medicated creams were no more effective than nonmedicated creams in preventing skin breakdown. Nonmedicated creams should be thick and should not easily absorb into the skin. Pubic hair also has a protective role in cyclists' vulvar health and its removal is not recommended. An unpublished study found that female cyclists eliminated their saddle concerns by avoiding pubic hair removal in a 6-month time frame.[80] Freshly shaved skin can also be a risk factor for the development of saddle sores.[77] Ensuring good hygiene by choosing clean clothing and quickly removing this clothing at the end of a ride is another important preventive measure.

Commercially available pressure-sensing technologies exist to evaluate areas of excess pressure. In the absence of technology, examination of the saddle to evaluate for uneven wear may provide insight into the sitting position and resulting biomechanics. Although it may be impractical to evaluate the saddle fit of a cyclist in the office, a rudimentary method to obtain a measurement of the ischial tuberosity width is to have a patient sit onto floral foam blocks, let ball-bearings settle into the depressions left behind, and measure the width between the ball bearings.[43] Once this measurement is obtained, it can be compared with the saddle to assess for discrepancies. This assessment measure may help to further characterize the concern of the patient and provide possible solutions with regard to their saddle. If the width between the ischial tuberosities does not match the widest part of the saddle, it suggests that the cyclist is using a saddle that is not well-fitted to their body.

CLINICS CARE PEARLS

- When evaluating a cyclist, inquire about the volume of riding, type of bike they ride, and if multiple, the volume on each. Inquire about the position that they typically ride in and if they are on a road bike, if they switch hand positions, or are in the drops or the hoods more often.
- If a patient has reported that they have had a bike fit, inquire when it was last done. Many overuse injuries can be improved through physical therapy and bike fit modifications, and a repeat bike fit analysis may be indicated.
- When a patient presents with a traumatic breast injury, consider breast cancer in the differential.
- For patients seeking care for pelvic pain, labial hypertrophy, or pudendal neuralgia, inquire about the use of cut-out saddles and encourage patients to discontinue their use, as these can worsen these conditions.

SUMMARY

Although an office-based visit is not a substitute for a proper bike fit performed by a certified fitter, the treating practitioner will gain a greater understanding of the concern by understanding how the bicycle can affect the cyclist. Both traumatic and nontraumatic injuries can be impacted by a cyclist's gender, and it is important to understand how this variable influences a particular concern.

A survey of more than 3000 female cyclists is noted to be the largest study to date on this population.[100] However, it focused only on sexual and urinary dysfunction and did not address other conditions seen in female cyclists. To fully examine the impact that cycling has on female cyclists, and to strengthen the recommendations for prevention and treatment, large-scale studies that identify the magnitude of concerns in female cyclists should be undertaken. There is a lack of epidemiologic studies to identify the distribution of concerns among women cyclists, and this limits the ability to adequately strategize solutions within this population. The growth of women in cycling provides evidence that large-scale studies are possible and warranted. Cycling provides a wide array of health benefits, and the options for appropriate cycling equipment for many different body types continue to emerge. The continued pursuit of scientific inquiry will further the opportunity to hone equipment design for a wider breadth of options for all cyclists. Removing barriers to a physical activity that can be accessible to so many deserves the attention of the scientific community.

DISCLOSURE

Drs Barreveld, Plante, Rice, and Kotler have nothing to disclose. Rozanne Puleo is the co-owner of the Serotta International Cycling Institute and is a medical contractor for Team Novo Nordisk. No funding sources were used for this article.

REFERENCES

1. Kiersnowska B. Female cycling and the discourse of moral panic in Late Victorian Britain. Atlantis J Spanish Assoc Anglo-American Stud 2019;41(2):85–103.
2. PeopleForBikes. U.S. bicycle participation study. PeopleforBikes Website. 2018.
3. The 'Bicycle Face'. The Literary Digest. 1895;11(19):8.
4. Hallenbeck S. Riding out of bounds: women bicyclists' embodied medical authority. Rhetoric Rev 2010;29(4):327–45.

5. Oja P, Titze S, Bauman A, et al. Health benefits of cycling: a systematic review. Scand J Med Sci Sports 2011;21(4):496–509.

6. Heesch KC, Sahlqvist S, Garrard J. Gender differences in recreational and transport cycling: a cross-sectional mixed-methods comparison of cycling patterns, motivators, and constraints. Int J Behav Nutr Phys Act 2012;9(1):106.

7. Ayala EE, Waniger KJ, Faulkner KP, et al. Experiences that affect participation of women and gender diverse athletes in competitive cycling. J Outdoor Recreation, Educ Leadersh 2020;12(1).

8. Cornish L. Bike shops for everyone. 2015. Available at: https://www.bikeleague. org/sites/default/files/Bike_Shops_For_Everyone.pdf. . Accessed October 31, 2020.

9. Palmer-Green D, Burt P, Jaques R, et al. Epidemiological study of injury in British cycling: 2011-2013 (Abstract from IOC World Conference on Prevention of Injury & Illness in Sport, Monaco 2014). Br J Sports Med 2014;48(7):650.

10. Kotler DH, Babu AN, Robidoux G. Prevention, evaluation, and rehabilitation of cycling-related injury. Curr Sports Med Rep 2016;15(3):199–206.

11. Coronado VG, Haileyesus T, Cheng TA, et al. Trends in sports-and recreation-related traumatic brain injuries treated in US emergency departments: the National Electronic Injury Surveillance System-All Injury Program (NEISS-AIP) 2001-2012. J head Trauma Rehabil 2015;30(3):185–97.

12. Dick R. Is there a gender difference in concussion incidence and outcomes? Br J Sports Med 2009;43(Suppl 1):i46–50.

13. Covassin T, Moran R, Elbin R. Sex differences in reported concussion injury rates and time loss from participation: an update of the National Collegiate Athletic Association Injury Surveillance Program from 2004–2005 through 2008–2009. J athletic Train 2016;51(3):189–94.

14. Wessels KK, Broglio SP, Sosnoff JJ. Concussions in wheelchair basketball. Arch Phys Med Rehabil 2012;93(2):275–8.

15. Brown DA, Elsass JA, Miller AJ, et al. Differences in symptom reporting between males and females at baseline and after a sports-related concussion: a systematic review and meta-analysis. Sports Med 2015;45(7):1027–40.

16. Kerr ZY, Register-Mihalik JK, Kroshus E, et al. Motivations associated with nondisclosure of self-reported concussions in former collegiate athletes. Am J Sports Med 2016;44(1):220–5.

17. McCrea M, Hammeke T, Olsen G, et al. Unreported concussion in high school football players: implications for prevention. Clin J Sport Med 2004;14(1):13–7.

18. Cottle JE, Hall EE, Patel K, et al. Concussion baseline testing: preexisting factors, symptoms, and neurocognitive performance. J athletic Train 2017;52(2): 77–81.

19. Covassin T, Swanik CB, Sachs M, et al. Sex differences in baseline neuropsychological function and concussion symptoms of collegiate athletes. Br J Sports Med 2006;40(11):923–7.

20. Creighton P, Olivier J. 248 Systematic review and meta-analysis of bicycle helmet efficacy to mitigate head, face and neck injuries. BMJ Publishing Group Ltd 2016;22:A90–1.

21. Avelar LET, Cardoso MA, Bordoni LS, et al. Aging and sexual differences of the human skull. Plast Reconstr Surg Glob Open 2017;5(4):e1297.

22. Lillie EM, Urban JE, Lynch SK, et al. Evaluation of skull cortical thickness changes with age and sex from computed tomography scans. J Bone Miner Res 2016;31(2):299–307.

23. Ruan J, Prasad P. The effects of skull thickness variations on human head dynamic impact responses. Stapp Car Crash J 2001;45.

24. Smith LJ, Eichelberger TD, Kane EJ. Breast injuries in female collegiate basketball, soccer, softball and volleyball athletes: Prevalence, type and impact on sports participation. Eur J Breast Health 2018;14(1):46.

25. Gatta G, Pinto A, Romano S, et al. Clinical, mammographic and ultrasonographic features of blunt breast trauma. Eur J Radiol 2006;59(3):327–30.

26. Dellon AL, Cowley RA, Hoopes JE. Blunt chest trauma: evaluation of the augmented breast. J Trauma Acute Care Surg 1980;20(11):982–5.

27. Suganthan N, Ratnasamy V. Mondor's disease–a rare cause of chest pain: a case report. J Med Case Rep 2018;12(1):1–3.

28. Scofield KL, Hecht S. Bone health in endurance athletes: runners, cyclists, and swimmers. Curr Sports Med Rep 2012;11(6):328–34.

29. Female athlete issues for the team physician: a Consensus Statement—2017 Update. Curr Sports Med Rep 2018;17(5):163–71.

30. Nagle KB, Brooks MA. A systematic review of bone health in cyclists. Sports health 2011;3(3):235–43.

31. Medelli J, Shabani M, Lounana J, et al. Low bone mineral density and calcium intake in elite cyclists. J Sports Med Phys fitness 2009;49(1):44.

32. Nichols JF, Rauh MJ. Longitudinal changes in bone mineral density in male master cyclists and nonathletes. J Strength Conditioning Res 2011;25(3):727–34.

33. Mcveigh JA, Meiring R, Cimato A, et al. Radial bone size and strength indices in male road cyclists, mountain bikers and controls. Eur J Sport Sci 2015;15(4):332–40.

34. Sherk VD, Barry DW, Villalon KL, et al. Bone loss over one year of training and competition in female cyclists. Clin J Sport Med 2014;24(4):331.

35. Beshgetoor D, Nichols JF, Rego I. Effect of training mode and calcium intake on bone mineral density in female master cyclists, runners, and non-athletes. Int J Sport Nutr Exerc Metab 2000;10(3):290–301.

36. Baker BS, Reiser RF. Longitudinal assessment of bone mineral density and body composition in competitive cyclists. J Strength Conditioning Res 2017;31(11):2969–76.

37. Mountjoy M, Sundgot-Borgen JK, Burke LM, et al. IOC consensus statement on relative energy deficiency in sport (RED-S): 2018 update. Br J Sports Med 2018;52(11):687–97.

38. Barry DW, Kohrt WM. Acute effects of 2 hours of moderate-intensity cycling on serum parathyroid hormone and calcium. Calcified Tissue Int 2007;80(6):359–65.

39. Yang J, Tibbetts AS, Covassin T, et al. Epidemiology of overuse and acute injuries among competitive collegiate athletes. J Athletic Train 2012;47(2):198–204.

40. Hewett TE, Myer GD, Ford KR, et al. Biomechanical measures of neuromuscular control and valgus loading of the knee predict anterior cruciate ligament injury risk in female athletes: a prospective study. Am J Sports Med 2005;33(4):492–501.

41. Weeks BK, Carty CP, Horan SA. Effect of sex and fatigue on single leg squat kinematics in healthy young adults. BMC Musculoskelet Disord 2015;16(1):271.

42. Powers CM. The influence of abnormal hip mechanics on knee injury: a biomechanical perspective. J Orthopaedic Sports Phys Ther 2010;40(2):42–51.

43. Sauer JL, Potter JJ, Weisshaar CL, et al. Influence of gender, power, and hand position on pelvic motion during seated cycling. Med Sci Sports Exerc 2007; 39(12):2204.

44. Boling M, Padua D, Marshall S, et al. Gender differences in the incidence and prevalence of patellofemoral pain syndrome. Scand J Med Sci Sports 2010; 20(5):725–30.

45. Fulkerson JP, Arendt EA. Anterior knee pain in females. Clin Orthopaedics Relat Res 2000;372:69–73.

46. Johnston TE, Baskins TA, Koppel RV, et al. The influence of extrinsic factors on knee biomechanics during cycling: a systematic review of the literature. Int J Sports Phys Ther 2017;12(7):1023.

47. Petersen W, Ellermann A, Gösele-Koppenburg A, et al. Patellofemoral pain syndrome. Knee Surg Sports Traumatol Arthrosc 2014;22(10):2264–74.

48. Segal NA, Felson DT, Torner JC, et al. Greater trochanteric pain syndrome: epidemiology and associated factors. Arch Phys Med Rehabil 2007;88(8): 988–92.

49. Nakagawa TH, Moriya ÉT, Maciel CD, et al. Trunk, pelvis, hip, and knee kinematics, hip strength, and gluteal muscle activation during a single-leg squat in males and females with and without patellofemoral pain syndrome. J Orthopaedic Sports Phys Ther 2012;42(6):491–501.

50. Wadsworth DJ, Weinrauch P. The role of a bike fit in cyclists with hip pain. a clinical commentary. Int J Sports Phys Ther 2019;14(3):468.

51. Patterson JMM, Jaggars MM, Boyer MI. Ulnar and median nerve palsy in long-distance cyclists: a prospective study. Am J Sports Med 2003;31(4):585–9.

52. Akuthota V, Plastaras C, Lindberg K, et al. The effect of long-distance bicycling on ulnar and median nerves: an electrophysiologic evaluation of cyclist palsy. Am J Sports Med 2005;33(8):1224–30.

53. Uzunkulaoglu A, Afsar SI, Karatas M. Association between gender, body mass index, and ulnar nerve entrapment at the elbow: a retrospective study. J Clin Neurophysiol 2016;33(6):545–8.

54. Mondelli M, Giannini F, Giacchi M. Carpal tunnel syndrome incidence in a general population. Neurology 2002;58(2):289–94.

55. Lleva JMC, Munakomi S, Chang KV. Ulnar neuropathy. In: StatPearls. Treasure Island (FL): StatPearls Publishing Copyright © 2021, StatPearls Publishing LLC.; 2021.

56. Colorado BS, Osei DA. Prevalence of carpal tunnel syndrome presenting with symptoms in an ulnar nerve distribution: a prospective study. Muscle & nerve 2019;59(1):60–3.

57. Jett R, Chabra S, Carver T. When to share product platforms: an anthropometric review. Corporate research review.

58. Lukas S. Where have all the women's bikes gone? A look inside an everchanging market. 2019. Available at: https://cyclingtips.com/2019/10/wherehave-all-the-womens-bikes-gone-a-look-inside-an-ever-changing-market/. Accessed March 3, 2021.

59. Swart J, Holliday W. Cycling biomechanics optimization—the (r) evolution of bicycle fitting. Curr Sports Med Rep 2019;18(12):490–6.

60. Potter JJ, Sauer JL, Weisshaar CL, et al. Gender differences in bicycle saddle pressure distribution during seated cycling. Med Sci Sports Exerc 2008;40(6): 1126–34.

61. Larsen AS, Larsen FG, Sørensen FF, et al. The effect of saddle nose width and cutout on saddle pressure distribution and perceived discomfort in women during ergometer cycling. Appl Ergon 2018;70:175–81.

62. Chen Y-L, Liu Y-N. Optimal protruding node length of bicycle seats determined using cycling postures and subjective ratings. Appl Ergon 2014;45(4):1181–6.

63. Rodano R, Squadrone R, Sacchi M, et al. Saddle pressure distribution in cycling: comparison among saddles of different design and materials. Paper presented at: ISBS-Conference Proceedings Archive. Caceres, July 1-5, 2002.

64. Verma R, Hansen EA, de Zee M, et al. Effect of seat positions on discomfort, muscle activation, pressure distribution and pedal force during cycling. J Electromyogr Kinesiol 2016;27:78–86.

65. De Bruyne G, Aerts JM, Berckmans D. Efficiency of Cycling Pads in Reducing Seat Pressure During Cycling. In: Rebelo F, Soares M, editors. Advances in Ergonomics in Design. AHFE 2018. Advances in Intelligent Systems and Computing, vol 777. Springer, Cham. https://doi.org/10.1007/978-3-319-94706-8_5.

66. Prather H, Camacho-Soto A. Musculoskeletal etiologies of pelvic pain. Obstet Gynecol Clin 2014;41(3):433–42.

67. Gyang A, Hartman M, Lamvu G. Musculoskeletal causes of chronic pelvic pain: what a gynecologist should know. Obstet Gynecol 2013;121(3):645–50.

68. Barreveld A, Adler A, Argoff C. Which neurological problems can lead to pelvic pain?. In: De E, Stern T, editors. Facing pelvic pain: a guide for patients and their families. Boston: Massachusetts General Hospital Psychiatry Academy; 2020.

69. Baran C, Mitchell GC, Hellstrom WJ. Cycling-related sexual dysfunction in men and women: a review. Sex Med Rev 2014;2(3–4):93–101.

70. Guess MK, Partin SN, Schrader S, et al. Women's bike seats: a pressing matter for competitive female cyclists. J Sex Med 2011;8(11):3144–53.

71. Trofaier M-L, Schneidinger C, Marschalek J, et al. Pelvic floor symptoms in female cyclists and possible remedies: a narrative review. Int Urogynecol J 2016;27(4):513–9.

72. Charon R. Narrative medicine: a model for empathy, reflection, profession, and trust. Jama 2001;286(15):1897–902.

73. Bressel E, Bliss S, Cronin J. A field-based approach for examining bicycle seat design effects on seat pressure and perceived stability. Appl Ergon 2009;40(3): 472–6.

74. Guess MK, Connell K, Schrader S, et al. Women's sexual health: Genital sensation and sexual function in women bicyclists and runners: are your feet safer than your seat? J Sex Med 2006;3(6):1018–27.

75. Partin SN, Connell KA, Schrader S, et al. The bar sinister: does handlebar level damage the pelvic floor in female cyclists? J Sex Med 2012;9(5):1367–73.

76. Bury K, Leavy JE, Lan C, et al. Saddle sores among female competitive cyclists: a systematic scoping review. J Sci Med Sport 2020;24(4):357–67.

77. Miller MG, Berry DC. Back in the saddle again: how to prevent cycling saddle sores. Athletic Ther Today 2007;12(4):19.

78. Bateman C, Dilke-Wing G. Saddle sores presenting to a genitourinary medicine department. BMJ 2015;350 :H2247.

79. McElhinney B, Horner T, Dinsmore W, et al. Exercise bicycle-induced bilateral vulval abscesses. Int J STD AIDS 1993;4(3):174–5.

80. Pidd H. How scientific rigour helped Team GB's saddle-sore cyclists on their medal trail. The Guardian; 2016. Available at: https://www.theguardian.com/

sport/blog/2016/aug/15/team-gb-cycling-saddle-sore-medals. Accessed 1/14/2021.

81. Makhanya NZ, Velleman M, Suleman FE. A case of cyclist's nodule in a female patient. South Afr J Sports Med 2014;26(3):93–4.
82. McCluggage WG, Smith JH. Reactive fibroblastic and myofibroblastic proliferation of the vulva (cyclist's nodule): a hitherto poorly described vulval lesion occurring in cyclists. Am J Surg Pathol 2011;35(1):110–4.
83. Norman M, Vitale K. "Bumpy" ride for the female cyclist: a rare case of perineal nodular induration, the ischial hygroma. Int J Surg Case Rep 2020;73:277–80.
84. Van de Perre S, Vanhoenacker FM, Vanstraelen L, et al. Perineal nodular swelling in a recreational cyclist: diagnosis and discussion. Skeletal Radiol 2009;38(9):933–4.
85. De Cima A, Pérez N, Ayala G. MR imaging findings in perineal nodular induration ("cyclist' s nodule"): a case report. Radiol Case Rep 2020;15(7):1091–4.
86. Peacock J, Cobley J, Patel B. Urological issues in cyclists. J Clin Urol 2020. 2051415820964982.
87. Leibovitch I, Mor Y. The vicious cycling: bicycling related urogenital disorders. Eur Urol 2005;47(3):277–87.
88. Baeyens L, Elston MA, Vermeersch E, et al. Bicyclist's vulva: observational study. Commentary: Attitudes to women's bicycling have changed. BMJ 2002; 325(7356):138–9.
89. Coutant-Foulc P, Lewis FM, Berville S, et al. Unilateral vulval swelling in cyclists: a report of 8 cases. J Lower Genital Tract Dis 2014;18(4):e84–9.
90. Humphries D. Unilateral vulval hypertrophy in competitive female cyclists. Br J Sports Med 2002;36(6):463–4.
91. Grouin A, Rouquette S, Saïdani M, et al. Bicyclist's vulva: diagnostic and therapeutic aspects. J Gynecol Obstet Hum Reprod 2018;47(6):223–5.
92. Laufer M, Reddy J. Labia minora hypertrophy. UpToDate 2021.
93. Motakef S, Rodriguez-Feliz J, Chung MT, et al. Vaginal labiaplasty: current practices and a simplified classification system for labial protrusion. Plast Reconstr Surg 2015;135(3):774–88.
94. Oranges CM, Sisti A, Sisti G. Labia minora reduction techniques: a comprehensive literature review. Aesthet Surg J 2015;35(4):419–31.
95. Reddy J, Laufer MR. Hypertrophic labia minora. J Pediatr Adolesc Gynecol 2010;23(1):3–6.
96. Female genital mutilation. In. 18 U.S.C 1662015. US Code of laws website. Available at: law.cornell.edu/UScode//text/18/116.
97. Liao LM, Michala L, Creighton SM. Labial surgery for well women: a review of the literature. BJOG 2010;117(1):20–5.
98. Rouzier R, Louis-Sylvestre C, Paniel B-J, et al. Hypertrophy of labia minora: experience with 163 reductions. Am J Obstet Gynecol 2000;182(1):35–40.
99. Weiss BD. Skin cream for alleviating seat pain in amateur long-distance bicyclists. Res Sports Med An Int J 1993;4(1):27–32.
100. Gaither TW, Awad MA, Murphy GP, et al. Cycling and female sexual and urinary function: results from a large, multinational, cross-sectional study. J Sex Med 2018;15(4):510–8.
101. Scheltinga M, Roumen R. Anterior cutaneous nerve entrapment syndrome (ACNES). Hernia 2018;22(3):507–16.
102. Labat JJ, Riant T, Robert R, et al. Diagnostic criteria for pudendal neuralgia by pudendal nerve entrapment (Nantes criteria). Neurourol Urodyn 2008;27(4): 306–10.

Triathlon Considerations

Daniel M. Cushman, MD[a],*, Nathan Dowling, PT[b], Meredith Ehn, DO[a],
Dana H. Kotler, MD[c]

KEYWORDS

- Cycling • Road biking • Running • Swimming • Time trial • Ironman

KEY POINTS

- Although triathlon includes swimming, cycling, and running, the sport should be seen as a whole. Injuries relating to cycling can have a direct relationship with the other 2 segments of the sport and vice versa.
- There are numerous risk factors related to injury in triathlon, both intrinsic and extrinsic.
- Clinicians should be aware of the 3 disciplines in triathlon, as well as the distances required for standard triathlons.
- Clinicians also should be aware of common scenarios relating to injuries to the triathlete.

INTRODUCTION

Triathlon is a relatively new sport, beginning in 1974, and has shown significant increase in popularity since its inception. Although difficult to calculate, more than 2 million athletes (1 athlete per one race) participated annually in triathlons in recent years in the United States alone.[1] The sport consists of 3 separate activities, performed in succession, with the overall goal of completing the race in the shortest amount of time. A standard triathlon consists of swimming, cycling, and running, performed in that particular order. Variations on triathlons have gained popularity as well, including duathlon (run, cycle, run), aquathlon (run, swim, run), aquabike (swim, cycle), and off-road triathlons (swim, mountain bike, trail run). The successive nature of the sport, in particular, the bike-run sequence, is often related to differences in performance and injury patterns.

TRIATHLON DISTANCES

There are several distances in the sport, as noted in **Table 1**. Recreational races may alter distances due to the logistical challenges related to setting up a race. Importantly, particularly for the recreational athlete, who may be new to triathlon, many participants

^a Division of Physical Medicine and Rehabilitation, University of Utah, 590 Wakara Way, Salt Lake City, UT 84108, USA; ^b Department of Physical Therapy, University of Utah, 590 Wakara Way, Salt Lake City, UT 84108, USA; ^c Department of Physical Medicine and Rehabilitation, Harvard Medical School, 25 Shattuck Street, Boston, MA 02115, USA
* Corresponding author. 590 Wakara Way, Salt Lake City, UT 84108, USA.
E-mail address: dan.cushman.work@gmail.com

Phys Med Rehabil Clin N Am 33 (2022) 81–90
https://doi.org/10.1016/j.pmr.2021.08.006
1047-9651/22/© 2021 Elsevier Inc. All rights reserved.

pmr.theclinics.com

Table 1			
Standard distances for triathlon; distances may vary based on the race			
Race Type	Swim Distance (km)	Cycling Distance (km)	Run Distance (km)
Sprint	0.75	20	5
Olympic	1.5	40	10
Half-Ironman (70.3)	1.9	90	21.1
Ironman (140.6)	3.9	181	42.2

underestimate the cumulative nature of these races. For example, for an Olympic-distance triathlon, although someone may be able to complete a 40-km ride, when adding it after a long swim and before a long run, the added exertion may pose more of a challenge than expected. Many novice participants will view the distances in isolation, when they should be viewed as a whole. Importantly, the cycling portion of the triathlon tends to be the most time intensive. Depending on the distance, cycling makes up approximately half of the total time for a triathlete; in other words, cycling takes as much time as swimming and running combined.[2] This can also vary depending on the athlete's comfort level, background, and experience. Thus, for performance and injury prevention, incorporation of appropriate cycling training and equipment is of the utmost importance.

TRIATHLON BICYCLES

The cycling portion of the triathlon always follows a swim and precedes a run, and thus has differences from standard cycling races. The cycling portion has been shown to be the most predictive of the lowest overall race time for elite Ironman athletes.[2,3] Although some decreased performance has been shown from swim-to-bike,[4,5] most of the difference is proceeding from the bike to the run, as both are predominantly lower extremity exercises. Drafting is allowed in some professional competitions, but most recreational races do not allow drafting. Thus, triathletes will often prefer time-trial–style bicycles to allow for improved individual aerodynamics. This position encompasses a steeper seat tube angle, which has many effects, including a more forward body position,[6] increasing anterior pelvic tilt,[7] increased rectus femoris activation during the upstroke,[7,8] decreased activation of hamstrings,[9] and alteration of the timing of muscle firing.[10] This steeper seat tube angle has been associated with relatively faster post-cycling running,[11] particularly for the first 5 km. It is not fully clear why this advantage is conferred, but may relate to an altered running kinematics seen post-cycling (increased stride length and frequency) caused by an increased similarity to running seen in the steeper seat tube angle. However, it has been shown that regardless of the bike, running economy suffers from a preceding bout of cycling,[12–15] and soleus activation in the preferred limb is diminished.[16]

THE BICYCLE FIT

Although bike fit, position, and posture have a significant effect on performance, comfort, and injury risk on any bicycle,[17] in many ways the stakes are higher with the triathlete. The concept of fitting the bicycle appropriately to the athlete is commonly practiced, although primary literature is lacking.[18,19] The concept of an individualized bike fit is exactly that: individualized; thus, it is less conducive for research that tends to be protocolized and affects numerous individuals.

Without sacrificing power or comfort, the primary objective of most triathlon-specific bike fits is to maximize aerodynamics. And with good reason: an aerodynamic position on a triathlon bike can have significant effects on overall drag,[20] thus increasing speed.[21] A secondary objective is minimizing end range hip flexion range of motion at the top of the pedal stroke. Also for good reason, as the triathlete still needs to run with appropriate hip extension after being on the bike for up to several hours. The problem is that these are contradictory objectives. To reduce frontal area and reduce wind drag, triathletes tend to use a time-trial–like bike, which allows the athlete to lean forward to the handlebars with forearms resting on pads and hands positioned well in front with aerobar extensions.[21] The subsequent trunk angle can be nearly horizontal. But the more the trunk leans forward, the more the hip is "closed down" (has an increase in baseline hip flexion). Fortunately, the modern triathlon bike helps to remedy this by increasing the seat tube angle closer to vertical, which moves the saddle forward relative to the pedals and center of the bicycle. By moving the saddle and thus the pelvis forward, hip flexion demand is decreased. Although there are other methods for "opening" the hip angle, most have limitations: saddle height is limited by leg length and hamstring flexibility, and trunk angle can be decreased but at the expense of aerodynamics. An increasingly common option is to use shorter crank arms than typical (160–165 mm vs a more standard 170–175 mm). Recent evidence has refuted the long-held belief that shorter crank arms would sacrifice power output.[22,23] Often the combination of a triathlon-specific/time-trial bicycle in combination with shorter crank arms will enable the triathlete to achieve an aerodynamic position without exceeding available hip flexion range of motion.

Effectively opening the hip angle will also allow for a greater amount of anterior pelvic tilt on the saddle. Although an anteriorly tilted pelvis will further close the hip angle and must be monitored during the bike fitting process, it will help facilitate 2 very desirable goals: maintenance of a neutral spine and activation of the gluteal muscles. Although it is unrealistic to expect a fully neutral spine in an aerodynamic position, allowing for an overly flexed spine can add adverse load on the lumbar spine, deactivate core and postural musculature, inhibit respiration, impair scapulothoracic stability, and increase the required cervical range of motion to look down the road. Optimizing recruitment of the gluteals will not only add power and efficiency to the pedal stoke, but also contribute to proximal femoral control and therefore knee tracking and stability. Furthermore, appropriate neuromuscular control of the lumbo-pelvic structures may help address low back pain,[24] a commonly occurring cycling-related injury.

A triathlon bike fit should also factor the nature of the race itself. In shorter distances, the triathlete may be able to tolerate a more aggressive, performance-oriented position. However, in full Ironman races, in which average cycling times are several hours, the triathlete needs to be in a sustainable position. The intended aerodynamic position becomes moot if the triathlete is frequently sitting up to rest. Furthermore, the bike leg of the race presents the best opportunity to consume calories and fluids, which is ideally done while in the aero position. If balance, stability, and bike handling skills are overly compromised while in the aerobars, the costs begin to outweigh the rewards. As noted in the following scenarios, an "ideal" position for an elite triathlete is not necessarily the "ideal" position for a recreational triathlete. Flexibility, muscular endurance, body type, injury history, and goals all need to be taken into account to maximize comfort, aerodynamics, and, ultimately, performance.

COMMON SCENARIOS IN THE BIKE FIT FOR TRIATHLETES

"Can I just put aerobars on my road bike?" This is a common question from the novice triathlete. It undoubtedly is the less expensive alternative; however, the road bike geometry with a less vertical seat tube angle will limit the ability to position the saddle far enough forward for both appropriate reach to the aerobars and adequate hip clearance. The resulting, compromised, solution is to sit on the front edge of the saddle, which provides less stability and drastically increases pressure on perineal structures. Similarly, the altered body position can compromise the handling of the bike because of the athlete's position over the handlebars. Although aerobars on a road bike can be accomplished in some cases, it is generally a less-than-ideal setup for the triathlete.

The Novice Triathlete

Assuming that the novice triathlete is also a novice cyclist (one should inquire before one assumes), the bike fit goals will likely be to maximize stability, bike handling, and comfort over performance: the same goals as with a novice cyclist in general. In general, aerodynamics matter less when speed is lower. Time-trial/triathlon bikes tend to have the triathlete farther forward on the bike, which moves the center of gravity farther forward from the rear wheel, which tends to decrease stability and handling. From a progressive loading standpoint, the novice triathlete is ideally starting with sprint or Olympic distances in which the cycling may be performed on a standard road bike anyway. The novice should be encouraged to progressively increase training hours, bicycle-specific strength, and bike handling skills before advancing to a triathlon bicycle, which tends to be more challenging to ride due to body position and its required muscular endurance.

The Overweight Triathlete

The primary concern in this population is lack of potential hip flexion due to soft tissue approximation. This often leads to compensatory hip abduction and external rotation such that the knees track outside of foot-knee-hip neutral alignment while pedaling. Of the previously mentioned strategies for decreasing hip flexion angle, raising the bars and thus decreasing the trunk angle, is frequently the most effective. If knee tracking remains compromised, 20-mm pedal spacers can help to place the foot more laterally under the knee, decreasing varus.

The Older Triathlete

Never underestimate the older athlete; age and years in the sport come with their own considerations with regard to performance, motivation, flexibility, or injury risk. Get to know this athlete, their experiences, and their capabilities. Physical examination of the triathlete's mobility and stability will dictate the bike fit no differently than with any other population.

The "Latest-and-Greatest" Triathlete Who Is Neither the Latest Nor Greatest

Odds are, this triathlete is attempting to ride in a very aggressive, aerodynamic position that their body cannot fully tolerate. The bike fit priority becomes more about education than adjustments to the bike. In fact, the bike fitter will likely be unable to get a wrench anywhere near the bike without this triathlete understanding, appreciating, and ultimately acknowledging the adverse effects of trying to fit a square peg in a round hole. However, after trust is gained and appropriate bike fit adjustments are made (often raising the bars), this triathlete will often see an increase in power output because the hips are no longer binding at the top of the pedal stroke and the glutes are more actively recruited due to a newfound ability to anteriorly rotate the pelvis. Some aerodynamic advantage may be lost, although "lower is not always better," but the gains in power are likely to compensate.

The Triathlete with Neck Pain

Also one of the more common locations of pain,[25,26] neck pain in the triathlete generally requires a more global view of the athlete. The strategies are top-down and bottom-up; however, both are based on the same premise: neutral spine, or at least close to it. This may be related directly to bike fit, or to neuromuscular postural control. From the top down, increased thoracic kyphosis will automatically require an increased amount of cervical extension to look ahead. The more aggressive the aero position, the more this is exacerbated. It is important to note where the issue is coming from: for example, excessive thoracic kyphosis, overaggressive positioning requiring excessive neck extension, or poor lumbar flexibility. In addition, appropriate scapular stability, not an overreliance on the upper trapezius, should be facilitated. Again, the importance of a neutral spine is extremely important. From the bottom up, a pelvis that is posteriorly tilted, due to restricted hip flexion, saddle height exceeding hamstring flexibility, adverse saddle pressure, or lack of postural awareness, leads directly to thoracolumbar flexion and compensatory cervical extension demand. Education regarding appropriate posture, then positioning the saddle to facilitate anterior pelvic rotation will allow a more neutral spine and decreased cervical extension, thereby decreasing neck pain.

The Triathlete with Low Back Pain

See the preceding section, "The Triathlete with Neck Pain." Low back pain has been demonstrated to be a common injury in triathletes,[26–28] but may be less common compared with other sports.[29] Postural education, correction of underlying imbalances in neuromuscular control, and a bike fit that facilitates anterior pelvic rotation will address a large percentage of symptoms in this population. However, there are multiple other factors on the bike that can be grouped into *contact point stability*. It has been said that "you can't fire a cannon from a canoe." To generate power through the pedals, the legs must have a stable platform from which to push.[30] If adequate stability is not present, then load will eventually exceed the body's tolerance. From a bike fit perspective, contact point stability may be affected though cleat position, insoles/orthotics, saddle position, saddle shape and width, and handlebar position: most adjustments to position influence one or more contact points. From an off-the-bike perspective, this triathlete may need to include individualized core and hip girdle strength training that mimics the demands of cycling posture: quadruped and prone plank exercises are typically beneficial. Importantly, there is not a "one-size-fits-all" approach to this athlete: positioning and therapy regimens must address biomechanical, flexibility, neuromuscular, and endurance deficits while addressing physiologic demands, preexisting pathology, and tolerance.

INJURIES TO TRIATHLETES

Injuries to triathletes appear to be higher than those who participate in only swimming, cycling, or running,[31] with a widely variable report of incidence of injuries, ranging from 15% to 91%.[28,31] Most appear to be related to overuse injuries.[32,33] It has been well-established that lower extremity injuries are the most common for triathletes,[31] and it is unclear whether cycling or running accounts for most of these. In many ways, cycling-related and running-related injuries cannot be separated, as triathletes routinely

Table 2
Intrinsic and extrinsic risk factors related to injuries in triathletes

Risk Factor	Risk
Intrinsic risk factors	
Previous injury	Increased risk
Supinated foot type	Increased risk
Pronated foot type	Decreased risk
Bike position	Decreased risk
Extrinsic risk factors	
Number of races participated	Increased risk
Training time (swimming)	Decreased risk
Training time (cycling)	Decreased risk
Training time (running)	Decreased risk
Weight training (risk for acute injuries only)	Increased risk
Cycling pace	Increased risk
Presence of a coach	Decreased risk
Stretching	Decreased risk
Softer running surface	Decreased risk
Participation in an Ironman distance	Increased risk
Use of paddles with swimming	Increased risk

Data from - Gosling CM, Gabbe BJ, Forbes AB. Triathlon related musculoskeletal injuries: The status of injury prevention knowledge. J Sci Med Sport. 2008;11(4):396 to 406.; - Schorn D, Vogler T, Gosheger G, et al. Risk factors for acute injuries and overuse syndromes of the shoulder in amateur triathletes - A retrospective analysis. PLoS One. 2018;13(6):e0198168.

perform these two activities back-to-back. Furthermore, it is challenging to say if the increased likelihood of cycling-related or running-related injuries are a result of the activities themselves, or as a result of the aforementioned greater exposure time spent with these activities. Achilles, knee, and low back injuries are commonly related to cycling.[34] **Table 2** lists risk factors related to injury for triathletes. Shaw and colleagues[35] found an increased risk of injury for triathletes who performed too much or too little training with cycling or running. Finally, the vast majority of health care professionals believe that poor cycling technique or setup is related to injury.[36] Common injuries can be seen in **Box 1**.

LESS COMMON DIAGNOSES

Importantly, several less common injuries can be seen in triathletes, related to cycling. Some of these are noted in **Box 1**. In a triathlete with nonresponsive hip pain that radiates into the quadriceps, iliac artery endofibrosis should remain on the differential. Repeated kinking of the iliac artery can eventually lead to vasospasm and fibrosis that can result in claudication to the affected leg.[37] Similarly, popliteal artery entrapment can have claudicatory symptoms down into the calf[38]; a deep vein thrombosis should always be ruled out in these cases as well.[39] Knee pain that does not respond to conservative measures also should raise suspicion for less common diagnoses, such as a synovial plica or prepatellar friction syndrome,[40] both of which can be exacerbated by the repetitive knee flexion involved with cycling.

Box 1
Common and uncommon injuries noted for triathletes, related to cycling

Common injuries

Axial neck pain (often related to inadequate thoracic/core strength and/or inappropriate bike fit)

Axial low back pain (often related to inadequate core strength and/or inappropriate bike fit)

Lumbar radiculopathy

Greater trochanteric pain syndrome

Iliopsoas tendinopathy

Femoroacetabular impingement

Iliotibial band syndrome at the hip or knee

Patellofemoral pain syndrome

Quadriceps tendinopathy

Patellar tendinopathy

Achilles tendinopathy

Posterior tibialis tendinopathy

Metatarsalgia and/or sesamoiditis

Bone stress injuries

Osteoarthritis

Myofascial pain

Uncommon injuries

Ischiofemoral impingement

Iliac artery endofibrosis

Popliteal artery entrapment

Chronic exertional compartment syndrome

Deep vein thrombosis

Gluteal tendinopathy at the iliac crest

Flexor hallucis longus tendinopathy

Plica syndrome

Prepatellar friction syndrome

SUMMARY

In conclusion, the popular sport of triathlon involves numerous athletic disciplines, performed in succession. The cycling portion of triathlon is performed directly before running, and may put athletes at risk of injury because of the cumulative nature of the lower extremity overload. The importance of bike fit, appropriate neuromuscular training, and appropriate equipment are tantamount for injury prevention and improved performance. Appropriate knowledge and observation of the kinetic chain is required to help diagnose and treat cycling-related injuries in triathletes. Finally, triathletes must be treated differently from cyclists, given the differences in equipment, bike position, and importantly, their requirement for subsequent running after cycling.

CLINICS CARE POINTS

- Always identify the experience, background, and goals of the injured triathlete.
- Consider a bicycle fit with an experienced physical therapist to aid in the diagnosis and treatment.
- Always consider contributing factors from swimming and running for the triathlete with pain related to cycling.

DISCLOSURE

All authors have no commercial or financial conflicts of interest for this article. No funding sources were used for this article.

REFERENCES

1. Sports & Fitness Industry Association. Triathlon (Traditional/Road) Participation Report 2019. SFIA. Available at: https://www.sfia.org/reports/781_Triathlon-%28Traditional-Road%29-Participation-Report-2019. Accessed February 14, 2021.
2. Figueiredo P, Marques EA, Lepers R. Changes in contributions of swimming, cycling, and running performances on overall triathlon performance over a 26-year period. J Strength Cond Res 2016;30(9):2406–15.
3. Sousa CV, Barbosa LP, Sales MM, et al. Cycling as the best sub-8-hour performance predictor in full distance triathlon. Sport (Basel) 2019;7(1):24.
4. Rothschild J, Sheard AC, Crocker GH. Influence of a 2-km swim on the cycling power-duration relationship in triathletes. J Strength Cond Res 2020. [Epub ahead of print].
5. Rothschild J, Crocker GH. Effects of a 2-km swim on markers of cycling performance in elite age-group triathletes. Sport (Basel) 2019;7(4):82.
6. Bini RR, Hume PA, Croft J. Cyclists and triathletes have different body positions on the bicycle. Eur J Sport Sci 2014;14(Suppl 1):S109–15.
7. Silder A, Gleason K, Thelen DG. Influence of bicycle seat tube angle and hand position on lower extremity kinematics and neuromuscular control: implications for triathlon running performance. J Appl Biomech 2011;27(4):297–305.
8. Bini RR, Hume PA, Lanferdini FJ, et al. Effects of body positions on the saddle on pedalling technique for cyclists and triathletes. Eur J Sport Sci 2014;14(Suppl 1): S413–20.
9. Ricard MD, Hills-Meyer P, Miller MG, et al. The effects of bicycle frame geometry on muscle activation and power during a Wingate anaerobic test. J Sport Sci Med 2006;5(1):25–32.
10. Duggan W, Donne B, Fleming N. Effect of seat tube angle and exercise intensity on muscle activity patterns in cyclists. Int J Exerc Sci 2017 10(8):1145-1156.
11. Garside I, Doran DA. Effects of bicycle frame ergonomics on triathlon 10-km running performance. J Sports Sci 2000;18(10):825–33.
12. Hausswirth C, Bigard AX, Guezennec CY. Relationships between running mechanics and energy cost of running at the end of a triathlon and a marathon. Int J Sports Med 1997;18(5):330–9.
13. du Plessis C, Blazevich AJ, Abbiss C, et al. Running economy and effort after cycling: effect of methodological choices. J Sports Sci 2020;38(10):1105–14.

14. Olcina G, Perez-Sousa MÁ, Escobar-Alvarez JA, et al. Effects of cycling on subsequent running performance, stride length, and muscle oxygen saturation in triathletes. Sport (Basel) 2019;7(5):115.
15. Weich C, Jensen RL, Vieten M. Triathlon transition study: quantifying differences in running movement pattern and precision after bike-run transition. Sport Biomech 2019;18(2):215–28.
16. Jacques T, Bini R, Arndt A. Running after cycling induces inter-limb differences in muscle activation but not in kinetics or kinematics. J Sports Sci 2021;39(2):154–60.
17. Kotler DH, Babu AN, Robidoux G. Prevention, evaluation, and rehabilitation of cycling-related injury. Curr Sports Med Rep 2016;15(3):199–206.
18. Wadsworth DJS, Weinrauch P. The role of a bike fit in cyclists with hip pain. A clinical commentary. Int J Sports Phys Ther 2019;14(3):468–86.
19. Priego Quesada JI, Pérez-Soriano P, Lucas-Cuevas AG, et al. Effect of bike-fit in the perception of comfort, fatigue and pain. J Sports Sci 2017;35(14):1459–65.
20. García-López J, Rodríguez-Marroyo JA, Juneau C-E, et al. Reference values and improvement of aerodynamic drag in professional cyclists. J Sports Sci 2008;26(3):277–86.
21. Crouch TN, Burton D, LaBry ZA, et al. Riding against the wind: a review of competition cycling aerodynamics. Sport Eng 2017;20(2):81–110.
22. Barratt PR, Martin JC, Elmer SJ, et al. Effects of pedal speed and crank length on pedaling mechanics during submaximal cycling. Med Sci Sports Exerc 2016;48(4):705–13.
23. Barratt PR, Korff T, Elmer SJ, et al. Effect of crank length on joint-specific power during maximal cycling. Med Sci Sports Exerc 2011;43(9):1689–97.
24. Van Hoof W, Volkaerts K, O'Sullivan K, et al. Comparing lower lumbar kinematics in cyclists with low back pain (flexion pattern) versus asymptomatic controls - field study using a wireless posture monitoring system. Man Ther 2012;17(4):312–7.
25. Deakon RT. Chronic musculoskeletal conditions associated with the cycling segment of the triathlon; prevention and treatment with an emphasis on proper bicycle fitting. Sports Med Arthrosc 2012;20(4):200–5.
26. Villavicencio AT, Burneikienë S, Hernández TD, et al. Back and neck pain in triathletes. Neurosurg Focus 2006;21(4):1–7.
27. Manninen JS, Kallinen M. Low back pain and other overuse injuries in a group of Japanese triathletes. Br J Sports Med 1996;30(2):134–9.
28. Egermann M, Brocai D, Lill CA, et al. Analysis of injuries in long-distance triathletes. Int J Sports Med 2003;24(4):271–6.
29. Fett D, Trompeter K, Platen P. Back pain in elite sports: a cross-sectional study on 1114 athletes. In: Smith B, editor. PLoS One 2017;12(6):e0180130.
30. McDaniel J, Subudhi A, Martin JC. Torso stabilization reduces the metabolic cost of producing cycling power. Can J Appl Physiol 2005;30(4):433–41.
31. Gosling CM, Gabbe BJ, Forbes AB. Triathlon related musculoskeletal injuries: the status of injury prevention knowledge. J Sci Med Sport 2008;11(4):396–406.
32. Burns J, Keenan A-M, Redmond AC. Factors associated with triathlon-related overuse injuries. J Orthop Sports Phys Ther 2003;33(4):177–84.
33. Schorn D, Vogler T, Gosheger G, et al. Risk factors for acute injuries and overuse syndromes of the shoulder in amateur triathletes - a retrospective analysis. PLoS One 2018;13(6):e0198168.
34. Vleck VE, Bentley DJ, Millet GP, et al. Triathlon event distance specialization: training and injury effects. J Strength Cond Res 2010;24(1):30–6.

35. Shaw T, Howat P, Trainor M, et al. Training patterns and sports injuries in triathletes. J Sci Med Sport 2004;7(4):446–50.
36. Gosling CM, Donaldson A, Forbes AB, et al. The perception of injury risk and safety in triathlon competition: an exploratory focus group study. Clin J Sport Med 2013;23(1):70–3.
37. Hinchliffe RJ, D'Abate F, Abraham P, et al. Diagnosis and management of iliac artery endofibrosis: results of a Delphi consensus study. Eur J Vasc Endovasc Surg 2016;52(1):90–8.
38. Hameed M, Coupland A, Davies AH. Popliteal artery entrapment syndrome: an approach to diagnosis and management. Br J Sports Med 2018;52(16):1073–4.
39. Kean J, Pearton A, Fell JW, et al. Deep vein thrombosis in a well-trained masters cyclist, is popliteal vein entrapment syndrome to blame? J Thromb Thrombolysis 2019;47(2):301–4.
40. Claes T, Claes S, De Roeck J, et al. Prepatellar friction syndrome: a common cause of knee pain in the elite cyclist. Acta Orthop Belg 2015;81(4):614–9.

Return to Cycling Following Brain Injury

A Proposed Multidisciplinary Approach

Dana H. Kotler, MD[a,*], Mary Alexis Iaccarino, MD[a],
Sarah Rice, PhD, DPT[b], Seth Herman, MD[c]

KEYWORDS

- Cycling • Traumatic brain injury • Concussion • Crash

KEY POINTS

- Traumatic brain injury is a heterogeneous process with sequelae including physical, cognitive, emotional, and behavioral deficits.
- Cycling provides known health benefits, and is an important form of exercise, recreation, and community mobility.
- Bike handling, or the ability to control the bicycle both in a straight line and around obstacles, comes with practice, experience, and training, and can be altered in the setting of traumatic brain injury.
- A multidisciplinary approach involving physicians and therapists with knowledge of cycling, as well as bike fitters can be used to identify and address residual deficits, as well as optimize strength, balance, bike setup, and decision making in cycling.

INTRODUCTION

After traumatic brain injury (TBI), patients desire to return to work, driving, and recreational activities. There is a body of literature identifying and outlining assessments of the key domains determining safe return to driving, including attention, visuospatial, and executive function.[1,2] In contrast, other modes of transportation and recreation such as cycling, have been largely ignored. Cycling is a widely used form of nonimpact exercise and recreation, and for some, an essential component of community mobility. Cycling has substantial health benefits with respect to cardiovascular fitness, which have been shown to outweigh the risks of cycling in an American

[a] Department of Physical Medicine and Rehabilitation, Harvard Medical School, Boston, MA, USA; [b] Athletico Physical Therapy, Chicago, IL, USA; [c] California Rehabilitation Institute, Los Angeles, CA, USA
* Corresponding author. Spaulding Outpatient Center - Wellesley, 65 Walnut Street, Suite 250, Wellesley, MA 02481.
E-mail address: dkotler@mgh.harvard.edu
Twitter: @DanaKotlerMD (D.H.K.); @iaccarinomd (M.A.I.)

Phys Med Rehabil Clin N Am 33 (2022) 91–105
https://doi.org/10.1016/j.pmr.2021.08.007
pmr.theclinics.com
1047-9651/22/© 2021 Elsevier Inc. All rights reserved.

urban environment.[3] No current guidelines exist for return to outdoor cycling following brain injury, in spite of the increased vulnerability of cyclists compared with other road users.

We propose that a thorough medical assessment is important for patients returning to cycling after an initial TBI, given the risks of further devastating losses resulting from potential reinjury. As cycling is characterized as a collision sport, and crash-related injuries tend to primarily affect the upper extremity and head,[4] the risk of sustaining another head injury can be significant. Overlapping brain injuries can pose risk for more severe deficits and prolonged recovery.[5] Riders with a history of crash and injury have a higher risk of recurrent crash involvement,[6] which is likely multifactorial in nature and may relate to riding habits, including location, time of day, and speed, as well as personality, behavior, risk-taking, and mental health. Cycling parallels driving in that it requires a broad set of motor, visual-spatial, cognitive, and behavioral skills; therefore, it is reasonable to follow a similar approach to return to driving. The neuro-cognitive, neuro-physical, neuro-behavioral, and neuro-emotional deficits common after TBI may interfere or compromise safe return to cycling. In addition to these intrinsic factors, cycling has a host of unique extrinsic factors, including equipment, bike fit, road conditions, weather, and infrastructure, which must also be taken into consideration in the assessment. The following text aims to discuss the many intrinsic and extrinsic factors and clinically relevant challenges faced by patients and providers in supporting a safe return to this sport. We identify several domains to consider in assessment and patient education to maximize safety in return to outdoor cycling, and present 2 cases applying this approach.

TRAUMATIC BRAIN INJURY RISK AND SURVEILLANCE IN CYCLING

The risk of TBI from cycling is high relative to most other sports. Emergency department records surveyed by the National Electronic Injury Surveillance System All Injury Program found that among female individuals, cycling was the most common sports or recreation-related cause of a TBI diagnosis. Among male individuals, cycling was second only to football.[7] In fact, cycling was validated as a significant risk factor for clinically significant head or neck injury in the original version of the "Canadian C-Spine Rules," a clinical prediction rule for identifying patients who require imaging for potential fractures of the head and neck.[8]

Heightened awareness of concussion/TBI in youth and collegiate sport organizations has led to improved concussion surveillance, including both baseline and sideline testing using outcome measures such as the Immediate Post-Concussion Assessment and Cognitive Test (ImPACT),[9] and athlete/coach/parent education. Baseline symptoms and testing performance are highly variable with changes for athletes of different ages or sexes.[10] Because of this variability, assessment of deficits resulting from an event and affecting return to sport may be precluded if the baseline is unknown. Sideline assessment and criteria for both removal and return to play are being established in 11 professional sports,[11] and laws regarding concussion education, surveillance, and return to play criteria for organized youth sports and recreational activities have been enacted in most states.[12]

Cycling is most frequently a loosely organized recreational activity; therefore, application of formal testing, return to sport guidelines, and education, while technically feasible, has been a challenge to implement. A recent survey of cyclists experiencing injuries from crashes identified multiple likely concussion events, experienced in and out of organized competition, with little or no medical follow-up.[13] This is particularly worrisome given that the most common sequelae of concussion/TBI are likely to increase the risk of reinjury in cycling. We encourage interested clinicians to engage in concussion awareness outreach activities, potentially targeting adult and youth members of recreational cycling and triathlon clubs as well as participants in organized cycling activities, such as triathlons, century rides, and bike-to-work events.

RETURN TO SPORTS ACTIVITY AFTER TRAUMATIC BRAIN INJURY

TBIs are characterized as a disruption of brain function due to a direct blow or indirect jolting or jostling of the head. Injuries are heterogeneous in severity and recovery. Although some injuries may have mild symptoms with full recovery in hours to days, more severe injuries can present with persistent alteration of consciousness and devastating impairments in physical and cognitive functions that last a lifetime. In recovery from TBI, sports can play an important role as both rehabilitation tools and recreational activity. Cycling is an enjoyable leisure activity as well as a source of aerobic exercise that can be used as part of TBI recovery and post-TBI recreation. For the brain-injured patient, cycling can help improve cardiovascular fitness, challenge dynamic balance and coordination, and test reaction time and response to the external environment. However, depending on one's injury severity and residual deficits, engaging in cycling may pose challenges.

Given the heterogeneous nature of brain injuries, the clinical requirements for consideration of return to cycling may vary. For those with mild TBI, in which full recovery is anticipated, return to outdoor cycling should occur after complete resolution of symptoms and completion of a return to exercise and sport progression. Over the past decade or more, return to sports after concussion has consisted of a consensus-based, stepwise, return-to-activity progression designed to allow symptom monitoring, increase endurance, and facilitate safe return to play (**Table 1**).[14,15] A stationary bike or trainer may be used as part of the aerobic exercise stage; volume and intensity can be increased over time, and cadence and resistance varied as part of resistance training. Evaluation by a medical provider with experience in concussion is recommended to help guide return to activity progression and gauge recovery.

For individuals with moderate and severe brain injuries, for which residual persistent deficits are likely, clinical considerations for return to activity should include resolution or stabilization of intracranial hemorrhage or edema, assessment of skull integrity for those with skull fracture or neurosurgical instrumentation, resolution or acceptable control of posttraumatic seizures, and stabilization of posttraumatic physical, cognitive, and psychological sequelae. These individuals also frequently experience reduced aerobic and pulmonary capacity, related to factors such as hospital-acquired deconditioning, fatigue as a symptom of TBI, sedentary lifestyle, and neuromotor and autonomic dysfunction. The corresponding physical activity intolerance appears to increase the risk of cardiorespiratory-related comorbidities and mortality. Fortunately, there is evidence that exercise training has the potential to improve outcomes and quality of life in patients post-TBI,[16] highlighting the importance of thoughtful return-to-sport progressions for these individuals.

AN INTEGRATED APPROACH FOR SAFE RETURN TO CYCLING

To support a safe return to cycling and prevent recurrent injury, it is imperative to address the modifiable factors to reduce the risk of a crash. We address how typical deficits occurring in the setting of mild to severe brain injuries may create barriers to

Table 1
Sample return to cycling protocol

Stage[a]	General Activity Guidance	Example of Cycling-Specific Activity
1. Relative rest/symptom limiting	Daily nonsport activities that do not cause symptoms	Same as general activity guidance
2. Light aerobic exercise	Brisk walking, light jogging	Stationary cycling at low intensity and short durations without use of rollers
3. Moderate aerobic exercise/sport-specific exercise	Increase intensity and duration of aerobic exercise; add lateral motion; incorporate sport related drills (eg, foot work, stick work, or ball drills)	Riding without a group on a road, track, or trail at low intensity and short duration[b]
4. All other noncontact exercise: aerobic and anaerobic	Noncontact sport-specific practice; rigorous aerobic exercise; introduce resistance and strength training	Riding without a group on a road, track, or trail with increased level of intensity and duration[b]
5. Contact drills and practice	Incorporate all sport-specific activities, including full-contact practice	Riding in a group and incorporating sprints, climbs, and pacelines
6. Game Play	Resume all normal sport activities, including game play	Return to competition

[a] A minimum of 24 hours is recommended between stages.
[b] Riding on a track, trail, or road may be considered a contact environment, as a fall could risk head injury; these guidelines may be most appropriate for advanced-level and competitive cyclists and should be discussed with a physician.

(Data from [14,15] McCrory et al, *Consensus statement on concussion in sport—the 5th international conference on concussion in sport held in Berlin October 2016,* Br J Sports Med 2018;51:838–847 Abramson A, Brayley J, Broglio S. Concussion in Cycling Consensus Statement 2012. Medicine of Cycling. https://www.medicineofcycling.com/wp-content/uploads/2012/01/ConcussionsInCyclists2012.pdf Accessed March 30, 2021.

safe return to cycling. In planning for return to cycling following TBI, it is essential to consider the type of riding in which an individual participates and note the potential for crash in each of these settings. Riding on country roads, bike paths, city streets, or more technical terrain each have unique risks and challenges, some of which have been quantified in prior epidemiologic research.[17] Riding at higher speeds, in groups, or in competition presents additional cognitive, visual, and motor demands. Depending on the environment, the complexity of these demands will vary, but the principles described as follows remain the same. In this article, we focus primarily on cycling for recreation and fitness; individuals wishing to ultimately return to activities such as racing, mountain biking, group riding, and city riding should weigh the potential risks with their physician. If the inability to participate in these activities causes a significant detriment to the individual's quality of life, efforts should be made to use these strategies to progress them to the riding they wish to pursue.

Bicycle safety and crash prevention is dependent on many factors, both extrinsic and intrinsic to the rider.[18] Typical extrinsic factors (infrastructure, road conditions, motor vehicles, weather, daylight) are not easily modifiable, whereas intrinsic factors (the rider and the rider's ability to control the bicycle) may be more readily addressed. Cognitive, behavioral, and motor skills are essential to cycling, and may be impaired as a result of TBI. Potential cognitive deficits after TBI are presented in **Box 1**. Interventions to address these factors take many forms; bicycles can be adjusted, fitness and riding skill may be trained, and decisions including route choices, speed, and risk-taking behavior can be targeted through education.

An initial evaluation of a cyclist desiring to return after TBI should start with a thorough understanding of the patient's preinjury status such as medical history, physical capabilities, and cognitive and behavioral status. In addition, preinjury sport and recreational history, including prior cycling experience, volume, and discipline (road, commuting, mountain biking) should be considered. A thorough history ensures that no medical, physical, cognitive, or behavioral issues that may play a role in safe return to cycling are missed due to the immediate focus of clinical care on the traumatic injury and subsequent deficits.

Medical clearance includes assessment of potential barriers to safe return to cycling, such as seizure, vision issues including acuity, field cuts and neglect, metabolic disturbances, vestibular dysfunction, medication side effects, and psychiatric or behavioral issues that may preclude or limit participation in cycling. Consultation with Neurology, Ophthalmology, and Psychiatry to evaluate and address these issues is recommended. Severe visual deficits (field cuts, double vision), balance or vestibular dysfunction, cognitive deficits or dementia, and seizure disorders without aura or warning signs are all conditions that may preclude independent participation in bicycling. In these cases, adaptive cycling or use of tricycles or tandem riding may be an alternative. Once medical clearance is obtained, we can target the broad range of intrinsic and extrinsic factors required for cycling, including persistent deficits. We propose evaluating the intrinsic factors using a similar approach to predriving assessments of neuropsychological skills, which are currently performed by specialty trained physical or occupational therapists. Therapists trained in assessment of the cyclist can then evaluate the patient's strength, flexibility, and balance, and the bicycle configuration and equipment, and collaborate with trained bike fitters to optimize fit and setup, and provide education on extrinsic factors including route, clothing, attire, and lighting choices to maximize safety on return to cycling.

INTRINSIC FACTORS: MOTOR AND NEUROPSYCHOLOGICAL ASSESSMENT

Riding a bicycle involves the integration of many abilities, including vision, motor functioning, physical fitness, and cognitive function, some of which may be compromised in the setting of TBI. Wierda and Brookhuis[19] described 3 levels of the cycling task: the

---

Box 1
Cognitive Deficits after Traumatic Brain Injury

Attention (sustained, divided, alternating)
Concentration
Distractibility
Visual-spatial processing
Memory (immediate, delayed, and working)
Processing speed
Executive functioning (judgment, planning, organization)

strategic level, in which one weighs the risks and benefits of a trip by bicycle, the maneuvering level, including decisions about course, tactics, speed, and obstacle avoidance, and the control level, involving maintenance of balance, direction, and control of the bicycle. As the adage suggests, this coordination of visual, proprioceptive, and vestibular input with motor function, once established, is "just like riding a bike." The experienced cyclist relies on automatic sequences of action that do not require specific attention or mental effort, in contrast to the novice cyclist, who needs to actively think about controlling their bicycle.[19] Because of this "muscle memory," the experienced cyclist's attention can be directed toward areas that require it, including avoidance of obstacles or reaction to events.

The skill of "bike handling" encompasses the ability to control the bicycle, negotiate around obstacles, and ride in a steady straight line when desired. The bicycle is controlled through steering with the handlebar, leaning the body, rolling the bicycle laterally using the pelvis, and moving the knees laterally, all while continuing to pedal to ensure forward motion. Although cardiovascular fitness and endurance are important for cycling, bike handling skill is not a reflection of fitness, and is often the product of experience.[20] Moreover, the seemingly simple act of riding in a straight line can in fact be used as a screening test to differentiate expert cyclists from novice cyclists.[21] These skills are developed with time and repetition, typically many hours on the bike over years. In a postinjury setting, supervised indoor training using bicycle rollers as a training tool can help challenge balance and simulate road biking. In contrast to a stationary trainer, to which the bicycle clamps and is held in place, rollers require the rider to balance on top of metal drums while pedaling (similar to a treadmill), and require balance, attention, training, and skill to ride successfully.

Vision is a primary sensory domain that is required to operate a bicycle safely. It is incumbent on the rider to process visual and vestibular input, determine errors, and correction of the movement or position to keep the bicycle upright and going in the correct direction.[20] The spectrum of visual deficits in TBI includes but is not limited to visual acuity, field of vision, visual processing speed, depth perception, and associated attentional deficits.[22,23] It is recommended that each of these aspects of vision be evaluated to ensure that they are functioning within an acceptable manner for a safe to return to cycling.

Motor function must be considered in return to cycling, including optimal range of motion, strength, muscle power, balance, and tone to adequately control and maneuver the bicycle. These domains of motor function may be impaired after TBI such that weakness, spasticity, contractures, decreased range of motion, and balance and vestibular function will interfere with safe return to biking. A more detailed discussion of bike fit and accommodation of strength and flexibility imbalances seen after TBI will follow in the bike fitting section later in this article. A thorough evaluation of the previously mentioned motor skills is recommended to ensure one can operate the bicycle safely. There may be a role for adaptive strategies or equipment, such as recumbent, 3-wheeled, or tandem bicycle, to allow safe return to cycling.

TBI has also been demonstrated to affect cognitive-motor integration. The widespread injury seen in concussion or more severe TBI is thought to impair task performance through a failure to communicate between brain networks. After mild TBI, individuals may demonstrate more subtle changes in oculomotor function, gait, and balance, which can become more pronounced when they are challenged with multitasking or integration.[24]

Cognitive deficits, including domains of visual-spatial processing, memory, attention, verbal fluency, and language are quite common sequelae post-TBI that can compromise optimal function.[25,26] **Box 1** shows the common cognitive deficits following TBI that will interfere with safe return to cycling. Based on the negative impact these deficits are known to have on the operation of a motor vehicle, a detailed neuropsychological assessment to assess residual cognitive abilities before engaging in cycling, especially on the road, is recommended. Concerns include slowed processing speed and associated reaction time, as well as distractibility, decision making, and judgment, all of which can be a major barrier for safe operation of a bicycle. There is no recognized test that can predict safe return to cycling; however, standard neuropsychological measures such as Trail Making, Digit Span, Stroop, and other tests commonly used are recommended.[27] The addition of bicycle-specific challenges or on-the-road testing to supplement precycling evaluation is important, especially given that there is no definitive test to determine one's fitness for return to cycling. On the rollers, tests may include turning the head to look back or retrieving a water bottle from the cage and drinking without veering or losing balance. Additional considerations include the brain-injured patient's preinjury personality; cognitive function; and visual, motor, and cognitive and behavioral capacity in the assessment, and other factors like level of energy, fatigue, endurance, and emotional system such as impulsivity, aggression, agitation, anger, irritability, and anxiety, which can play a role in the safe operation of bicycle.

EXTRINSIC FACTORS: INFRASTRUCTURE AND CONDITIONS

For our patients recovering from TBI, strategies for safe cycling may vary by community; with respect to route choices, optimal routes minimize shared space with fast-moving traffic. Prior research on cycling injury and fatality, including the League of American Bicyclists' "Every Bicyclist Counts Project," has found that urban arterial roads were the most common location for fatality.[17] Other factors associated with crashing include cycling in regions with lower level of active travel,[28] where drivers may not be used to the presence of cyclists.

There is a growing body of evidence that purpose-built bicycle-specific infrastructure (such as separated bike lanes and dividers) reduce crashes and injuries among cyclists.[18] Although the timing of bicycle-commuting may not be flexible, fitness and recreational rides should be taken during daylight non–rush hours if possible to maximize visibility and minimize traffic. During evening hours or weather with poor visibility, lights and bright/reflective clothing are helpful (and in many cases lights are required, white in front, red in rear). In addition, attention must be paid to road conditions, including potholes, cracks, gravel, and other potential hazards including railroad tracks. Depending on location, weather may be a factor in crashes, including wet, oily, or slippery roads (often worse when crossing over painted lines).

Prior studies of cycling safety have mainly focused on helmet design, regulation, and implementation to mitigate injury from a crash, but this approach has neglected injury prevention through increased ridership and bicycle-specific urban design. Prior research has shown that increased ridership rates are associated with a decrease in injury rates.[29,30] The percentage of short trips made by bicycle is far lower in North America (approximately 1%) compared with Europe (10%–20% or more), particularly the Netherlands and Denmark.[31] Studies have also shown a higher risk of injury associated with cycling in North America compared with Europe,[32] and this perceived lack of safety has been shown to be a deterrent to cycling, creating an unfortunate feedback loop.

Although it has been established that improved cycling infrastructure reduces the risk of crashes and injuries sustained during cycling,[18,33] many other factors influencing cycling safety may not be straightforward. Research has shown that driver passing distance is smaller and speed is higher on roads with bicycle lanes compared with those without.[34] Other research on cycling injury and mortality has revealed that regardless of the season, bicyclist deaths occurred most often between 6 and 9 PM, most frequently in urban areas compared with rural areas, and are higher for male than female cyclists (8 times higher in 2017 data). Alcohol was involved in 37% of all fatal bicyclist crashes in 2017.[35]

Considering these factors, cyclists may be cleared to ride under certain conditions initially, from daylight and dry conditions in empty parking lots or private property, to minimal-traffic roads, paths, and eventually city roads or more technical terrain. Clearance to ride in a progressive fashion may help to mitigate the risk posed by these extrinsic factors, similar to returning to work with restrictions or modified duty. The National Highway Traffic Safety Administration (NHTSA) on their Bicycle Safety Web site generally recommends careful route planning, choosing routes with less traffic and slower speeds.[36,37] They also recommend using bike lanes or bike paths, although these may in fact be shared by more people in closer proximity particularly during warmer months. For the cyclist with impairments in attention or processing speed, consider that these routes may have additional potential interactions, including dogs and children, which pose a different and unpredictable challenge compared with road traffic.

BIKE FIT AND COMPONENT SELECTION

The aim of bike fitting is to adjust the bicycle to a comfortable and safe position for the cyclist, reducing pain and potential for injury, and optimizing performance. First and foremost for our patients is ensuring that the bicycle is in good working order, the rider has easy access to the brakes and shifters, and that the bike is configured for steady handling. Mechanical failure is a relatively uncommon cause of bicycle crashes, and is generally preventable through routine maintenance, as well as bike handling skill. As specified on the NHTSA fact sheet: "Ride a bike that works—it really doesn't matter how well you ride if the brakes don't work."[38] Tire blowout, or failure of a crank, derailleur, or chain have the potential to cause a crash, and bicycle parts such as forks can be subject to recall for manufacturing defects. Regular maintenance by a bike shop, cleaning and lubricating regularly, and inflating the tires to the recommended pressure make these issues less likely to occur.[39]

The configuration of the bicycle itself plays a role in ease of handling and thereby crash avoidance. Bicycles possess self-stabilizing or gyroscopic properties, and generally become more stable at higher velocities, whereas at slower velocity a bicycle will start to oscillate laterally.[20,40] The handling and stability of a bicycle is governed by the geometry of the frame in conjunction with the components on the front of the bike. The combination of head tube angle, fork rake, and offset measurements make up the measurement of trail, reflecting distance from the bottom bracket to the front axle. Longer trail will slow the steering, allowing for a bike that performs better in a straight line (like a bus), whereas shorter trail will allow the bike to turn more quickly with less input from the rider (like a sports car). Bringing the handlebars closer to the frame or raising them excessively will also influence handling, making the bike "twitchier," less stable, and harder to control.[41] Although there is ample evidence that bike fit is associated with improvement in comfort[42] and performance,[43,44] there is little evidence that bike fit leads to a reduction in injury, either overuse or traumatic,[45] and this is an important direction for future research.[46] Factors that may require accommodation in patients with TBI include spasticity, contractures, decreased range of motion related to the injury, and protracted recovery.

Although bike fitting for the racer or avid cyclist often involves small adjustments and subtle changes, the recreational cyclist may present with a bike with severe flaws in setup that, although well-intentioned, can compromise the handling of a bike and potentially lead to crash or injury, and this should be the low-hanging fruit for the bike fitter. For example, in an effort to find a more upright position, a rider who tinkers with their own bike may alter the setup of their stem and handlebars causing the bicycle to be very unsteady, or worse, to a point that the attachment is not secure and compromises the integrity of the fork, putting it at risk for failure.

Much of the focus of head injury in cycling research has related to the use of cycling helmets. Importantly, helmets have been shown to reduce the risk of head injury and death in a crash setting,[47,48] but do nothing to prevent crashes, which is the focus of this section. In most fatality cases researched by the League of American Bicyclists, the cyclist was wearing a helmet.[17] For patients recovering from brain injury, it is of course recommended to wear an approved cycling helmet, but specifically one that is within approximately 3 years of its manufacturing date (specified on the helmet), or an otherwise specified warranty, and has not been traumatized either through crashing or through repeatedly dropping the helmet, which may compromise its integrity.

ILLUSTRATIVE CASES

The following are 2 patients who wished to return to cycling following TBI (in both cases sustained while bicycling). In each case, the patient was medically cleared by their brain injury physiatrist, and was referred to Cycling Medicine Clinic for input on safely returning to outdoor cycling.

Case #1

A 57-year-old cyclist was referred to the cycling medicine clinic after a TBI 1.5 years prior, when he was hit by a motor vehicle while cycling. His TBI was characterized by subarachnoid hemorrhage, subdural hematoma, and diffuse axonal injury. Before his injury he was an avid cyclist, often riding with his wife; he also regularly commuted by bicycle and did charity rides nearly every year, riding up to 100 miles per week in the warmer months. Following his injury, he noted a decline in his balance and coordination. He ambulated without an assistive device and reported no falls but noted that activities such as descending stairs required extra attention. He also described residual difficulty with word-finding, memory of names, and occasionally directions. Treatment following his acute care hospitalization included extensive rehabilitation, both inpatient and outpatient. He progressed in activity tolerance, including indoor spin classes and gym workouts without any exacerbation of symptoms. He had not had any formal bike fitting. Although he was eager to return to cycling, he endorsed feelings of anxiety related to returning to cycling. Of note, he was on chronic anticoagulation for a remote history of pulmonary embolism.

On examination, he demonstrated a pronounced head-forward posture, with notable atrophy of cervical and shoulder girdle muscles, thoracic kyphosis, though without pain or substantial restriction of cervical range of motion. He had no pain or restriction with lumbar flexion or extension, or with hip flexion and rotation, but hamstrings, hip flexors, and iliotibial band (ITB) showed significant tightness, with pelvic rotation at approximately 30° on hip flexion. Upper and lower extremity muscle strength was intact, with the exception of the gluteus medius, which was 4/5 on the right and 4+/5 on the left. On balance testing, he had difficulty with standing with his feet together, with right-sided deviation when eyes were closed. Single-leg balance was fair but he required significant focus to perform a single-leg squat with fair control and correct deviations in balance. Gait showed a normal base, normal cadence and stride length, and was nonantalgic.

Examination of his cycling biomechanics showed an appropriately sized road bicycle, with a crank length of 175 mm. Saddle position was slightly low. Body position showed excessive reach, with brake hoods positioned low on the bars; he felt more comfortable sitting up straighter with his fingertips on top of the bars, an unsafe position for riding. His reported weight distribution as 50% seat, 50% handlebars, indicating excess pressure in the hands for the typical cyclist.

During our clinic visit, we discussed bicycle-specific biomechanics and the relationship of strength imbalances, flexibility, and bicycle fit to comfort, power generation, and safety. The visit included extensive discussion of mental and physical fatigue and its impact on attention and safety on the bicycle. We educated him on the importance of route selection, duration of riding, and time of day. His plan included a comprehensive bike fit addressing both safety (including handling), as well as comfort. We also recommended additional physical therapy specifically focused on balance exercise relevant to cycling, using bicycle rollers to improve and optimize balance before riding outdoors (**Fig. 1**). These balance skills translate to the ability of a rider to hold a straight line, and maintain smooth pedal stroke and good control of the bike on the road. In his case, the chronic anticoagulation was a particularly important factor warranting aggressive balance and skills training before return to outdoor cycling. In follow-up, he demonstrated improved balance, bike handling, confidence, and safety awareness, and returned successfully to outdoor riding over 3 to 4 months.

In follow-up, he reported that he rides regularly with his wife or a few friends around the neighborhood, but is not riding in the large groups or at the speeds that he used to ride. The most limiting factor since his TBI has been his vision, specifically the ability to quickly change his focus with movements of the eyes or head. The combination of visual input and motor control is challenging, and he feels a similar challenge with other activities, such as tennis. He found that due to neck muscle discomfort, a more upright position on the bike is more comfortable for him, and he now rides a fitness geometry bike rather than his prior road geometry bike. He finds the upright position allows him to turn his head with more ease, which in turn helps him be more aware of his surroundings. He continues to have some uneasiness and anxiety when on the bike in heavier traffic, closely passing cars, or close to the location where he was hit, and avoids busy streets and riding during rush hour. Although he has not returned to his previous volume or intensity of cycling, he does find his current riding to be gratifying. This case illustrates how for a patient with severe TBI, many goals are met through traditional rehabilitation approaches; however, the unique demands of cycling necessitate specific return-to-cycling strategies. For this athlete, balance training using rollers was very effective, and was perceived to be an essential late-stage component of his rehabilitation and return to cycling.

Case #2

A 59-year-old cyclist was referred to cycling clinic by his primary physiatrist for input on his return to cycling following TBI sustained in a cycling crash. He reportedly lost traction while riding over a wooden bridge, slid, and fell on his side. He does not have any recollection of the crash, but remembers another cyclist helping him up, and he rode home from the scene of the crash. He developed acute headache and aphasia the following week, and was found to have a left parietal/temporal subdural hematoma, initially managed conservatively but ultimately requiring evacuation for mass effect and midline shift. His treatment included inpatient rehabilitation where he improved functionally, followed by outpatient physical, occupational, and speech

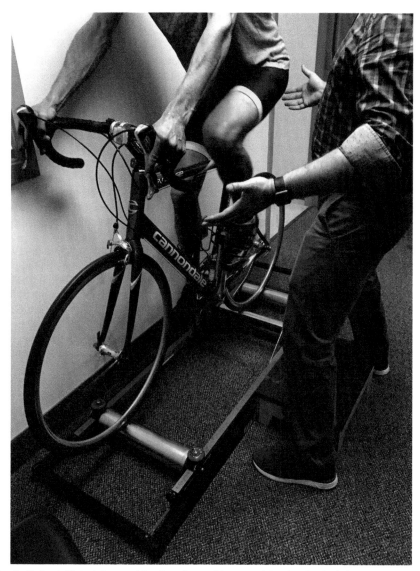

Fig. 1. Patient #2 training on bicycle rollers with supervision in physical therapy.

therapies. On discharge, he was treated with melatonin for sleep and amantadine for attention. He developed a deep venous thrombosis following discharge and was anti-coagulated with Eliquis (apixaban) short-term.

Since his injury, his concentration had improved greatly, and he returned to driving and to work. He had already made substantial progress on his balance training. Before injury he was an avid cyclist, riding for more than 20 years, primarily road cycling and touring, averaging 100 to 125 miles per week in the warm weather and 50 to 75 miles per week in the cold weather. Since the injury, he was concerned about riding by him-self, and was particularly nervous riding downhill. He did feel some initial headache with exertion on the bike, but this improved. His goals were to improve his confidence while riding, make sure his bike is adjusted properly, and return to riding to longer rides. He had never had a formal bike fit, but since his crash he had his bike assessed for damage, and some small repairs made.

On examination, he demonstrated relatively neutral posture, slightly head-forward without pain or restriction in cervical range of motion. He had mild tenderness to palpation of cervical paraspinal muscles and trapezius bilaterally. He had no pain with lumbar or hip flexion, and demonstrated restricted range on lumbar extension. Upper and lower extremity strength was full on manual muscle testing, with the exception of the gluteus medius, which was 4/5 right and 4−/5 left. He had a brisk right patellar reflex but otherwise reflexes were symmetric 2+. Hamstring flexibility was fair, with pelvic rotation at 50°, and modified Thomas test showed left hip flexor tightness and bilateral ITB tightness. Assessment of his cycling mechanics showed an appropriately sized fitness geometry bike, frame size L with 175-mm cranks. He used flat pedals with athletic shoes. Saddle position was low and forward, with knee slightly ahead of the pedal spindle, relatively neutral spine position, with appropriate reach and no excessive frontal plane motion.

We also recommended additional cycling-specific drills, including roller training with the goal of returning to road cycling with improved confidence and safety. Regarding bike fit, we recommended a comprehensive fit including adjustment of saddle position to improve comfort and position, consideration of a slightly wider handlebar for stability, and consideration of a clipless pedal system, such as an SPD mountain bike pedal for improved mechanics and safety/ease of use. We discussed how this type of pedal system, while often daunting for riders, promotes improved stability on the bike, and does not limit the rider in the ability to take the foot off the pedal quickly, as the spring tension can be adjusted for very easy release.

In follow-up, he reported substantial progress, having successfully returned to outdoor riding. He continued to ride his flat-bar hybrid bike, which he felt was the most stable and comfortable geometry for him. He had difficulty getting used to the clipless pedals, and ultimately returned to a flat pedal with toe cages, which he is comfortable with. He reported that his main limiting factor was confidence on maneuvering his bicycle, particularly slowing to a stop with control. Early in returning to cycling, he noted that objects or shadows moving in his peripheral vision were distracting, although this gradually resolved. Similar to the prior patient, he found quick head movements and changes of focus to be a challenge. He used exercises to "tease himself visually," such as quick head turns and changes of focal point, which made him more confident. He also noted that gaining improved flexibility of his neck was helpful in his comfort and confidence while riding. He tracks and maintains his cycling in a spreadsheet, trying to set achievable goals. He rode more than 2000 miles over the past year, primarily on suburban roads and bike paths and is pleased with his progress. Similar to Case #1, this athlete felt that the visual and cognitive demands of moving through space quickly on 2 wheels had not been fully addressed through traditional rehabilitation strategies, and reported substantial benefit from cycling-specific balance and visual exercises to gain confidence while riding.

CLINICS CARE POINTS

- Cycling requires a broad set of motor, visual-spatial, cognitive, and behavioral skills, many of which can be impaired in the setting of TBI.
- The sport of cycling encompasses a wide range of activities: riding for leisure at slow speed, racing at high velocity in a group, or riding over technical terrain, each with different degrees of risk.

- Return to cycling after brain injury involves a multidisciplinary team focused on optimization of motor function, vision, and cognition, adjustment of the bicycle for comfort and control, and education on safety strategies, including route choices to mitigate risk of recurrent injury.
- Focused balance training with cycling-specific balance drills is an important component of physical therapy before returning to the road, and has been felt by patients to be tremendously helpful.

SUMMARY

Given the understanding that TBI is a very heterogeneous disease process that results in a broad range of physical, cognitive, emotional, and behavioral deficits and unique medical sequelae, we recommend a collaborative, multidisciplinary approach, including physicians and therapists with knowledge of cycling, as well as bike fitters, to ensure safe return to cycling. In both cases presented, the clinic evaluation and subsequent training also provided reassurance to the patient and their family about their ability to safety return to cycling, which enhanced their overall quality of life. Our clearance strategy is rooted in the already established strategy for safe return to driving. Cycling can have a positive impact has on overall function, quality of life, mood and sleep, and has the potential to enhance cognition, coordination, and improve other known deficits seen in brain injury. We strongly encourage cycling as an optimal activity not only for leisure and fitness, but as a means to enhance recovery.

DISCLOSURE

All authors have no commercial or financial conflicts of interest for this article. No funding sources were used for this article.

REFERENCES

1. Saviola D, De Tanti A, Conforti J, et al. Safe return to driving following severe acquired brain injury: role of a short neuropsychological assessment. Eur J Phys Rehabil Med 2018;54(5):717–23.
2. Schanke AK, Sundet K. Comprehensive driving assessment: neuropsychological testing and on-road evaluation of brain injured patients. Scand J Psychol 2000; 41(2):113–21.
3. Johan de Hartog J, Boogaard H, Nijland H, et al. Do the health benefits of cycling outweigh the risks? Environ Health Perspect 2010;118(8):1109–16.
4. Perrin AE. Cycling-related injury. Conn Med 2012;76(8):461–6.
5. Guskiewicz KM, McCrea M, Marshall SW, et al. Cumulative effects associated with recurrent concussion in collegiate football players: the NCAA Concussion Study. Jama 2003;290(19):2549–55.
6. Tin Tin S, Woodward A, Ameratunga S. What influences the association between previous and future crashes among cyclists? A propensity score analysis. PloS one 2014;9(1):e87633.
7. Coronado VG, Haileyesus T, Cheng TA, et al. Trends in sports-and recreation-related traumatic brain injuries treated in US emergency departments: the National Electronic Injury Surveillance System-All Injury Program (NEISS-AIP) 2001-2012. J Head Trauma Rehabil 2015;30(3):185–97.
8. Stiell IG, Wells GA, Vandemheen KL, et al. The Canadian C-spine rule for radiography in alert and stable trauma patients. Jama 2001;286(15):1841–8.

9. Cottle JE, Hall EE, Patel K, et al. Concussion baseline testing: preexisting factors, symptoms, and neurocognitive performance. J Athl Train 2017;52(2):77–81.

10. Abeare CA, Messa I, Zuccato BG, et al. Prevalence of invalid performance on baseline testing for sport-related concussion by age and validity indicator. JAMA Neurol 2018;75(6):697–703.

11. Patricios JS, Ardern CL, Hislop MD, et al. Implementation of the 2017 Berlin Concussion in Sport Group Consensus Statement in contact and collision sports: a joint position statement from 11 national and international sports organisations. Br J Sports Med 2018;52(10):635–41.

12. Lowrey KM. Traumatic brain injury in youth sports: fact sheet. Summary matrix of state laws addressing concussions in youth sports. Edina: Network for Public Health Law; 2019.

13. Rice S, Iaccarino MA, Bhatnagar S, et al. Reporting of concussion-like symptoms after cycling crashes: a survey of competitive and recreational cyclists. J Athl Train 2020;55(1):11–6.

14. McCrory P, Meeuwisse W, Dvorak J, et al. Consensus statement on concussion in sport—the 5th international conference on concussion in sport held in Berlin, October 2016. Br J Sports Med 2017;51(11):838–47.

15. Abramson AK, Brayley J, Broglio S. Concussions in cycling consensus statement. Paper presented at: Medicine of Cycling 2012.

16. Hamel RN, Smoliga JM. Physical activity intolerance and cardiorespiratory dysfunction in patients with moderate-to-severe traumatic brain injury. Sports Med 2019;49(8):1183–98.

17. League of American Bicyclists. Bicyclist safety must be a priority: findings from a year of fatality tracking – and the urgent need for better data. Washington, DC: League of American Bicyclists; 2014.

18. Reynolds CC, Harris MA, Teschke K, et al. The impact of transportation infrastructure on bicycling injuries and crashes: a review of the literature. Environ Health 2009;8:47.

19. Wierda M, Brookhuis KA. Analysis of cycling skill: a cognitive approach. Appl Cogn Psychol 1991;5(2):113–22.

20. Fonda B. Bicycle rider control: a balancing act [Doctoral Dissertation]. Birmingham: University of Birmingham; 2016.

21. Fonda B, Sarabon N, Lee F. A new test battery to assess bike handling skills of experienced and inexperienced cyclists. J Sci Cycling 2014;3(2):18.

22. Owsley C, McGwin G Jr. Vision impairment and driving. Surv Ophthalmol 1999; 43(6):535–50.

23. Owsley C, Wood JM, McGwin G Jr. A roadmap for interpreting the literature on vision and driving. Surv Ophthalmol 2015;60(3):250–62.

24. Sergio LE, Gorbet DJ, Adams MS, et al. The effects of mild traumatic brain injury on cognitive-motor integration for skilled performance. Front Neurol 2020;11:1060.

25. Barman A, Chatterjee A, Bhide R. Cognitive impairment and rehabilitation strategies after traumatic brain injury. Indian J Psychol Med 2016;38(3):172–81.

26. Sun H, Luo C, Chen X, et al. Assessment of cognitive dysfunction in traumatic brain injury patients: a review. Forensic Sci Res 2017;2(4):174–9.

27. McKay A, Liew C, Schönberger M, et al. Predictors of the on-road driving assessment after traumatic brain injury: comparing cognitive tests, injury factors, and demographics. J head Trauma Rehabil 2016;31(6):E44–52.

28. Tin Tin S, Woodward A, Ameratunga S. Incidence, risk, and protective factors of bicycle crashes: findings from a prospective cohort study in New Zealand. Prev Med 2013;57(3):152–61.
29. Jacobsen PL. Safety in numbers: more walkers and bicyclists, safer walking and bicycling. Inj Prev 2015;21(4):271–5.
30. Robinson DL. Safety in numbers in Australia: more walkers and bicyclists, safer walking and bicycling. Health Promot J Austr 2005;16(1):47–51.
31. Pucher J, Buehler R. Making cycling irresistible: lessons from the Netherlands, Denmark and Germany. Transport Rev 2008;28(4):495–528.
32. Pucher J, Dijkstra L. Promoting safe walking and cycling to improve public health: lessons from the Netherlands and Germany. Am J Public Health 2003;93(9):1509–16.
33. Teschke K, Frendo T, Shen H, et al. Bicycling crash circumstances vary by route type: a cross-sectional analysis. BMC Public Health 2014;14:1205.
34. Parkin J, Meyers C. The effect of cycle lanes on the proximity between motor traffic and cycle traffic. Accid Anal Prev 2010;42(1):159–65.
35. National Center for Statistics and Analysis. Bicyclists and other cyclists, 2017 data. National Highway Traffic Safety Administration; 2019.
36. National Highway Traffic Safety Administration. Bicycle safety. United States Department of Transportation. Available at: https://www.nhtsa.gov/road-safety/bicyclists. Accessed 3/7/21, 2021..
37. National Highway Traffic Safety Administration. Bicyclist and pedestrian safety. In: Administration NHTS. US Department of Trasnportation; 2019.
38. National Highway Traffic Safety Administration. 2016 Bicyclists and other cyclists traffic safety fact sheet. NHTSA's National Center for Statistics and Analysis; 2018.
39. Hymas R. Bicycle accidents, road safety for bikes, Utah bicycle accidents. Available at: https://www.utahbicyclelawyers.com/mechanical-problems-that-may-lead-to-bicycle-crashes. Accessed 2/8/2021.
40. Schwab A, Meijaard J. A review on bicycle dynamics and rider control. Vehicle Syst Dyn 2013;51(7):1059–90.
41. Wilson DG, Papadopoulos J, Whitt FR. Bicycling Science. Cambridge: MIT Press; 2004.
42. Salai M, Brosh T, Blankstein A, et al. Effect of changing the saddle angle on the incidence of low back pain in recreational bicyclists. Br J Sports Med 1999;33(6):398–400.
43. Peveler WW, Pounders JD, Bishop PA. Effects of saddle height on anaerobic power production in cycling. J Strength Cond Res 2007;21(4):1023.
44. Swart J, Holliday W. Cycling biomechanics optimization—the (r) evolution of bicycle fitting. Curr Sports Med Rep 2019;18(12):490–6.
45. Priego Quesada JI, Kerr ZY, Bertucci WM, et al. The association of bike fitting with injury, comfort, and pain during cycling: An international retrospective survey. Eur J Sport Sci 2019;19(6):842–9.
46. Bini RR. The need for a link between bike fitting and injury risk. J Sci Cycling 2016;5(1):1–2.
47. Olivier J, Creighton P. Bicycle injuries and helmet use: a systematic review and meta-analysis. Int J Epidemiol 2016;46(1):278–92.
48. Rivara FP, Thompson DC, Thompson RS. Epidemiology of bicycle injuries and risk factors for serious injury. Inj Prev 2015;21(1):47–51.

Fear, Anxiety, and Return to Sport After Cycling Crashes

A Survey of Cyclists

Dana H. Kotler, MD[a,b,c,d,*], Daniel M. Cushman, MD[e],
Sarah Rice, PhD, DPT[f], Christopher Gilbert, AM[g],
Saurabha Bhatnagar, MD[a,b,h], C. Greg Robidoux, PT[c],
Mary Alexis Iaccarino, MD[a,b,i]

KEYWORDS

- Bicycle • Trauma • Injury • Psychological • Concussion

KEY POINTS

- Cycling injuries are complex, sharing characteristics with both sports injuries and traffic collisions, both of which have been associated with post-traumatic symptoms.
- Psychological factors impact injury occurrence, rehabilitation, and return to play, and should be identified and addressed by sports medicine clinicians.
- In this survey, fear and anxiety after cycling crashes were reported commonly, but treated infrequently.
- Factors influencing the development of fear or anxiety after a crash include gender, a history of depression, and the severity of the crash.
- Symptoms of head injury overlap with the psychological effects of trauma and careful assessment for head injury must be done to ensure appropriate treatment.

[a] Department of Physical Medicine and Rehabilitation, Harvard Medical School, Boston, MA, USA; [b] Spaulding Rehabilitation Hospital, Boston, MA, USA; [c] Spaulding Outpatient Center-Wellesley, Wellesley, MA, USA; [d] Newton-Wellesley Hospital, Newton, MA, USA; [e] Division of Physical Medicine and Rehabilitation, University of Utah, 590 Wakara Way, Salt Lake City, UT 84108, USA; [f] Athletico Physical Therapy, Chicago, IL, USA; [g] Harvard University Extension, 51 Brattle Street, Cambridge, MA 02138, USA; [h] US Department of Veterans Affairs, 1722 I St NW, Washington, DC, USA; [i] Massachusetts General Hospital, Boston, MA, USA
* Corresponding author. Spaulding Outpatient Center – Wellesley, 65 Walnut Street, Suite 250, Wellesley, MA 02481.
E-mail address: dkotler@mgh.harvard.edu
Twitter: @DanaKotlerMD (D.H.K.); @thecyclingpt (C.G.R.); @iaccarinomd (M.A.I.)

Phys Med Rehabil Clin N Am 33 (2022) 107–122
https://doi.org/10.1016/j.pmr.2021.08.008

INTRODUCTION

Bicycling is sustainable throughout a lifetime thanks to its tremendous versatility, including its adaptability to the needs of individuals with medical and musculoskeletal conditions.[1] Cycling has also become increasingly popular for transportation and fitness. The number of bicycle commuters has increased by 51% in the United States over the past decade to 877,995.[2,3] Simultaneously, cycling events, including triathlons, *gran fondos*, and charity rides are increasing in popularity, often with thousands of cyclists at a time participating in these events.[4] This increasing number of cyclists carries with it a potential increase in bicycle crashes and resulting injuries. Bicycle crashes can be caused by any combination of poor infrastructure or road conditions, mechanical failure, and a lack of bike-handling skill. Because serious crashes can occur when cyclists are forced to share roadways with fast-moving traffic, strategies to improve cycling infrastructure have decreased cycling crashes and injuries.[5] Crashes are also common in competitive cycling, where riders travel at high speeds in close proximity to one another; incidental contact between riders can lead to a larger crash involving multiple riders.

When evaluating the injured cyclist, clinicians must also consider the psychological repercussions of a crash. Emotional injury may be related to the psychological distress of the crash itself or as a response to a physical injury that occurred during the crash. Having both physical injuries and emotional distress after a crash may impact injury recovery and return to sport. Research has already demonstrated this link in athletes with anterior cruciate ligament rupture,[6] specifically that athletes with depression and anterior cruciate ligament rupture have been shown to have poorer functional outcomes after surgery than those without depression.[7] Moreover, the psychological ramifications of injury, including a lack of confidence and fear of reinjury, can have a profound impact on return to sport.[8] The purpose of this study was to (1) characterize bicycle crashes and cyclist injuries in recreational and competitive cyclists, (2) examine self-reported fear and anxiety after cycling crashes, and (3) evaluate cyclist-related and crash-related factors most commonly associated with emotional symptoms. We hypothesized that fear or anxiety would be a commonly reported symptom, and associated with markers of severe crashes and concussive symptoms.

METHODS

We performed a public, online cross-sectional survey of cyclists aged 18 and older, entitled Injury Issues in the Cycling Community using REDCap software,[9] institutional review board exemption. This study was hosted by Mass General Brigham, formerly Partners Healthcare (IRB project #2014P002211). The survey was distributed to the cycling community throughout the United States via email, social media, and a cycling health-related website, administered from January 24, 2015, through May 3, 2016. An estimated response rate cannot be calculated because it is unknown how many potential participants viewed the link.

To evaluate postcrash fear or anxiety, a relevant subset of the survey database was analyzed, as outlined in Appendix 1. We examined data from individuals who reported a cycling crash within the past 2 years for relevant factors within their medical history, as well as other variables associated with fear or anxiety when returning to cycling. For respondents reporting postcrash fear or anxiety that affected their return to cycling, we assessed whether they received treatment for these symptoms, as well as the time to return to their previous level of cycling. If they had sustained more than 1 crash in the last 2 years, participants were asked to report only their most serious crash.

We used the χ^2 test to compare categorical demographic variables. A logistic regression analysis was used to identify variables associated with anxiety after a crash. Predictor variables included age, gender, years of riding, estimated warm-weather mileage, estimated cold weather mileage, competing in bicycle racing, and history of anxiety, concussion, and depression. A second analysis examined crash-related factors, namely, involvement of a motor vehicle, head injury, absence of injury, immediate confusion, dizziness, or amnesia, more than cosmetic damage to the bicycle, more than cosmetic damage to the helmet, requiring medical care after the crash, and length of time to return to previous level of cycling. A subset of concussive symptoms from the 22-item symptom checklist of the SCAT3[10] was initially included in the logistic regression analysis but these symptoms showed collinearity with other non–concussion-related variables. Therefore, a third analysis was performed on selected concussion symptoms, namely, headache, head pressure, neck pain, nausea/vomiting, dizziness, blurred vision, balance problems, photophobia, phonophobia, feeling slowed down, and feeling "in a fog." P values were considered a priori to be significant at a P value of .05 or less.

RESULTS

A total of 781 participants from 32 states in the United States (with 4 participants outside of the United States) completed the survey; the states with the most responses were Massachusetts, Connecticut, Illinois, New York, California, Pennsylvania, and New Hampshire. There were 404 respondents (mean age 41 ± 14 years) who had sustained a crash within the last 2 years. Demographic information is reported in **Table 1**; those who sustained a crash seem to ride more mileage and are more likely to participate in racing compared with those who have not sustained a crash. Although more than one-half of the respondents competed in competitive racing in both the full study population and the crash subset, there was a significantly higher proportion of racers in the crash subset than those who had not crashed.

Table 2 lists factors relating to the crashes. Most crashes occurred on training rides. Although there were multiple causes for crashes, collision with a motor vehicle was the most common primary etiology of the crash (22.0%). Other causes of crashes occurring at similar frequency were collision with another cyclist, change in road surface, unforeseen obstacles such as potholes, or rider error. Of the crashes reported, 23.8% involved a motor vehicle (although collision with a motor vehicle may not have been the primary cause of the crash). The upper body was the most commonly injured region. Although the head was involved in only 19.6% of the injuries, helmets sustained major damage in 30.5% of crashes. Most participants returned to their previous level of cycling within 1 week or less. **Fig. 1** outlines the time-frame of return.

Of the 404 cyclists who had a crash in the last 2 years, approximately 1 in 4 riders (107%, 26.5%) reported the presence of fear or anxiety after the crash. Logistic regression revealed the following cyclist-associated factors with postcrash anxiety: female gender (odds ratio [OR], 1.78; 95% confidence interval [CI], 1.07–2.96; $P = .026$) and a history of depression (OR, 2.34; 95% CI, 1.11–4.93; $P = .025$). The crash-related factors associated with postcrash fear or anxiety were major damage to bike (OR, 2.12; 95% CI, 1.22–3.67; $P = .007$) and requiring medical treatment (OR, 2.04; 95% CI, 1.16–3.59; $P = .014$). Of the SCAT3 symptom checklist, the only concussive symptom associated with postcrash fear or anxiety was headache (OR, 2.07; 95% CI, 1.05–4.10; $P = .036$).

Only a small fraction of the 107 riders who expressed fear or anxiety; 13 individuals (12.1%) reported receiving formal treatment for these symptoms (5.6% of the 107

Table 1
Demographic information of cyclists included in study

		All Participants (n = 781)		Cyclists Who Crashed (n = 404)		
		No.	%	No.	%	P Value
Female		250	32.0%	122	30.2%	.524
Regular use of helmet		766	98.1%	400	99.0%	.227
Compete in racing		397	50.8%	266	65.8%	<.001
Majority of riding is solo		504	64.5%	252	62.4%	.464
Cycling experience	<1 y	5	0.6%	4	1.0%	.850
	1–5 y	147	18.8%	76	18.8%	
	5–10 y	179	22.9%	104	25.7%	
	10–20 y	178	22.8%	94	23.3%	
	More than 20 y	272	34.8%	126	31.2%	
Warm-weather riding (April–September)	0–50 mi/wk	96	12.3%	29	7.2%	.002
	51–100 mi/wk	233	29.8%	102	25.3%	
	101–150 mi/wk	252	32.3%	137	33.9%	
	Over 150 mi/wk	200	25.6%	136	33.7%	
Cold weather riding (October–March)	0–50 mi/wk	390	49.9%	159	39.4%	.002
	51–100 mi/wk	249	31.9%	141	34.9%	
	101–150 mi/wk	94	12.0%	65	16.1%	
	Over 150 mi/wk	48	6.2%	39	9.7%	

P values refer to intergroup differences between cyclists who did not crash (not listed) and cyclists who crashed.

riders seeking therapy, and 2.8% of the 107 riders seeking physician evaluation). Most of the cyclists addressed their symptoms by reaching out to friends, teammates, or colleagues (47.7% of 107 riders).

DISCUSSION

The results of this survey-based study of bicycle crashes found that bicycle crashes occur frequently and are more common for competitive cyclists during training rides and in high mileage riders. Motor vehicles were the most frequent cause of bicycle crashes either through direct impact with the bicycle or indirectly causing the cyclist to crash. Physical injuries were most likely to occur in the upper extremity and helmet damage was also common. Psychological symptoms of fear and anxiety were more common in women, cyclists with premorbid depression, and when there was damage to the bicycle or physical injury requiring medical treatment. With the exception of headache, there were no specific concussive symptoms associated with lingering fear or anxiety.

Our findings that bicycle crashes occurred frequently within our sample, and that they often involved motor vehicles, may be in part related to the increased popularity of cycling and the shortcomings of current cycling infrastructure. Research has demonstrated that cycling confers substantial health benefits, including improved fitness and a decrease in all-cause mortality, cardiovascular disease, colon cancer morbidity, and obesity.[11] Active transportation (also including walking and public transportation) further correlates with decreased rates of obesity,[12] increased physical

Table 2
Factors associated with crashes reported in the survey. (n = 404 cyclists who had sustained a crash)

		No.	%
Timing of crash	Race	118	29.2
	Training ride	181	44.8
	Commute/city ride	105	26.0
Cause	Collision with motor vehicle	89	22.0
	Collision with another rider	78	19.3
	Collision with pedestrian, stroller, or jogger.	5	1.2
	Mechanical failure (ie, flat tire, dropped chain)	13	3.2
	Unforeseen obstacle (ie, pothole, dog)	61	15.1
	Change in road surface (ie, gravel, sand, dirt)	84	20.8
	Multitasking (ie, drinking water, checking watch, computer)	4	1.0
	Rider error	69	17.1
Involved motor vehicle (not necessarily collision with motor vehicle)	No	308	76.2
	Yes	96	23.8
Involved area(s)	Upper body	205	50.7
	Lower body	139	34.4
	Skin	125	30.9
	Head	79	19.6
	Spine	17	4.2
	No significant injury	66	16.3
	Other	12	3.0
Additional factor	Immediate concussive symptoms after the crash	86	21.3
	[a]Major, noncosmetic bike damage	118	29.2
	Major, non-cosmetic helmet damage	123	30.5
	[a]Received medical care after crash	205	50.7
	Since crash, returned to previous level of cycling	377	93.3
	Fear or anxiety after crash impacting return to cycling	107	26.5

[a] Association with postcrash fear or anxiety.

activity, and a concomitant net decrease in mortality.[13] Even when weighed against the mortality effect of air pollution and traffic accidents, active transportation nonetheless confers a net gain in longevity of 3 to 14 months. Furthermore, a study conducted in Copenhagen, Denmark, determined that car transport carries society-wide costs more than 6 times those of cycling (through accidents, climate change, health impacts, and travel time).[14] A modal shift, including decreasing the number of short automobile trips, can be practically implemented through policies and programs improving safety and accessibility of active transport.[15] As cities plan their transit infrastructure, the individual health benefits of cycling often dovetail with both public health and transportation goals.

Other crash-related factors evaluated in our study include weekly mileage, participation in competitive cycling, and body region injured. Although our sample did contain a large proportion of competitive cyclists, most reported crashes occurred outside of competition. This raises concerns about risk awareness for cyclists and highlights the importance of maintaining alertness during what might be an otherwise routine activity. The participants in our sample were also more likely to ride greater weekly mileage than those who did not crash; this finding could merely be a function of increased exposure, because those training for competition may ride longer

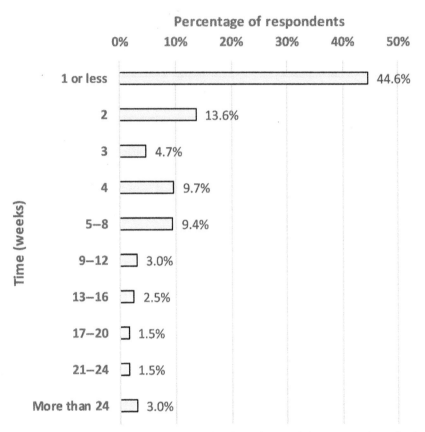

Fig. 1. Timeline of return to previous level of cycling after crash (n = 404 cyclists who had sustained a crash). A total of 27 riders (6.7%) were unable to return to their previous level of cycling.

distances and ride more frequently, which is challenging to fully quantify. In addition, cycling injuries are particularly complex; for example, cycling crashes can share characteristics with sports injuries, traffic collisions, and may include head trauma. In contrast with the overuse injuries of cyclists, which tend to affect the lower body, bicycle crashes tend to affect the upper extremity and the head,[16–19] which is consistent with our findings.

Fear and anxiety were commonly reported among cyclists that had crashes (approximately one-quarter of cyclists who had crashed), but few cyclists received treatment for these symptoms. Psychological factors impact injury occurrence, rehabilitation, and return to play, and therefore must be identified and addressed by sports medicine clinicians.[20] Research has documented post-traumatic symptoms, such as fear and anxiety, in both athletes after injury[21] and individuals sustaining injuries from traffic accidents,[22] and has also described stages of psychological recovery.[23] Although advances in sports medicine may allow athletes to return to play more quickly, psychological recovery may lag behind physical recovery after an injury from a cycling crash. Problematic responses to injury can carry an emotional cost, impact rehabilitation, long-term functioning,[20] and mortality. Moreover, severe athletic injuries and the associated depression have been linked to suicide attempts in young athletes.[24]

Using major damage to the bike and physical injuries requiring medical treatment as proxies for crash severity, we observed that a more severe crash was significantly associated with development of subsequent fear or anxiety. Injury severity has been shown to be a predictor of post-traumatic stress symptoms after traffic accidents.[22] With regard to the psychological toll of cycling crashes specifically, Craig and colleagues[25] documented higher scores on measures of psychological and trauma-related distress in cyclists after a crash, which improved over time. Greater perceived danger of death, including collisions with motor vehicles, has been associated with the development of post-traumatic stress disorder (PTSD), which can manifest in part as increased anxiety.[25] For cyclists and other less protected occupants of the road, the involvement of a motor vehicle may increase the perceived danger of a crash (by adding more than a ton of mass to the equation), even if it does not cause greater physical injury, or even if it does not result in a collision directly with the motor vehicle. Interestingly, in comparison to car occupants, cyclists display better psychological health in spite of similarly severe injuries, including lower rates of distress, pain catastrophizing, and PTSD, possibly an effect of the benefits of physical activity on psychological health.[25]

Female gender was significantly associated with the self-reported presence of fear or anxiety after a cycling crash. Our findings are consistent with what is known about symptom reporting in female athletes, and differences in self-reported behaviors of anxiety and fear between genders.[26] In a prospective study of transport and recreational cyclists in Australia, which accounted for exposure, female cyclists had higher rates of crashes and crash-related injuries requiring medical attention.[27] Similarly, female gender has been described as a predictive factor for persistent PTSD 6 months after road traffic accidents, though this was not limited to bicycles.[22] However, because more men cycle than women,[3,28] and men are typically less likely to seek medical care,[29] there is limited exposure-based research on the gender differences in cycling crashes and injuries.

Cyclists reporting a history of depression were more likely to develop fear or anxiety after a crash. Prior study in this area is outlined in the 2010 consensus statement by Wiese-Bjornstal[30] indicating that premorbid negative mood has a substantial impact on injury occurrence in high-intensity athletes, and that psychological interventions benefit athlete recovery and rehabilitation. Depressed mood also affects rehabilitation; patients with major depressive disorder undergoing anterior cruciate ligament reconstruction reported lower functional scores at baseline and 1 year after surgery.[7] In the management of the injured cyclist, including those with chronic pain or functional limitation, this finding speaks to the importance of the biopsychosocial model including management of the underlying disorder as well as its manifestations. Social support, such as from friends, family, and athletic staff, is recognized as an effective psychological intervention for injured athletes, improving coping, motivation, and focus during rehabilitation, as well as reducing depression or anxiety upon return to play.[31] In our sample, many of the cyclists reporting fear or anxiety addressed it through reaching out to friends, teammates or colleagues.

Although concussion symptoms are frequently seen after cycling crashes,[32,33] and head injuries may result in physical, cognitive, emotional, and sleep-related symptoms, our data did not show an association between reported head injury or immediate neurologic symptoms and the development of fear or anxiety after a crash. Additionally, of the SCAT3 symptom checklist, the only symptom associated with the presence of fear or anxiety in our study was headache. Other studies have shown head or neck injury to be an important predictor of trauma-related, as well as general psychological distress.[25] Research has also demonstrated that concussed athletes report greater incidences of PTSD symptoms than healthy controls.[21] Our finding that self-reported head injury or immediate neurologic symptoms after the crash were not associated with the development of fear or anxiety may reflect underreporting of head injury, or the unique and complex nature of cycling injuries. It is well known that head injuries tend to be underreported, as can be gleaned from the discrepancy in numbers between participants who reported a head injury (19.6%) and those who reported major damage to the helmet (30.5%). Despite the lack of correlation between fear or anxiety and reported head injury, predictors of postcrash fear or anxiety in our study overlap with predictors of protracted recovery in athletes with concussion, including female sex, depression, anxiety, and history of psychiatric illness.[34,35] In addition, non-head-injured cyclists also endorse emotional and sleep-related symptoms,[32] further highlighting the overlap of symptoms of head injury with psychological effects of trauma.[36]

Several limitations exist for this study. The data were collected using a voluntary online survey of past bicycle crashes, and thus may be prone to errors owing to symptom over-reporting,[37] recall bias, and self-selection bias. Fear and anxiety are defined by self-report as part of a larger symptom questionnaire. Our survey participant demographics are not perfectly representative of cyclists within the United States, potentially limiting its generalizability. Notably, a large percentage (more than one-half) of our participants participated in racing. Our study contained more males than females, which parallels cycling demographics (as of 2016 females composed 28% of bicycle commuters,[3] and 15% of racing license holders[38]); however, this ratio is not ideal for comparing between genders. Finally, more severe injuries may not have been included within our sample, because these athletes may have been less likely to respond to the survey owing to injury or disability. Future research should use specific psychological self-report scales to better characterize psychological distress caused by bicycle crashes.

CLINICS CARE POINTS

- Cycling crashes are common, frequently involving a motor vehicle and resulting in upper extremity and head injury.
- Cycling injuries are complex, sharing characteristics with both sports injuries and traffic collisions, both of which have been associated with post-traumatic symptoms.
- Fear and anxiety after cycling crashes are commonly reported, but infrequently treated.
- Symptoms of head injury overlap with the psychological effects of trauma and careful assessment for head injury must be done to ensure appropriate treatment.
- Female cyclists, those with a history of depression, and those involved in more severe crashes are more likely to develop fear or anxiety after a crash.
- Social support can be an effective intervention for injured athletes, with an impact on depression and anxiety.
- Providers caring for cyclists should identify and address psychological factors after crashes, as they can impact injury occurrence, rehabilitation, and return to sport.

SUMMARY

Our survey data demonstrate that the development of fear or anxiety after a cycling crash is not uncommon. Cyclists in our survey reported that fear and anxiety have been infrequently addressed after cycling crashes, reflecting a lack of appropriate treatment which could impede return to sport. Factors associated with development of fear or anxiety after a crash include female gender, a history of depression, and greater crash severity. In guiding return to sport, it is important to understand the progression of psychological recovery.[23] Fear and lack of confidence have been identified as prominent emotional responses, which can negatively impact rehabilitation and return to sport,[8,39–41] although positive psychological responses (motivation, confidence, and low fear) have been associated with a higher rate of return to sport, faster return to sport, and greater likelihood of returning to the preinjury level of participation.[41,42] Coaches, trainers, teammates, and the cycling community should be included as part of a comprehensive team to encourage conversation about fear or anxiety after a crash, because the mental health of cyclists is equally important to their physical health for optimal performance and quality of life.

ACKNOWLEDGMENTS

The authors thank Dr Ross Zafonte, Dr Mark Greve, the Medicine of Cycling organization, and Dr Marilou Shaughnessy for their assistance and support with this article.

DISCLOSURE

All authors have no commercial or financial conflicts of interest for this article. No funding sources were used for this article.

REFERENCES

1. Kotler DH, Babu AN, Robidoux G. Prevention, evaluation, and rehabilitation of cycling-related injury. Curr Sports Med Rep 2016;15(3):199–206.
2. League of American Bicyclists. Where we ride: analysis of bicycling in American cities, annual American community survey data report for 2016. Washington, DC: League of American Bicyclists; 2016.
3. United States Census Bureau. Table B08006 – Sex of Workers By Means of Transportation To Work. In. American Community Survey. American FactFinder2016.
4. Pan-Mass Challenge Fact Sheet. pmc.org2019.
5. Reynolds CC, Harris MA, Teschke K, et al. The impact of transportation infrastructure on bicycling injuries and crashes: a review of the literature. Environ Health 2009;8:47.
6. Padaki AS, Noticewala MS, Levine WN, et al. Prevalence of Posttraumatic Stress Disorder Symptoms Among Young Athletes After Anterior Cruciate Ligament Rupture. Orthop J Sports Med 2018;6(7). 2325967118787159.
7. Garcia GH, Wu H-H, Park MJ, et al. Depression symptomatology and anterior cruciate ligament injury: incidence and effect on functional outcome—a prospective cohort study. Am J Sports Med 2016;44(3):572–9.
8. Kvist J, Ek A, Sporrstedt K, et al. Fear of re-injury: a hindrance for returning to sports after anterior cruciate ligament reconstruction. Knee Surg Sports Traumatol Arthrosc 2005;13(5):393–7.
9. Harris PA, Taylor R, Thielke R, et al. Research electronic data capture (REDCap)—a metadata-driven methodology and workflow process for providing translational research informatics support. J Biomed Inform 2009;42(2):377–81.
10. Guskiewicz KM, Register-Mihalik J, McCrory P, et al. Evidence-based approach to revising the SCAT2: introducing the SCAT3. Br J Sports Med 2013;47(5):289–93.

11. Oja P, Titze S, Bauman A, et al. Health benefits of cycling: a systematic review. Scand J Med Sci Sports 2011;21(4):496–509.
12. Bassett DR, Pucher J Jr, Buehler R, et al. Walking, cycling, and obesity rates in Europe, North America, and Australia. J Phys Activity Health 2008;5(6):795–814.
13. Johan de Hartog J, Boogaard H, Nijland H, et al. Do the health benefits of cycling outweigh the risks? Environ Health Perspect 2010;118(8):1109–16.
14. Gössling S, Choi AS. Transport transitions in Copenhagen: comparing the cost of cars and bicycles. Ecol Econ 2015;113:106–13.
15. Maibach E, Steg L, Anable J. Promoting physical activity and reducing climate change: opportunities to replace short car trips with active transportation. Prev Med 2009;49(4):326–7.
16. De Bernardo N, Barrios C, Vera P, et al. Incidence and risk for traumatic and over-use injuries in top-level road cyclists. J Sports Sci 2012;30(10):1047–53.
17. Palmer-Green D, Burt P, Jaques R, et al. Epidemiological study of injury in British cycling: 2011-2013 (Abstract from IOC World Conference on Prevention of Injury & Illness in Sport, Monaco 2014). Br J Sports Med 2014;48(7):650.
18. Perrin AE. Cycling-related injury. Conn Med 2012;76(8):461–6.
19. Rivara FP, Thompson DC, Thompson RS. Epidemiology of bicycle injuries and risk factors for serious injury. Inj Prev 2015;21(1):47–51.
20. Psychological issues related to injury in athletes and the team physician: a consensus statement. Med Sci Sports Exerc 2006;38(11):2030–4.
21. Brassil HE, Salvatore AP. The frequency of post-traumatic stress disorder symptoms in athletes with and without sports related concussion. Clin Transl Med 2018;7(1):25.
22. Chossegros L, Hours M, Charnay P, et al. Predictive factors of chronic post-traumatic stress disorder 6 months after a road traffic accident. Accid Anal Prev 2011;43(1):471–7.
23. Clement D, Arvinen-Barrow M, Fetty T. Psychosocial responses during different phases of sport-injury rehabilitation: a qualitative study. J Athl Train 2015;50(1):95–104.
24. Smith AM, Milliner EK. Injured athletes and the risk of suicide. J Athl Train 1994;29(4):337.
25. Craig A, Elbers N, Jagnoor J, et al. The psychological impact of traffic injuries sustained in a road crash by bicyclists: a prospective study. Traffic Inj Prev 2017;18(3):273–80.
26. Stoyanova M, Hope DA. Gender, gender roles, and anxiety: perceived confirmability of self report, behavioral avoidance, and physiological reactivity. J Anxiety Disord 2012;26(1):206–14.
27. Poulos R, Hatfield J, Rissel C, et al. An exposure based study of crash and injury rates in a cohort of transport and recreational cyclists in New South Wales, Australia. Accid Anal Prev 2015;78:29–38.
28. USA Cycling Active Member Demographics. 2019. Available at: https://legacy.usacycling.org/corp/demographics.php. Accessed January 27, 2019.
29. Galdas PM, Cheater F, Marshall P. Men and health help-seeking behaviour: literature review. J Adv Nurs 2005;49(6):616–23.
30. Wiese-Bjornstal DM. Psychology and socioculture affect injury risk, response, and recovery in high-intensity athletes: a consensus statement. Scand J Med Sci Sports 2010;20:103–11.
31. Yang J, Schaefer JT, Zhang N, et al. Social support from the athletic trainer and symptoms of depression and anxiety at return to play. J Athl Train 2014;49(6):773–9.

32. Rice SE, Iaccarino MA, Bhatnagar S, et al. Reporting of concussion-like symptoms following cycling crashes: a survey of competitive and recreational cyclists. J Athl Train 2020;55(1):11–6.

33. Coronado VG, Haileyesus T, Cheng TA, et al. Trends in sports-and recreation-related traumatic brain injuries treated in US emergency departments: the National Electronic Injury Surveillance System-All Injury Program (NEISS-AIP) 2001-2012. J head Trauma Rehabil 2015;30(3):185–97.

34. Morgan CD, Zuckerman SL, Lee YM, et al. Predictors of postconcussion syndrome after sports-related concussion in young athletes: a matched case-control study. J Neurosurg Pediatr 2015;15(6):589–98.

35. Iverson GL, Gardner AJ, Terry DP, et al. Predictors of clinical recovery from concussion: a systematic review. Br J Sports Med 2017;51(12):941–8.

36. Covassin T, Crutcher B, Bleecker A, et al. Postinjury anxiety and social support among collegiate athletes: a comparison between orthopaedic injuries and concussions. J Athl Train 2014;49(4):462–8.

37. Iverson GL, Brooks BL, Ashton VL, et al. Interview versus questionnaire symptom reporting in people with the postconcussion syndrome. J head Trauma Rehabil 2010;25(1):23–30.

38. USA Cycling. Active Member Demographics. In. Vol 2018. usacycling.org2017:-Membership infographics.

39. Hsu C-J, Meierbachtol A, George SZ, et al. Fear of reinjury in athletes: implications for rehabilitation. Sports health 2017;9(2):162–7.

40. Ardern CL, Taylor NF, Feller JA, et al. A systematic review of the psychological factors associated with returning to sport following injury. Br J Sports Med 2013;47(17):1120–6.

41. Czuppon S, Racette BA, Klein SE, et al. Variables associated with return to sport following anterior cruciate ligament reconstruction: a systematic review. Br J Sports Med 2014;48(5):356–64.

42. Sonesson S, Kvist J, Ardern C, et al. Psychological factors are important to return to pre-injury sport activity after anterior cruciate ligament reconstruction: expect and motivate to satisfy. Knee Surg Sports Traumatol Arthrosc 2017;25(5):1375–84.

APPENDIX 1: SELECTED SURVEY QUESTIONS.

1. What is your age?
   a. 18 to 100 or older
2. What is your gender?
   a. Male
   b. Female
   c. Transgender male
   d. Transgender female
   e. Genderqueer/nonbinary
3. In which state do you currently reside? Non-US residents (including Puerto Rico and other US territories), select "International."
   a. List of 50 US states and "International"
4. Do you have a history of any of the following medical conditions? Please check all that apply to you.
   a. Anxiety
   b. Asthma
   c. Cancer

   d. Cardiac arrhythmias
   e. Carpal tunnel syndrome
   f. Concussion
   g. Coronary artery disease/atherosclerosis
   h. Depression

   i. Erectile dysfunction

   j. Hypertension
   k. Inflammatory arthritis (rheumatoid, gout)
   l. Low back pain

   m. Major limb amputations

   n. Neck pain
   o. Osteoarthritis

   p. Other psychiatric disorders (bipolar disorder, schizophrenia, etc.)

   q. Pelvic pain

   r. Sleep disorder/Insomnia

   s. Stress fractures

   t. Thyroid disorder

   u. None
5. In which types of cycling do you routinely participate?
   a. Road
   b. Cyclocross
   c. Mountain
   d. BMX
   e. Triathlon
   f. Commuting
   g. Touring
   h. Leisure, recreation, I ride to get ice cream
6. For how many years have you been riding a bicycle on a regular basis?
   a. Less than 1 year
   b. 1 to 5 years
   c. 5 to 10 years
   d. 10 to 20 years
   e. More than 20 years
7. Please estimate your total cycling mileage per week in the warm-weather months
   (approximately April to September).
   a. Less than 25 miles/wk
   b. 25 to 50 miles/wk
   c. 51 to 75 miles/wk
   d. 76 to 100 miles/wk
   e. 101 to 125 miles/wk
   f. 126 to 150 miles/wk

g. More than 150 miles/wk
8. Please estimate your total cycling mileage per week in the cold weather months (approximately October to March). Include indoor cycling miles in the total.
   a. Less than 25 miles/wk
   b. 25 to 50 miles/wk
   c. 51 to 75 miles/wk
   d. 76 to 100 miles/wk
   e. 101 to 125 miles/wk
   f. 126 to 150 miles/wk
   g. greater than 150 miles/wk
9. Do you tend to ride alone or with others?
   a. Alone
   b. With 1 other person
   c. With a group
10. On the majority of your rides, do you tend to wear an approved cycling helmet?
    a. Yes
    b. No
11. Have you been in a cycling crash in the past 2 years? If you have had more than 1 crash, please pick the crash you would rate as the most serious one.
    a. Yes
    b. No
12. What were the circumstances of your crash?
    a. Race
    b. Training ride
    c. Commute/city ride
13. Which best describes the cause of your crash?
    a. Collision with motor vehicle
    b. Collision with another rider
    c. Collision with pedestrian, stroller, or jogger. Mechanical failure (ie, flat tire, dropped chain) Unforeseen obstacle (ie, pothole, dog)
    d. Change in road surface (ie, gravel, sand, dirt) Multitasking (ie, drinking water, checking watch, computer)
    e. Rider error
14. Was there a motor vehicle involved?
    a. Yes
    b. No
15. Please check the following boxes as applicable to describe the areas of injury directly resulting from your crash.
    a. Upper body (shoulder, collar bone, hand, wrist elbow, etc.)
    b. Lower body (hip, knee, leg, ankle, foot)
    c. Skin only
    d. Head
    e. Spine
    f. No significant injury
    g. Other (please specify)
16. Was there a period of time IMMEDIATELY AFTER your crash where you were confused, dazed or off-balance, or a period of time that you are unable to remember?
    a. Yes
    b. No
17. Please check all of the following that you experienced after your crash.

a. Headache
b. "Pressure in head"
c. Neck pain
d. Nausea or vomiting
e. Dizziness
f. Blurred vision
g. Balance problems
h. Sensitivity to light
i. Sensitivity to noise
j. Feeling slowed down
k. Feeling like "in a fog"
l. "Don't feel right"
m. Difficulty concentrating
n. Difficulty remembering
o. Fatigue or low energy
p. Confusion
q. Drowsiness
r. Trouble falling asleep
s. More emotional
t. Irritability
u. Sadness
v. Nervous or anxious
w. Seizure
x. Loss of consciousness (told to you by another person)
y. Loss of memory at the time of the crash
z. I did not experience any of these

18. Was there major (noncosmetic) damage to your bicycle resulting from this crash?
    a. Yes
    b. No
19. Was there major (noncosmetic) damage to your helmet resulting from this crash?
    a. Yes
    b. No
    c. I was not wearing a helmet
20. Did you receive any medical care after your crash?
    a. Yes
    b. No
21. Please select the medical care you received after the crash.
    a. Emergency medical services on site
    b. Emergency department visit at the time of the crash emergency department visit, delayed after the crash, primary care doctor visit (nonemergent)
    c. Specialist visit
    d. Other (please specify)
22. What type of specialist did you seek treatment from after your crash? (Check all that apply.)
    a. Orthopedic surgeon
    b. Neurologist
    c. Osteopath
    d. Sports medicine physician (nonsurgical)
    e. Physiatrist (physical medicine and rehabilitation specialist)
    f. Other (specify)
23. If you received medical care after the crash, check any treatment you received.

    a. Physical examination

    b. Imaging (radiograph, MRI, CT scan, ultrasound examination)

    c. Medications

    d. Wound care

    e. Referral to specialist

    f. Surgery

    g. Physical therapy

    h. Occupational therapy

    i. Psychology/therapy/counseling

    j. Other (please specify)

    k. No treatment received

24. Since your crash, have you been able to return to cycling at your previous level?

    a. Yes

    b. No

25. After your crash, how long, in weeks, did it take you to return to cycling at your previous level?

    a. Less than 1

    b. 2

    c. 3

    d. 4 (1 month)

    e. 5

    f. 6

    g. 7

    h. 8 (2 months)

    i. 9

    j. 10

    k. 11

    l. 12 (3 months)

    m. 13

    n. 14

    o. 15

    p. 16 (4 months)

    q. 17

    r. 18

    s. 19

    t. 20 (5 months)

    u. 21

    v. 22

    w. 23

    x. 24 (6 months)

    y. More than 24 weeks (6 months)

26. Were you satisfied with the medical care you received after your crash?

    a. Yes

    b. No

27. Please elaborate on why you were satisfied with the medical care you received after your crash.

28. Please elaborate on why you were NOT satisfied with the medical care you received after your crash.

29. Since your crash, have you experienced any fear or anxiety that has affected your ability to return to cycling at your previous level?

    a. Yes

    b. No

30. Have you pursued any treatment for the fear or anxiety related to your crash?
    a. Yes
    b. No

31. If you have experienced anxiety related to your crash, please check any of the following that you have pursued.
    a. Speaking with physician
    b. Therapy or counseling
    c. Speaking with friends, colleagues, or teammates
    d. Medications
    e. Other (specify)
    f. None

Infrastructure and Injury Prevention in Cycling

Kevin Rix, PhD, MPH[a,b,*], Isabell Sakamoto, MS, CHES[c]

KEYWORDS

- Injury prevention • Trauma • Pediatric injury • Adult injury • Cycling

KEY POINTS

- Cycling injuries can be reduced by both behaviors of the individual and environmental changes.
- Injury prevention strategies to reduce cycling-related injuries have historically relied solely on the individual to undertake personal safety behaviors to keep them safe while riding.
- Although important, these strategies are not sufficient to keep a bicycle rider safe while riding.
- In addition, understanding the role the environment has on cycling injuries and strategies that can be implemented to keep riders safe outside of individual behaviors is critical moving forward to give riders the most protection.

INTRODUCTION

In the United States, cycling is not only a popular form of leisure and physical activity but also a rapidly growing form of transportation especially in urban communities.[1–6] In 2016, approximately 12.4% of Americans cycled on a regular basis, and as of 2017, the number of cyclists had grown to approximately 47.5 million riders.[7] A June 2020 report by the *Union Cycliste Internationale*, the world governing body of cycling, reported that, during the global COVID-19 pandemic in 2020, cycling in some areas of the United States increased by 253%.[8,9]

The rapid increase in bicycle usage creates a double-edged sword for clinicians and public health professionals. The growth of cycling represents a net positive for increased physical activity rates but innately creates the opportunity for larger numbers of cycling-related injuries, especially for those riders using bicycles in geographic locations without proper infrastructure to protect a rider from injury. The

[a] Penn Injury Science Center, University of Pennsylvania, 423 Guardian Dr. Blockley Hall, Rm. 937 Philadelphia, PA 19146, USA; [b] Trauma Services, Dell Seton Medical Center at the University of Texas, 1500 Red River Street, Austin, TX 78701, USA; [c] Seattle Children's Hospital, Community Health & Benefit, Seattle, WA 98105, USA
* Corresponding author.
E-mail address: Kevin.Rix@pennmedicine.upenn.edu
Twitter: @kcrix (K.R.)

Phys Med Rehabil Clin N Am 33 (2022) 123–134
https://doi.org/10.1016/j.pmr.2021.08.009
1047-9651/22/© 2021 Elsevier Inc. All rights reserved.

National Highway Traffic Safety Administration reported 857 cyclist deaths in 2018, whereas in the same year the Centers for Disease Control and Prevention (CDC) reported that 306,133 individuals were treated in hospital emergency departments for unintentional bicycle injuries.[10,11] The total number of bicycle-related injuries has trended downward over the previous 5 years; however, there is still much work that can be done to reduce these injuries further. Bicycle injuries remain not only a physical burden to those sustaining them but also an additional economic strain, resulting in nearly 10 billion dollars in medical costs and productivity loss per year.[6]

One issue that persists with more cyclists on the road in the United States is that most urban environments were built for the use of motor vehicles as opposed to bicycles or other forms of transportation.[12] Previous work has found that streets with improved bicycle infrastructure, particularly divided bicycle lanes with a physical barrier between cyclists and the motor vehicles, are most effective at reducing cycling injuries.[13] When assessing risk in cycling, it is important to consider the built environment, especially in urban areas, including how the road, lighting, and speed limits impact these risks.[14]

To reduce bicycle injuries, a multifaceted approach should be explored. This begins with examining how current environments are designed, and what modifications should be made as roads and paths are reworked, completed through policy efforts and city/town planning initiatives. These efforts should be done in combination with public health professionals and community safety advocates implementing evidence-informed community-based programming aimed at influencing the individual behaviors of cyclists for safe cycling. In a comprehensive system, local health care systems are engaged in the process from inception until a project's completion. This allows clinicians to have the information not only to treat patients who have sustained a bicycle injury but also to be equipped with the necessary information to provide a level of tertiary prevention, including education and behavioral recommendations to reduce the likelihood of reinjury after treatment. Clinicians can also play a critical role in influencing and informing policymakers by being able to share their experiences in practice and advocating for community level change.

This article focuses on 4 separate aspects of prevention that play a role in reducing injuries among cyclists across adult and pediatric populations. First, this article describes the current burden of cycling-related injuries in both pediatric and adult populations. Second, this article explores the role the built environment has on injury prevalence for cyclists and discusses the need for improved infrastructure. Third, this article discusses some of the individual-level behaviors that protect cyclists but should be used in harmony with environmental change. Finally, this article identifies critical items of importance for clinicians to be aware of when treating patients for bicycle-related injuries and their role in acting in a tertiary role to prevent further injury to cyclists after recovery, as well as the role clinicians can play in advocating for safer roadways for all. A comprehensive system focusing not only on individual cyclist behaviors but also on their environment and the care they may receive should an injury occur, will allow for continued safe expansion in the number of riders on the road.

EPIDEMIOLOGY AND RISK FACTORS FOR CYCLING INJURIES
Pediatric Cycling Injury Epidemiology

In 2019, there were an estimated 117,923 bicycle-related nonfatal emergency department visits for children aged 1 to 18 in the United States with a distinctly high injury rate among children aged 10 to 14.[15] Nationwide, bicycle-related injuries are the most common sport and recreational injury type for children and send more children to emergency departments than any other recreational activity.[16,17] Most bicycle-related injuries in children result from falls or collision with a fixed or moving object, with the most serious injuries and fatalities caused by collisions with motor vehicles.[18] Studies have found that bicycle-related injuries in children may be more common in the summer months, which could be attributed to seasonal increases in bicycling in general and typically occur in streets or at home.[19–21]

In pediatric populations, male riders are more likely to be involved in collisions involving motor vehicles than their female counterparts.[19,21] Among adolescent riders, no helmet use while riding has been identified as a risk factor for severe injuries, such as traumatic brain injuries (TBIs).[19,21–23] As children age, differences in sex-specific rates of bicycle-related head injuries (ie, boys being more commonly injured) may become less pronounced; however, this difference may be attributed to lower bicycle-riding rates as children age in general.[19] In the United States, bicycle-related injuries in children most commonly affect the upper extremities, followed by the lower extremities, face, and head and neck.[20,21] Although the most common types of bicycle injuries in children are bruises, scrapes, and cuts, soft tissue injuries, fractures, abdominal injury, and TBIs are common causes of emergency department visits and hospitalizations.[18,20] TBIs and injuries to the head and neck appear to be common among patients aged 10 to 14 years and non-helmet users.[20] TBIs are particularly concerning considering being a major cause of death and disability and may require special attention upon presentation to a health care treatment facility.

Adult Cycling Injury Epidemiology

The CDC identified 216,120 total emergency department bicycle injuries in 2019 for riders 18 years and older.[15] Among these injuries, individuals aged 50 to 59 years old suffered from the highest death rate associated with bicycles.[15]

As in pediatric populations, adult cyclists are more frequently injured in the summer months and in the afternoon compared with colder months and the early morning.[24] The most common traumatic injuries suffered by adult riders are extremity injuries, and male riders have been found to be more likely to be injured than female riders in adult populations.[25–27] Although motor vehicles are the most common cause of crashes resulting in injury, other obstructions, such as train tracks, surface features (ie, fire hydrants, signs), infrastructure, and pedestrians, have been documented to be injury-causing hazards for adult riders as well.[28,29]

Alcohol has also been shown to play a role in bicycle-related crashes in adult populations.[27,29] Cyclists injured while under the influence are often less experienced, are less likely to wear a helmet while cycling, and more likely to ride at night and on city streets.[27] Cyclists injured after drinking have also be shown to be more likely to suffer moderate and severe injury as documented by hospital injury severity scores.[29]

Beyond traumatic injuries, adult cyclists are also more likely to suffer from overuse injuries than their pediatric counterparts. Most often these overuse injuries present in the lower extremities or the back.[30–32] These injuries are most common in riders 50 years old or older, as well as in competitive and professional adult cyclists who spend an extended amount of time riding.[33] These overuse injuries also regularly present in recreational cyclists with extended exposure to bicycle riding.[34] Although not traumatic in nature, repetitiveness of motion may lead to tendonitis, hip pain, iliotibial band syndrome, stress fractures, and compartment syndrome among other conditions requiring medical intervention, warranting cycling practice conversations with the patient's provider.[35,36]

CYCLING AND THE ENVIRONMENT

Prevention efforts often aim to modify the behavior of the individual. However, growing evidence suggests efforts should also be placed on understanding the environment's impact on both cycling usage and its relationship to injury risk, particularly in urban environments.[13,14,37] Previous work has found that up to 20% of riders who cycle in urban environments will experience a traumatic event while cycling, and these traumatic events were not associated with the riders' personal characteristics, safety practices, or their experience.[38] The presence alone of bicycle-specific infrastructure has been documented to increase the overall usage of bicycles in a community, as well reduce bicycle-specific injuries and crashes.[13] Street design, road hazards, proximity to motor vehicles, and other aspects of infrastructure need to be addressed when considering how to most efficiently prevent injuries to cyclists. In countries such as Sweden and Denmark, cycling infrastructure has been built into many city and town planning initiatives for decades.[39–41] In contrast, in the United States, overall bicycle-specific infrastructure is limited, even in larger metropolitan areas where cycling may be common.[40–42] Dedicated cycling lanes are rare, and when present, they often do not adequately separate cyclists from motor vehicles. Improving this infrastructure could reduce bicycle crashes and injury. In addition, the presence of adequate cycling infrastructure has been shown to increase the usage of bicycles in a community.

Types of Cycling Infrastructure

Depending on the area in which a cyclist is riding, the options for types of riding surface types and infrastructure may be extremely varied. Although not encompassing all road types, common riding environments for cyclists include the following:

- Protected cycle tracks/bicycle lanes: Dedicated on-street separated lanes with a physical barrier between motor vehicle traffic and cyclists, such as concrete barriers, street bollards, or manicured plants and shrubs.
- Unprotected cycle tracks/bicycle lanes: On-street dedicated lanes that designate through painted roadways lanes in which bicycles are to travel within, without physical separation from motor vehicle traffic.
- Shared road: Streets in which no lanes have been dedicated for bicycles or other nonmotorized modes of transportation.
- Sidewalk: Paved or cemented path dedicated for on-foot pedestrian traffic.
- Off-road: Any pathway of natural environment with no paved or cemented surface.

Examples of riding surface types and infrastructure are shown in **Figs. 1** and **2**.

Cycling Infrastructure Impact on Injury

Riding infrastructure identified in this article focuses on environments in which the general populace may be riding a bicycle. Competitive and professional cycling competitions are often completed on closed courses in a variety of terrain and may not be as applicable to the injury risks associated with the public environment.

Slight environmental changes in riding environments may play a larger role in whether a rider is at increased risk of injury while riding. In a case cross-over study conducted by Teschke and colleagues[37] that examined 14 different route types, riders using cycle tracks had approximately one-ninth the risk of injury compared with the reference group of those riding on major streets with parked cars and no bicycle-specific infrastructure. One study that examined bicycle crashes and infrastructure in London from 2012 to 2013 identified that the frequency of bicycle crashes

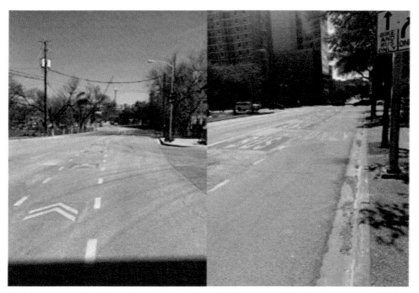

Fig. 1. Unprotected cycle track and shared road. (*Courtesy of* Kevin Rix, Austin, TX.)

correlated with the road density in which cyclists most used.[12] This study also identified that the effects of bicycle-specific infrastructure on crashes varied by season. Overall, bicycle usage increased in warmer months (May through October), with a greater number of crashes (1680 vs 1115) reported compared with colder months, suggesting a potential temporal relationship for cycle infrastructure use and crashes. This study also identified that placement of upgraded bicycle infrastructure, specifically a bicycle-specific highway, had a negative correlation to bicycle crashes in winter months.

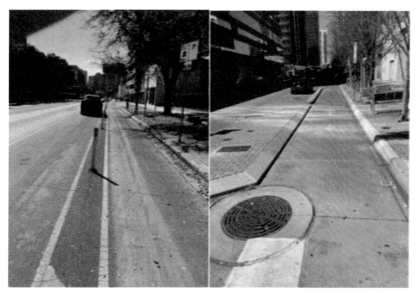

Fig. 2. Protected lanes. (*Courtesy of* Kevin Rix, Austin, TX.)

The presence of bicycle infrastructure may also play a role in reducing the severity of an injury if a crash with a motor vehicle does occur. In New York City from 2008 to 2014, a level 1 trauma center identified that the addition of painted bicycle lanes reduced injury risk nearly 90% (Incidence Density Ratio = 0.09, 95% confidence interval: 0.02–0.33).[43] Cycling infrastructure reduces the incidence of bicycle injuries on the roadway; however, when infrastructure is breached, and injury still occurs, the outcomes are more likely to be severe.[43] This is consistent across the literature, as a review of 23 peer-reviewed papers related to transportation infrastructure and cyclists safety found that in papers that examined infrastructure at intersections, multilane roundabouts posed significantly increased risk of injuries to cyclists when no infrastructure was present compared with roads with any amount of infrastructure present.[14] This study also identifies that cyclists were at highest risk of injury when using mixed-use trails and sidewalks shared by both pedestrians and bicycles and were at lowest risk when using bicycle-specific infrastructure.[14]

The Role of Cycling Infrastructure and Improving Health

People are using bicycles now more than ever; however, there is still much to be learned about the effects of bicycle-specific infrastructure on safety. This is due to a lack of cycling-specific infrastructure in the United States, outside of a few major cities and college environments.[6,44] Pucher and Buehler[44] identified how positive changes in bicycle infrastructure in European countries, including the introduction of "cycle superhighways," made cycling quicker as riders could go at higher speeds and also kept motorized transportation away from the cyclists. These "cycle superhighways" illustrate the point that not all bicycle infrastructure is the same. In a multicity study in the United States, although protected bicycle lanes had varied success in their ability to reduce the risk of injuries to riders, lanes with the most separation from motor vehicle traffic had the largest decrease in injury risk.[45] The further cyclists can be away from all other traffic, both motorized and pedestrian, the safer cyclists can be while riding.

Cycling infrastructure and pathways should be carefully considered before being implemented. Bicycle riders report that access to bicycle-specific infrastructure contributes to whether they ride a bicycle, and to their perceived safety while riding.[42,46–49] In general, areas with bicycle-specific infrastructure that physically separate cyclists from motorized vehicles are preferred by cyclists, as opposed to street designs in which the cyclists are expected to ride without a physical barrier.[46] Cycling infrastructure has also been associated with reducing the disparities in the types of riders who use bicycles for transportation. In Melbourne, Australia, where only approximately 20% of riders are women, women riders preferred to use paths with maximum separation from motorized vehicles.[50] Similarly, for older adults, when routes were perceived to be safer for travel, including the presence of a separated bicycle lane, older adults were more likely to ride a bicycle.[51] Comparatively, male and younger riders are predicted more frequently to perceive urban cycling as a safe activity.[42] Introduction of bicycle-specific infrastructure may narrow these disparities in bicycle usage, while increasing actual safety measures for all. The more that cities and other urban environments can create physical separations from motorized traffic, the more individuals may recognize cycling as a safe modality of transportation.

INDIVIDUAL-LEVEL BEHAVIORAL INJURY PREVENTION

When worn consistently and correctly, helmets can provide some protection against severe brain injury and potential death resulting from a bicycle crash, yet less than half of children regularly wear a bicycle helmet.[52–56] Child helmet ownership and use tend to increase with parental income and education level, but decrease with the child's age.[19,21,57] One recent study found that poor fit and physical discomfort of bicycle helmets are the main barriers to helmet use in children.[58] Proper fit of bicycle helmets can contribute to comfort and thus increase the odds that children will actually wear the helmet.[59] There is evidence that community-based educational programs aimed to promote helmet wearing in children can be effective.[18] Policy changes must also work in conjunction with these helmet-use initiatives. In areas where helmets are not required by law, pediatric patients who have sustained a head injury without wearing a helmet were more likely to also experience a brain injury (28.1%) compared with those wearing a helmet (13.8%).[19]

In adult populations, cycling helmets may have similar benefits to reducing the likelihood of head and brain injury.[59–62] Overall, bicycle helmets reduce brain injury by approximately 48% and serious head injuries by 60% and reduce the number of killed or seriously injured cyclists by nearly 34%.[28,59–62] In adult populations, legal requirements for helmet usage vary greatly by geographic location; evidence suggests that legally requiring helmets will increase helmet use and therefore decrease head injuries.[28] However, there is also evidence to suggest that even if helmets are mandated, helmets alone may not significantly reduce injuries.[63–78] These measures must be done in concert with improvements to bicycle-related infrastructure, as discussed above.

It is important to understand how some of these individual level factors play a role in protecting both children and adult riders from injuries. However, with greater variety of personal choices and requirements, a more effective strategy to reduce bicycle-related injuries across the entire population should focus on the changing the environments in which riders travel. Environmental adaptations, such as the implementation of dedicated cycling tracks and all infrastructure that separates the cyclist from other forms of transportation, provide greater levels of protection to the rider than individual modifications. These environmental adaptations are accomplished through policy change and community level decisions. Clinicians can influence these decisions, by advocating that these decisions are made in the best interest of patient health and to potentially reduce injury burdens placed on local cities and communities.

SUMMARY

Environmental changes to roadways and cycling pathways can provide the longest lasting impacts to reduce injury burdens for cyclists. Across current injury prevention literature regarding improving cyclist safety, the need for increased prevalence of bicycle-specific infrastructure and improvements in current infrastructure, particularly in the United States and across North America, is fundamentally important for reducing injuries and increasing the number of cyclists.[47,48,51]

However, it is important to recognize that these infrastructure changes need to be carefully planned in order to maximize their effectiveness. Separating cyclists from other modes of transportation, although ensuring the system remains connected and efficient, can optimize safety and increase usage. Combining environmental and policy changes with efforts to change individual-level cycling behaviors will provide a wholistic strategy for improving bicycle safety at the community level.

CLINICS CARE POINTS

- Bicycle usage is growing across the United States and the globe, particularly in urban environments, as an alternative to motor vehicle or public transportation.

- Clinicians, particularly those working in urban environments, should ask patients about their transportation habits and discuss injury prevention strategies with patients classifying as bicycle riders, including helping patients to identify safe riding pathways that include bicycle-specific infrastructure.
- Prevalence of bicycle injuries in pediatric populations is similar to adult populations, and these injuries commonly require clinical treatment.
- Environmental factors play a major role in the likelihood of injury while riding a bicycle, and clinicians should be aware of the infrastructure present in their service community to be prepared for appropriate treatment.
- Helmet use has been shown to reduce head and brain injury for both pediatric and adult riders after a bicycle crash and should be encouraged across all ages.
- Clinicians can advocate for their patients and for their communities to assist in policy and community planning change.

DISCLOSURE

The authors have nothing to disclose.

REFERENCES

1. Oja P, Vuori I, Paronen O. Daily walking and cycling to work: their utility as health-enhancing physical activity. Patient Educ Couns 1998;33:S87–94.
2. Foster CE, Panter JR, Wareham NJ. Assessing the impact of road traffic on cycling for leisure and cycling to work. Int J Behav Nutr Phys activity 2011; 8(1):1–5.
3. Fishman E. Cycling as Transport. Transport Reviews 2016;36(1):1-8.
4. Fishman E, Washington S, Haworth N. Bike share: a synthesis of the literature. Transport Rev 2013;33(2):148–65.
5. Heinen E, van Wee B, Maat K. Commuting by bicycle: an overview of the literature. Transport Rev 2009;30(1):59–96.
6. Pucher J, Buehler R. Making cycling irresistible: lessons from the Netherlands, Denmark and Germany. Transport reviews 2008;28(4):495-528.
7. Lange D. Cycling statistics & facts: reports from Statista. Cycling Dossier. 2020. Available at: https://www.statista.com/topics/1686/cycling/#: ~ :text=Cycling%2C %20also%20known%20as%20biking,to%2047.5%20million%20in%202017. Accessed January 22, 2021.
8. Union Cycliste Internationale. 2020 cycling boom in the USA. 2020. Available at: https://www.uci.org/news/2020/2020-cycling-boom-in-the-usa. Accessed January 22, 2021.
9. Laker L. The surprising reasons a biking boom is great for cities. 2020. Available at: https://www.huffpost.com/entry/cycling-lanes-safer-roads-coronavirus-bike-shortage_n_5ed11296c5b67c705dfc5d3. Accessed January 22, 2021.
10. National Highway Traffic Safety Administration. U.S. Department of Transportation. 2018 Fatal motor vehicle crashes: overview. 2019. Available at: https://crashstats.nhtsa.dot.gov/Api/Public/ViewPublication/812826. Accessed January 5, 2021.
11. Centers for Disease Control and Prevention. Web-based Injury Statistics Query and Reporting System (WISQARS). Non-Fatal Injury Reports. Atlanta, GA: Centers for Disease Control and Prevention, National Center for Injury Prevention

and Control. Available at: www.cdc.gov/injury/wisqars. Accessed January 21, 2021.

12. Ding H, Sze NN, Li H, et al. Roles of infrastructure and land use in bicycle crash exposure and frequency: a case study using Greater London bike sharing data. Accid Anal Prev 2020;144:105652.

13. Pedroso FE, Angriman F, Bellows AL, et al. Bicycle use and cyclist safety following Boston's bicycle infrastructure expansion, 2009–2012. Am J Public Health 2016;106(12):2171–7.

14. Reynolds CC, Harris MA, Teschke K, et al. The impact of transportation infrastructure on bicycling injuries and crashes: a review of the literature. Environ Health 2009;8(1):1–9.

15. Centers for Disease Control and Prevention. Web-based Injury Statistics Query and Reporting System (WISQARS). Pediatric Non-Fatal Injuries. Atlanta, GA: Centers for Disease Control and Prevention, National Center for Injury Prevention and Control. Available at: www.cdc.gov/injury/wisqars. Accessed June 13, 2021.

16. Rivara FP, Cummings P, Koepsell TD, et al, editors. Injury control: a guide to research and program evaluation. Cambridge University Press; 2009.

17. Nationwide Children's. "Make Safe Happen". 2020. Available at: https://makesafehappen.com/articles/bicycle-safety-kids. Accessed February 1, 2021.

18. Gill AC. Bicycle injuries in children: prevention 2020. Available at: https://www.uptodate.com/contents/bicycle-injuries-in-children-prevention. Accessed February 1, 2021.

19. Kaushik R, Krisch IM, Schroeder DR, et al. Pediatric bicycle-related head injuries: a population-based study in a county without a helmet law. Inj Epidemiol 2015; 2(1):1–9.

20. Nationwide Children's. Bicycle-related injuries send 25 children to emergency departments every hour. 2018. Available at: https://www.nationwidechildrens.org/newsroom/news-releases/2018/06/bike-injuries-study#: ~ :text=The%20study%2C%20published%20online%20in,day%20or%2025%20every%20hour. Accessed January 15, 2020.

21. McAdams RJ, Swidarski K, Clark RM, et al. Bicycle-related injuries among children treated in US emergency departments, 2006-2015. Accid Anal Prev 2018; 118:11–7.

22. Hagel BE, Romanow NT, Enns N, et al. Severe bicycling injury risk factors in children and adolescents: a case-control study. Accid Anal Prev 2015;78:165–72.

23. Mehan TJ, Gardner R, Smith GA, et al. Bicycle-related injuries among children and adolescents in the United States. Clin Pediatr 2009;48(2):166–73.

24. Siman-Tov M, Jaffe DH, Peleg K, Israel Trauma Group. Bicycle injuries: a matter of mechanism and age. Accid Anal Prev 2012;44(1):135–9.

25. Chaney RA, Kim C. Characterizing bicycle collisions by neighborhood in a large midwestern city. Health Promot Pract 2014;15(2):232–42.

26. de Waard D, Houwing S, Lewis-Evans B, et al. Bicycling under the influence of alcohol. Transp Res F Traffic Psychol Behav 2016;41:302–8.

27. Crocker P, Zad O, Milling T, et al. Alcohol, bicycling, and head and brain injury: a study of impaired cyclists' riding patterns R1. Am J Emerg Med 2010;28(1): 68–72.

28. Høye A. Bicycle helmets–to wear or not to wear? A meta-analyses of the effects of bicycle helmets on injuries. Accid Anal Prev 2018;117:85–97.

29. Sethi M, Heyer JH, Wall S, et al. Alcohol use by urban bicyclists is associated with more severe injury, greater hospital resource use, and higher mortality. Alcohol 2016;53:1–7.

30. Banks KP, Ly JQ, Beall DP, et al. Overuse injuries of the upper extremity in the competitive athlete: magnetic resonance imaging findings associated with repetitive trauma. Curr Probl Diagn Radiol 2005;34(4):127–42.
31. Silberman MR. Bicycling injuries. Curr Sports Med Rep 2013;12(5):337–45.
32. Piotrowska SE, Majchrzycki M, Rogala P, et al. Lower extremity and spine pain in cyclists. Ann Agric Environ Med 2017;24(4):654–8.
33. Pommering TL, Manos DC, Singichetti B, et al. Injuries and illnesses occurring on a recreational bicycle tour: the great Ohio bicycle adventure. Wilderness Environ Med 2017;28(4):299–306.
34. Wilber CA, Holland GJ, Madison RE, et al. An epidemiological analysis of overuse injuries among recreational cyclists. Int J Sports Med 1995;16(03):201–6.
35. Wanich T, Hodgkins C, Columbier JA, et al. Cycling injuries of the lower extremity. J Am Acad Orthop Surg 2007;15(12):748–56.
36. Safe Kids Worldwide. Bike. Available at: https://www.safekids.org/bike. Accessed March 28, 2021.
37. Teschke K, Harris MA, Reynolds CC, et al. Route infrastructure and the risk of injuries to bicyclists: a case-crossover study. Am J Public Health 2012;102(12):2336–43.
38. Hoffman MR, Lambert WE, Peck EG, et al. Bicycle commuter injury prevention: it is time to focus on the environment. J Trauma Acute Care Surg 2010;69(5):1112–9.
39. Martin E. Making a bicycle city: infrastructure and cycling in Copenhagen since 1880. Urban Hist 2019;46(3):493–517.
40. Bjornsson T. A Swedish bicycle plan. World Transport Pol Pract 2013;19(1):45–50.
41. Cushing M, Hooshmand J, Pomares B, et al. Vision Zero in the United States versus Sweden: infrastructure improvement for cycling safety. Am J Public Health 2016;106(12):2178–80.
42. Branion-Calles M, Nelson T, Fuller D, et al. Associations between individual characteristics, availability of bicycle infrastructure, and city-wide safety perceptions of bicycling: a cross-sectional survey of bicyclists in 6 Canadian and US cities. Transportation Res A Pol Pract 2019;123:229–39.
43. Wall SP, Lee DC, Frangos SG, et al. The effect of sharrows, painted bicycle lanes and physically protected paths on the severity of bicycle injuries caused by motor vehicles. Safety 2016;2(4):26.
44. Pucher J, Buehler R. Safer Cycling Through Improved Infrastructure. Am J Public Health 2016;106(12):2089-91.
45. Cicchino JB, McCarthy ML, Newgard CD, et al. Not all protected bike lanes are the same: infrastructure and risk of cyclist collisions and falls leading to emergency department visits in three US cities. Accid Anal Prev 2020;141:105490.
46. Caulfield B, Brick E, McCarthy OT. Determining bicycle infrastructure preferences–a case study of Dublin. Transp Res D Transp Environ 2012;17(5):413–7.
47. Dill J. Bicycling for transportation and health: the role of infrastructure. J Public Health Pol 2009;30(1):S95–110.
48. Moudon AV, Lee C, Cheadle AD, et al. Cycling and the built environment, a US perspective. Transp Res D Transp Environ 2005;10(3):245–61.
49. Barrero GA, Rodriguez-Valencia A. Asking the user: a perceptional approach for bicycle infrastructure design. Int J Sustainable Transportation 2020;1–17 [Epub ahead of print].

50. Garrard J, Rose G, Lo SK. Promoting transportation cycling for women: the role of bicycle infrastructure. Prev Med 2008;46(1):55–9.
51. Van Cauwenberg J, de Geus B, Deforche B. Cycling for transport among older adults: health benefits, prevalence, determinants, injuries and the potential of E-bikes. In: Geographies of Transport and ageing. Transportation. Cham (Switzerland): Palgrave Macmillan; 2018. p. 133–51.
52. American Academy of Pediatrics. Bicycle helmets. Pediatrics 2001;108(4): 1030–2.
53. Gleave J. and Officer S.S.T Cycle Helmets: The impacts of compulsory cycle helmet legislation on cyclist fatalities and premature deaths in the UK. Transport Planning Society; 2012.
54. Joseph B, Azim A, Haider AA, et al. Bicycle helmets work when it matters the most. Am J Surg 2017;213(2):413–7.
55. Strotmeyer S, Koff A, Honeyman JN, et al. Injuries among Amish children: opportunities for prevention. Inj Epidemiol 2019;6(1):1–6.
56. Stier R, Jehn P, Johannsen H, et al. Reality or wishful thinking: do bicycle helmets prevent facial injuries? Int J Oral Maxillofac Surg 2019;48(9):1235–40.
57. Carone L, Ardley R, Davies P. Cycling related traumatic brain injury requiring intensive care: association with non-helmet wearing in young people. Injury 2019;50(1):61–4.
58. Piotrowski CC, Warda L, Pankratz C, et al. The perspectives of young people on barriers to and facilitators of bicycle helmet and booster seat use. Child Care Health Dev 2020;46(5):591–8.
59. Olivier J, Creighton P. Bicycle injuries and helmet use: a systematic review and meta-analysis. Int J Epidemiol 2017;46(1):278–92.
60. Attewell RG, Glase K, McFadden M. Bicycle helmet efficacy: a meta-analysis. Accid Anal Prev 2001;33(3):345–52.
61. Elvik R. Publication bias and time-trend bias in meta-analysis of bicycle helmet efficacy: a re-analysis of Attewell, Glase and McFadden, 2001. Accid Anal Prev 2011;43(3):1245–51.
62. Elvik R. Corrigendum to: "Publication bias and time-trend bias in meta-analysis of bicycle helmet efficacy: a re-analysis of Attewell, Glase and McFadden, 2001"[Accid. Anal. Prev. 43 (2011) 1245–1251]. Accid Anal Prev 2013;60:245–53.
63. De Jong P. The health impact of mandatory bicycle helmet laws. Risk Anal An Int J 2012;32(5):782–90.
64. Asplund C, St Pierre P. Knee pain and bicycling: fitting concepts for clinicians. Phys Sportsmed 2004;32(4):23–30.
65. Holmes JC, Pruitt AL, Whalen NJ. Lower extremity overuse in bicycling. Clin Sports Med 1994;13(1):187–205.
66. Kotler DH, Babu AN, Robidoux G. Prevention, evaluation, and rehabilitation of cycling-related injury. Curr Sports Med Rep 2016;15(3):199–206.
67. Silberman MR, Webner D, Collina S, et al. Road bicycle fit. Clin J Sport Med 2005; 15(4):271–6.
68. Clarsen B, Krosshaug T, Bahr R. Overuse injuries in professional road cyclists. Am J Sports Med 2010;38(12):2494–501.
69. Ayachi FS, Dorey J, Guastavino C. Identifying factors of bicycle comfort: an online survey with enthusiast cyclists. Appl Ergon 2015;46:124–36.
70. Patel D, Magnusen E, Sandell JM. Prevention of unintentional injury in children. Paediatr Child Health 2017;27(9):420–6.
71. Watson MC, Errington G. Preventing unintentional injuries in children: successful approaches. Paediatr Child Health 2016;26(5):194–9.

72. Clements JL. Promoting the use of bicycle helmets during primary care visits. J Am Acad Nurse Pract 2005;17(9):350–4.
73. Johnston BD, Rivara FP, Droesch RM, et al. Behavior change counseling in the emergency department to reduce injury risk: a randomized, controlled trial. Pediatrics 2002;110(2):267–74.
74. Corden TE, Tripathy N, Pierce SE, et al. The role of the health care professional in bicycle safety. Wis Med J 2005;104(2):35–8.
75. Earnest MA, Wong SL, Federico SG. Perspective: physician advocacy: what is it and how do we do it? Acad Med 2010;85(1):63–7.
76. ABIM Foundation. American Board of Internal Medicine; ACP-ASIM Foundation. American College of Physicians-American Society of Internal Medicine; European Federation of Internal Medicine. Medical professionalism in the new millennium: a physician charter. Ann Intern Med 2002;136(3):243–6.
77. American Medical Association. Declaration of professional responsibility. Adopted by the AMA House of Delegates.. 2001. Available at: http://www.ama-assn. org/ama/pub/category/7491.html. Accessed May 28, 2021.
78. American College of Surgeons. Statement on bicycle safety and promotion of bicycle helmet use. 2014. Available at: https://www.facs.org/about-acs/statements/ 75-bicycle-safety. Accessed May 28, 2021.

Acute Cycling Injuries

Mark Greve, MD

KEYWORDS

- Sports injuries • Bicycling injuries • Traumatic brain injury • Sports medicine
- Blunt chest trauma • Burn management • Wound management

KEY POINTS

- Cycling collisions typically occur with mechanisms higher than traditional sports injuries. Most impacts are caused by rider collisions and mass casualties are common.
- The majority of cycling injuries are soft tissue and musculoskeletal. Upper extremities fractures are common, typically from a FOOSH mechanism or from shoulder impacts.
- Brain injuries are common in cycling. Severe brain injuries require focused management. Concussions are commonly missed.
- Road rash is nearly ubiquitous and should be treated like a burn. Early cleaning and wound exploration reduces infections, improves healing and cosmetics.

INTRODUCTION

Cycling mechanisms of injury are more similar to those from motor vehicle accidents than are traditional sports injuries. Clinicians providing medical coverage for cycling events should be advanced trauma life support (ATLS) practitioners. That is not to say that most cycling injuries are severe; the opposite is true—a vast majority of cycling injuries are minor and not associated with lasting disability.[1,2] Medical practitioners who care for cyclists, especially in the prehospital and competition settings, should be prepared to manage this broad range of injuries.[3] A unique aspect of cycling race medicine is that management often is performed on public roadways in close proximity to the athletes during competition. Medical staff, such as team and event physicians, are among a large supporting fleet of vehicles that accompany the race.[3] In professional cycling, the event does not stop for riders to be medically assessed or treated. Rider assessment and treatment generally are done with limited time and resources (**Fig. 1**).

This article's focus is on acute traumatic injuries to cyclists and the management of these injuries in the competition setting. Technologies, such as ultrasound imaging, point-of-care testing, and telemedicine, although highly valuable, are not standards of care as of this writing.

Department of Emergency Medicine, Division of Sports Medicine, Warren Alpert School of Medicine, Brown University, 55 Claverick Street, 2nd floor, Providence, RI 02903, USA
E-mail address: mark.greve@brownphysicians.org

Phys Med Rehabil Clin N Am 33 (2022) 135–158
https://doi.org/10.1016/j.pmr.2021.08.010
1047-9651/22/© 2021 Elsevier Inc. All rights reserved.

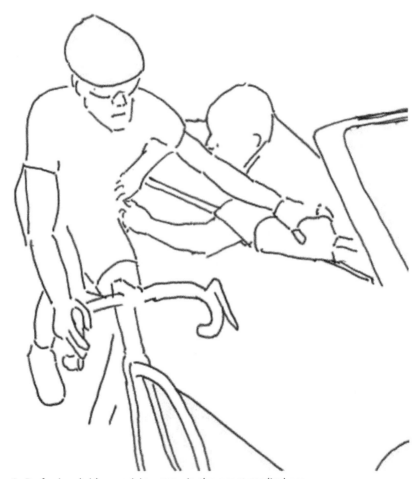

Fig. 1. Professional rider receiving care via the event medical car.

MECHANISM

Cyclists have little protection from injury—no seatbelts, crumple zones, or airbags. Competitive cycling occurs in many arenas. Cyclists often compete in austere environments, remote from medical facilities, at high speed and for hundreds of kilometers in all weather conditions.

The inciting event for a collision can be from a litany of factors but most commonly is from contact with another rider.[1] Collisions with motor vehicles are common both in and out of competition and a common cause of death[1,2] (**Fig. 2**).

Acute cycling injuries are sustained when there is an impact. Physics rule the day. Speed matters. What is struck matters. Helmets and other protective equipment matter. One rider falling easily can cascade into a mass casualty scene[1,2] (**Fig. 3**).

Riders who have impact with stationary objects, such as walls, guardrails, or cars, typically have more severe injuries compared with those who only strike the ground.[1] In the event of a loss of control, the cyclist commonly falls toward the 10 o'clock or 2 o'clock position. Falls on outstretched hands are common. Riders going over the handlebars are at high risk of head, face, and neck injuries. Riders going backwards

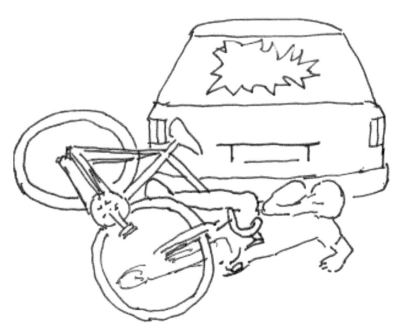

Fig. 2. Cycling mechanisms of injury are more similar to motor vehicle accidents than traditional sports injuries.

additionally are exposed to spine trauma. Striking the chest is common, potentially involving vital organs.[4] Abdominal trauma is less common.[1] Higher-risk injuries to the brain, spine, and thorax occur with higher speeds and mechanisms. Head injury is the leading cause of death for cyclists and cycling is a common cause of concussion.[4] Helmets reduce serious head injuries, but they do not prevent nor reduce concussion.[5,6]

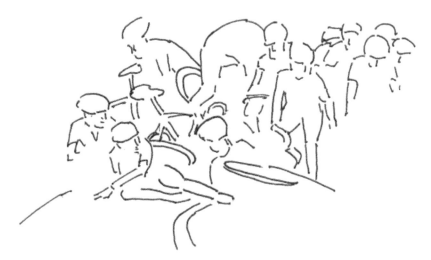

Fig. 3. Mass casualties are common in cycling.

Commonly reported sites of injury correspond to primary points of impact, including the hands/wrist, elbow, shoulder, hip, knee, and head. In most collisions, there are extensive abrasions, commonly called *road rash*.[1,2] Fractures of the upper extremities, typically the clavicle, are the most common reasons for a rider to withdraw from competition[2,7] (**Fig. 4**).

Central Nervous System Trauma

There are several challenges in the management of head-injured competitive cyclists, a leading one being the threat of serious injury. The potential of a rider crashing at a high rate of speed and/or striking a fixed object is very real. Higher-energy collisions carry a higher incidence of intercranial injury, especially bleeding. These are time-critical injuries. The standard neurologic assessment tool is a Glasgow Coma Scale (GCS).[8] Any abnormal score should require the withdrawal of the athlete (**Table 1**).

The standard of care in most sports is for the injured athlete to be removed from play for an appropriate examination.[9] But there are no time allowances in professional cycling for the assessment of injured riders. In professional road cycling, crashing is part of the sport, and this does not pause competition, even for mass casualties. Mechanics repair and replace equipment on the fly in a race to get the racers back into competition. If the riders can get back on their bike, they generally are allowed to continue with the event without medical assessment. Identifying riders with head injuries is a challenge in this setting. A stepwise approach may help to identify high-risk patients and remove them from play for more definitive assessment and treatment. Team physicians have developed, implemented, and published such a standardized approach[10] (**Figs. 5** and **6**).

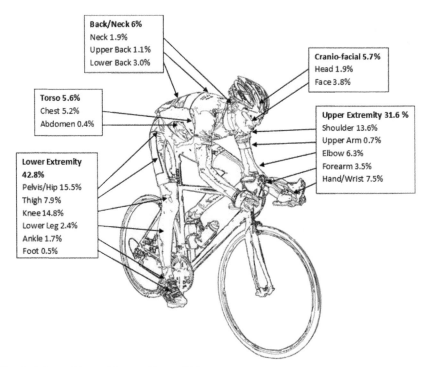

Fig. 4. Points of impact in a cycling collision.

Table 1 Glasgow Coma Scale is the standard neurologic assessment tool in the setting of traumatic brain injury	
Eye opening	
No eye opening	1
Eyes open to pain	2
Eyes open to speech	3
Eyes open spontaneously	4
Best verbal response	
None	1
Incomprehensible	2
Inappropriate words	3
Confused	4
Oriented	5
Best motor	
None	1
Extensor response to pain	2
Flexor response to pain	3
Withdraws from pain	4
Localizes to pain	5
Obeys commands	6
Severe TBI: GCS <9	
Moderate TBI: GCS 9–12	
Minor TBI: GCS ≥13	

The best responses are added up to give the total score. This score determines level of injury.

Severe traumatic brain injuries (TBIs) should in theory be hard to miss. These forms are injuries are associated with a very depressed GCS. Patients are either unresponsive or very confused.[11] Severe TBI has a close association with intercranial bleeding.[12] These time-critical lesions can expand, and the patient can decompensate in short course. Brain injuries can be described further as primary and secondary injuries. Primary injury is the direct physical effect on the brain tissue from trauma, for example, in penetrating trauma the blast effect of the missile creates the primary injury. That tissue is irrevocably lost. Secondary injuries are from the disruption of central nervous system (CNS) function on a cellular basis and primarily from hypoxia and hypoperfusion.[11,13] The field management of these injuries is to mitigate these secondary effects as aggressively as possible while executing a rapid medical transport to a facility with neurosurgical capabilities. This often requires advanced airway management, aggressive resuscitation, spinal precautions, and the use of parenteral medications to control CNS pressures.[12] The test of choice to identify pathology, especially intercranial bleeding, is computed tomography (CT) scan of the brain. There are several evidence-based tools for identifying which patients need a CT scan of the brain; one of the most widely accepted is the Canadian CT Head Rules.[14]

CT scan is required for patients with minor head injuries and any 1 of the following:

- High-risk features include GCS less than 15 at 2 hours postinjury, suspected open or depressed skull fracture, any signs of basal skull fracture, vomiting for greater than or equal to 2 episodes, and age greater than 65.

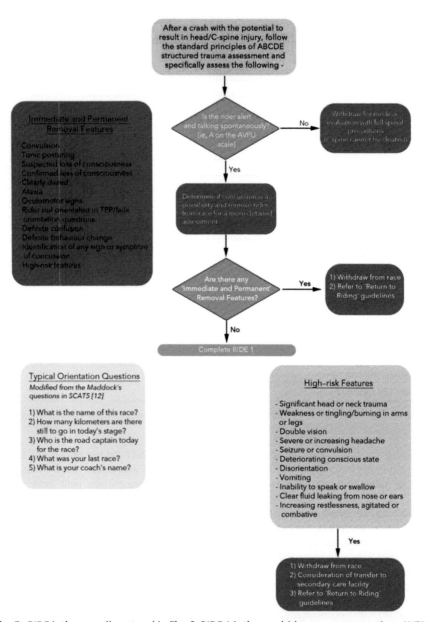

Fig. 5. RIDE is the overall protocol in **Fig. 6**. RIDE 1 is the roadside assessment portion. AVPU, level of consciousness (Alert, Verbal, Pain, Unresponsive); c spine, cervical spine; TTP, tender to palpation; Maddock, part of the SCAT questions and used to check orientation. (*From* Heron N, Elliott J, Jones N, Loosemore M, Kemp S. Sports-related concussion (SRC) in road cycling: the RoadsIde heaD Injury assEssment (RIDE) for elite road cycling. Br J Sports Med. 2020 Feb;54(3):127-128. https://doi.org/10.1136/bjsports-2019-101455. Epub 2019 Oct 25. PMID: 31653774.)

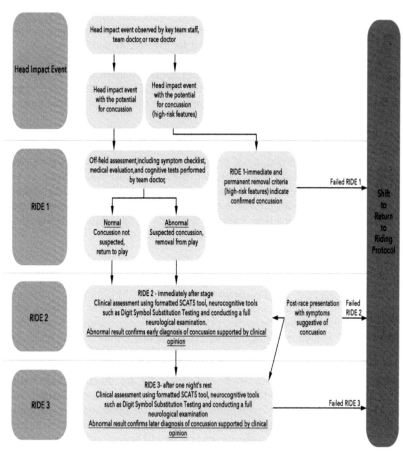

Fig. 6. Cycling RIDE protocol. (*From* Heron N, Elliott J, Jones N, Loosemore M, Kemp S. Sports-related concussion (SRC) in road cycling: the RoadsIde heaD Injury assEssment (RIDE) for elite road cycling. Br J Sports Med. 2020 Feb;54(3):127-128. https://doi.org/10.1136/bjsports-2019-101455. Epub 2019 Oct 25. PMID: 31653774.)

- Medium risks include amnesia before impact greater than 30 minutes and any dangerous mechanism.

Although a vast majority of minor and moderate TBIs require only monitoring, this monitoring is important, in particular for the first 4 hours after injury.[12] If a patient has been evaluated properly, serial examinations after this observational period are of limited yield.[15]

Concussions in cycling can be challanging to identify. Athletes may be neurologically injured despite having a normal GCS. Although loss of consciousness is considered a more concerning symptom for intercranial hemorrhage, riders being "dazed" often corresponds more to concussive injury.[15] The identification of riders with concussions is no easy task. Typically, if riders can remount, they are allowed to do so; although this may function as a screening tool for other forms of cycling injury, it is not well suited to head injuries. Concussed riders can be the least aware of their injuries and likely are physically able to get on their bike and propel it forward. The roadside head injury assessment (RIDE) protocol was developed to fill this gap and protocolize the assessment of the rider in the field. If this cannot be done in the field, the rider should be withdrawn from the event for medical evaluation.

Although developments, such as the RIDE protocol, and better appreciation of concussion in sport have been important and impactful there still is a large gap in the management of concussed cyclists. This extends beyond the race course and to cycling at large. Better science and technology for the diagnosis of concussed cyclists are of paramount importance.

Once off the bike, assessment of riders for concussive injuries is synonymous with that of other sports. The most accepted standard is Sports Concussion Assessment Tool 5 (SCAT5), but often this is not applicable to the professional cycling environment.[9,10] All sports organizations, including cycling, should have protocols for the management and return to sport for head-injured athletes. Athletes need standardized concussion testing, including baseline testing and access to medical resources, for the management of head injuries. Teams and events should require a return to baseline neurologic testing prior to returning to competition.

Spine Trauma

Spine trauma carries a significant risk of spinal cord injury. The higher the injury on the spine, the higher the potential level of disability, including the potential of paralysis and spinal shock. Cervical spine injuries are particularly worrisome for these reasons. Alteration of mental status in the setting of trauma is an independent indicator for spine immobilization.[16] Concurrent management of facial and dental trauma should focus on airway patency while avoiding disruption of the skeletal axis (**Fig. 7**).

Riders sustaining a crash with tenderness to the spinal area, in particular bony tenderness, should have full spinal immobilization.[16] Care should include full spinal precautions and an appropriate examination, including sensation, strength, and reflexes. Riders should be reassessed particularly after immobilization and during transport.[16] Those with any neurologic findings are high risk. Bleeding anywhere in the CNS space, including the spinal column, occurs in a closed space and can cause delayed or worsening symptoms.

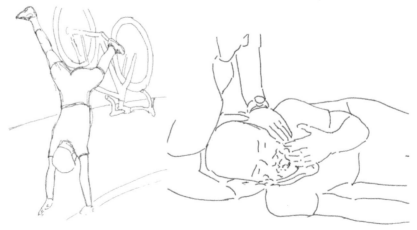

Fig. 7. Cyclists going over the bars are at risk for head, face and spine injuries (*left*). Riders with suspected brain injury should be immobilized with a rigid cervical collar (*right*). Dental and facial trauma management should focus on the integrity of the airway.

Neurogenic shock is loss of sympathetic outflow resulting in a bradycardic, vasoplegic hypotensive state. It can be challenging to discriminate neurogenic shock from other forms of shock on the bradycardia alone and all shock should be managed according to ATLS guidelines, including aggressive management of hypotension.[12]

Chest Trauma

Thoracic trauma can be serious business. Knowledge of ATLS is critical to the field management of these types of injuries. Penetrating and rapid deceleration injuries to the chest are associated with high morbidity and mortality. Considering the life critical structures in the chest—the heart, great vessels, lungs, and airway—careful attention should be paid to cyclists with chest trauma to assure proper cardiovascular function. Prolonged resuscitative efforts in traumatic cardiac arrest are futile.[12] Fortunately, this is rare and on the far end of the spectrum.

Penetrating trauma such as missile injuries are rare but being impaled is a reported injury to cyclist.[1] As a general rule, impaled objects should be removed only in a hospital setting. Penetrating trauma to the chest cavity is particularly concerning if it is within "the box,"[17] the superior margin being the clavicles; inferior margin, the lowest part of the ribs; and both lateral margins the nipple lines (**Fig. 8**).

Penetrating trauma to this zone is more likely to involve the heart and great vessels. Penetrating trauma can also create lower airway trauma and potentially compromise respiratory function.

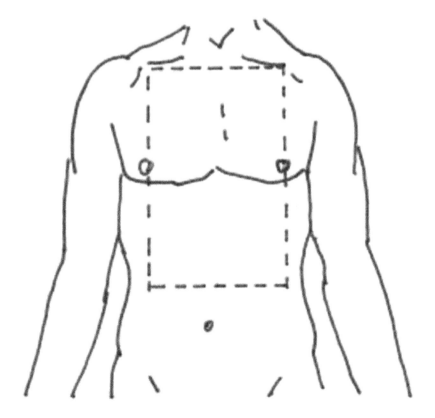

Fig. 8. Chest trauma box.

Penetrating wounds that violate the pleura can cause air and blood to accumulate in the chest cavity. These are classic battlefield injuries and accurately described as *sucking chest wounds*. These wounds can create a ball valve effect, resulting in increased intrathoracic pressures. These wounds should be covered upon discovery, if possible, by a dressing that mimics the ball valve effect but vents to the exterior environment. This can be with a nonocclusive dressing taped on 3 sides (**Fig. 9**).

A pneumothorax is extraplural air in the chest cavity. This can be created by air entering from the external environment (open pneumothorax) or blunt trauma causing air leakage typically from the lung pleura. Any pneumothorax can develop into a tension pneumothorax, and sucking chest wounds are especially well known for causing this. Small volumes of air and even larger volumes can be asymptomatic; as long as there is no shift in the mediastinum, they are a simple pneumothorax. The issue in a tension pneumothorax is that increasing intrathoracic pressures can displace mediastinal structures, compressing the heart and not allowing it to fill. Patients with a tension pneumothorax can rapidly develop obstructive shock. To stabilize, air is allowed to vent to the extrathoracic space to convert the tension pneumothorax to a simple. This technique dates back to ancient Greek times and is a fundamental skill in emergency medical services and combat medicine. The current technique for needle decompression of the chest recently has changed. The standard 5-cm angiocatheter is considered not as effective as an 8-cm angiocatheter. Current ATLS recommendations state "Cadaver studies have shown improved success in reaching the thoracic cavity when the fourth or fifth intercostal space midaxillary line is used instead of the second intercostal space midclavicular line in adult patients. ATLS now recommends this location for needle decompression in adult patients. Needle decompression can fail to improve clinical decompensation in patients who have hemothorax or in whom the angiocatheter has kinked. Performing a finger thoracostomy can ensure adequate decompression of the chest and eliminate tension pneumothorax as the cause of decompensation."[8] (**Fig. 10**).

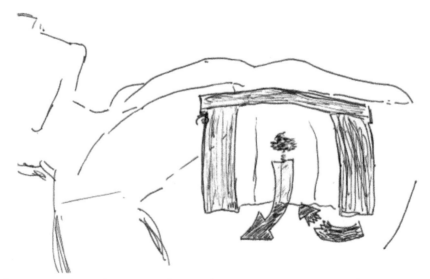

Fig. 9. Nonocclusive dressing taped on 3 sides is a standard treatment of a sucking chest wound.

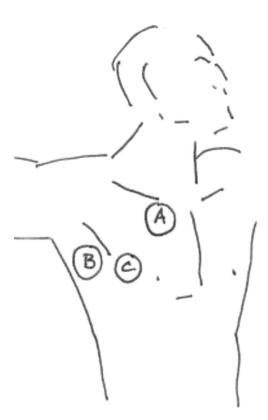

Fig. 10. ATLS recommendations for location of needle decompression of the chest: A, second intercostal (IC) midclavicular (old approach); B, fourth/fifth IC midaxillary (new approach); and C, fourth/fifth IC anterior axillary (new approach).

Definitive management of a pneumothorax often involves tube thoracostomy, which typically can wait until a patient is at a medical facility. A hemothorax is blood accumulating in the chest cavity and often occurs with a pneumothorax. The field management is equivalent, although a hemothorax is more likely to require a large bore thoracostomy.

Blunt cardiac injury can manifest in several ways. Arrhythmias and cardiac arrest should be managed per advanced cardiac life support protocol. One of the less common causes for patients decompensating from blunt cardiac trauma can be from a pericardial effusion. In these injuries, fluid, typically blood, accumulates in the sac around the heart. Small volumes may be asymptomatic but, if these effusions are large enough, they can prevent proper cardiac filling and put the patient in obstructive shock similar to a tension pneumothorax. Without the use of additional diagnostic tools, a pericardial effusion and a tension pneumothorax can be indistinguishable. Clinicians may perform double-needle decompressions on an unstable trauma patient for these reasons.[8] Many pericardial effusions can be temporized by aggressive intravenous resuscitation, given these lesions are preload-dependent. Definitive care for pericardial effusions, such as a pericardial drain, is not done in the field setting.

Rib fractures can be a challenge to distinguish from soft tissue injuries of the chest wall. Poorly localized mild pain is expected in cases of soft tissue injury. As long as no suspicion for other injuries, such as a pneumothorax, medical staff typically lets them continue.

Abdominal and Genitourinary Trauma

Abdominal trauma is comparatively rare in uncomplicated cycling collisions.[1–3] In blunt trauma, attention always should be paid to distinguish chest wall pain from abdominal pain. In particular, the lower ribs lie over the spleen and liver. These are danger zones for trauma; both these organs can rupture causing hemorrhagic shock.[8] Clinicians should assume violation of the peritoneum in penetrating wounds. Impaled objects should not be removed unless they prevent the extrication of patient. Duodenal hematomas and other spear handlebar injuries have been associated with cycling.[18] Traditional road handlebars, as required for mass start Union Cycliste Internationale events, do not have these exposed ends (**Fig. 11**).

Cycling has been associated with chronic genitourinary (GU) trauma, mostly through compressive forces on the perineal area causing compression of the pudendal artery and nerve. This has been associated with GU dysfunction in both male cyclists and female cyclists.[19,20] The actual incidence of acute GU trauma to road cyclists is infrequent, with the kidneys being most injured GU organ.[21] Straddle injuries occur with blunt trauma to the groin and inner thighs involving the genitals and often can be from impacting the bicycle during a crash. Penetrating trauma to the genitals also can occur, although infrequent penetrating trauma to the genitals often requires management by urologic specialist[21] (**Fig. 12**).

Skeletal Trauma

Skeletal trauma is common to cyclists, and, roadside, the most important decision often is whether there is a functional impairment. Riders who demonstrate proper function generally can be allowed to continue with medical supervision. Fractures or dislocations generally mean the withdrawal of an athlete.[7] Although the management of injuries depends in part on the experience of the clinician, compromised neurovascular function requires emergent reduction. These limbs are at imminent risk of amputation and there should be no delay in reestablishing neurovascular competence.[22]

Open fractures are fractures with exposed bone. These areas should be cleaned gently, covered with antiseptic impregnated gauze, and splinted. They should not be reduced unless there is compromised neurovascular function.[23]

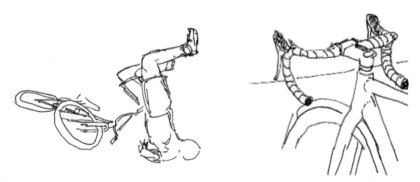

Fig. 11. Spear injuries may occur when the rider impacts the end of their handlebars during a coliision (*left*). The design of traditional road bars helps prevent this injury (*right*).

Upper extremity injuries are common to cyclists.[1,2,7] The upper extremity has many complicated articulating structures, such as the shoulder, wrist, and hand. Many of these bones and joints can have long-term complications if injuries are not diagnosed and treated properly. There are no diagnostic rules that can rule out fractures to the upper extremity based on clinical grounds. If there is a concern for fracture, radiographic imaging needs to be done. As a general rule, if it hurts when a bone is pushed on, it is more likely to be fractured. At the roadside, the rider should be able to operate the bicycle properly. A hand injury could mean a rider is not able to brake properly.

Clavicle fractures are the most common fractures.[1,2,7] For the most part, clavicle fractures are uncomplicated and associated with minor short-term disability during the healing process. The most common complication of clavicle fractures are pneumothoraxes. The clavicle does lie close to major nerves, and vascular structures and can be associated with more serious injury. For these, as for all fractures, neurovascular examinations should be performed at the time of injury, before and after splinting, and regularly during transport. Although most clavicle fractures can heal without intervention, it is becoming much more common to place internal fixation, especially for elite athletes. This generally improves recovery time, alignment, and function.[24] At the time of injury a standard sling is adequate, with the addition of a swathe should more stability be needed. Attention should be paid that shoulders should not be immobilized for prolonged periods, and, aside from the acute period, should have movement as tolerated every few hours. Butterfly or figure-of-8 dressings do not result in improved outcomes.[25] In field situations, a Ross sling can be fashioned

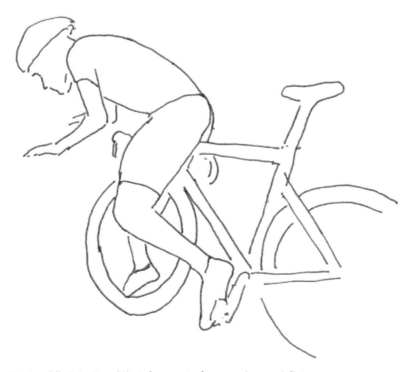

Fig. 12. Straddle injuries while infrequent often require specialist care.

by placing the arm in the standard sling position, pulling the bottom of a shirt/jersey up over the injured forearm and pinning the cloth to the shirt/jersey on the opposite side (riders' numbers are held with safety pins) (**Fig. 13**)

Acromioclavicular (AC) joint separations are graded by different systems according to the degree of separation, from tenderness on the joint with normal radiographs to being fully disarticulated. The higher the grade of separation, the more common the need for surgery. AC separations can be splinted in the same manner as clavicle fractures.

Sternomanubrial and sternoclavicular dislocations are rare but should be managed with the same level of concern as having a penetrating injury to the chest. Dislocated joints may tamponade damaged internal vascular structures and these generally are reduced operatively only with thoracic surgeon support because their reduction could result in intrathoracic bleeding.[26]

The scapula articulates with the humerus as well as the clavicle. This entire structure glides over the thoracic rib cage. The scapula is a comparatively strong bone and any fracture to the scapula should be considered high-energy thoracic trauma and require medical transport.

As riders are impacting the ground, a common reaction is to put the hand out to blunt the impact. Falls on an outstretched hand (FOOSH) mechanisms are common causes for injuries of the upper extremity, in particular the hand and wrist. Hand and wrist pain deserve special attention because these are more complicated structures with many small bones. Scaphoid fractures are notorious for occult fractures and have the potential for malunion. Clinicians cannot rule out fracture on clinical grounds. If riders are not disabled, then they can often be reassessed after the event (**Fig. 14**).

Lower Extremity Fractures

As a rule of thumb, riders need to be able to bear weight on the affected extremity to continue with the event. If they cannot, they should be removed from competition for diagnostic imaging. Many of the bones of the lower extremity, such as the pelvis and femur, take a significant amount of force to break and should be considered a high mechanism injury.

The pelvis is a ringlike structure. Higher mechanism trauma that interrupts the stability of the ring carries significant risk of uncontrolled pelvic bleeding. Compression forces rather than direct-impact injuries tend to cause fractures that may destabilize the pelvic ring. Stabilization of pelvic fractures with pelvic binders or sheets can temporarily stabilize the pelvis and control bleeding[27] (**Fig. 15**).

Stable pelvic fractures can occur with lower-energy mechanisms. Injuries, such as acetabular fractures, pubic rami, iliac wing, and avulsion fractures, are less likely to

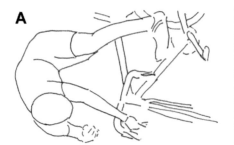
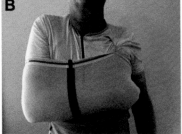

Fig. 13. (A) Shoulder injuries are common. (B). Ross sling and swath can be created by pulling the jersey over the arm and pinning to the adjacent shoulder.

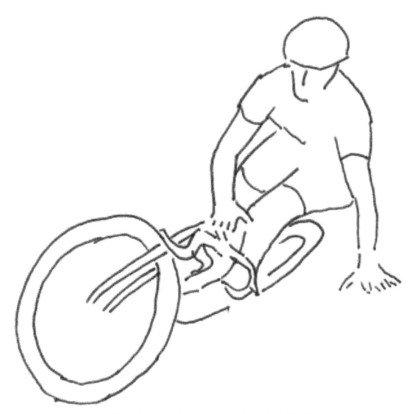

Fig. 14. Cyclists often put their hand out in response to a fall. FOOS are common causes for injuries to the hands and wrists.

cause internal bleeding. Many of these can be difficult to properly diagnose roadside, are very painful, and typically cause the withdrawal of the rider. Proper diagnosis generally require diagnostic imaging.

Hip injury is common to cyclists.[1] Many riders impact their hip during a bicycle collision. Missed fractures can lead to avascular necrosis of the hip and need for joint repair/replacement.[28] The challenge to roadside clinicians is which rider needs to get emergent imaging. Riders should be able to fully support their weight, including hopping on the leg unassisted to continue with the event. Plain films of the hip are considered inadequate to rule out fracture, given the high incidence of missed fracture. More advanced imaging, such as CT or magnetic resonance imaging (MRI), are indicated should there be persisting concern.[28]

Femurs are large bones. Femur fractures are very painful injuries that generally occur with high mechanism and can create a potential space for blood, leading to hypovolemic shock. Many femur factures can be placed into traction in the field, which can mitigate the hemodynamic complications, improve pain for the patient, and stabilize the fracture for extrication. The reality is that there often are many barriers to field application, including injury to adjacent joints.[29]

Injuries to the knee and ankle can be evaluated for fracture by the Ottawa ankle and knee rules.[30,31] Riders need to be able to bear weight and not have bony tenderness on examination. These rules do not apply to internal derangements, such as ligamentous and meniscal injuries, only to fractures. If riders are capable of continuing, these

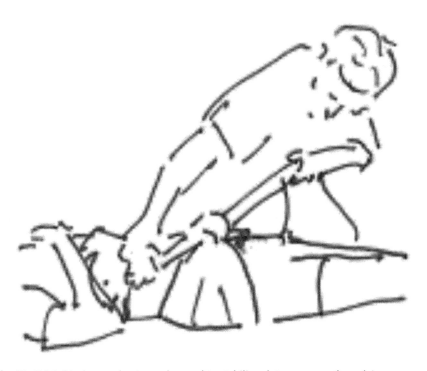

Fig. 15. Pelvic binders or sheets can be used to stabilize clot, compress the pelvic space, and reduce tissue damage.

can be deferred. Typically knee pain is tolerated poorly in competition. Often riders withdraw from competition because this may cause more lasting damage. Foot fractures are rare, presumably due to mechanism, but also may be a protective effect from their rigid footwear[1] (**Fig. 16**).

Soft Tissue Injury

Abrasions (road rash)

Road rash is clinically a burn. Severe road rash should include estimates on body surface area, depth, and management per ATLS protocol, including referral to the appropriate trauma center.[8]

Aside from these critical care concerns, the nature of a burn is a painful, wet, and a potentially large, complicated wound. Unlike most thermal burns, road rash has debris in the wound and needs aggressive cleaning. It is of paramount importance to start irrigating the wound as soon after injury as possible. Often, definitive care occurs at the end of the event.

Soft tissue injuries can include lacerations and involve deeper structures, such as bones, joints, nerves, and blood vessels. It is important to inspect and irrigate the wound soon after injury and assure the wounds are not complicated. If a cyclist is in motion, the rider often can do this themself by being provided water bottles from the team car. If they are hemostatic, wound care generally can be deferred until the end of the event (**Fig. 17**).

In the event they are not hemostatic or any concern for complicated wounds, then riders should be held for wound management. Tourniquets should be applied on discovery of arterial bleeding or any extremity wound causing uncontrolled bleeding.[8]

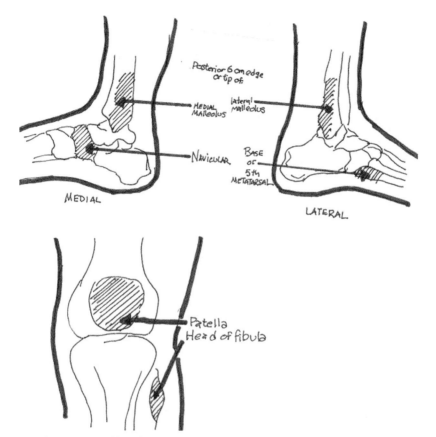

Fig. 16. The Ottawa ankle rules (*top*). Any tenderness on the distal or posterior aspects of the medial or lateral malleolus, on the base of the fifth metatarsal or the navicular bone warrants diagnostic imaging. (*top left and right*) The Ottowa knee rules (*bottom*) On the knee, tenderness of the patella or fibular head is an indicator for diagnostic imaging. As a golden rule, riders must be able to bear weight on injured extremities.

Tourniquets can be applied for 2 consecutive hours with little risk of ischemic damage. With a tourniquet applied emergent transport should be initiated, and wound care can occur during transport or at the medical center.

Water or other sterile solution should be applied under pressure to clean out debris. This improves wound assessment, reduces chances of infection, and improves cosmetics. Irrigation alone is inadequate, and wounds also should be scrubbed using antiseptic solution. Use of topical anesthetics on open wounds causes severe pain upon application and should be avoided. Embedded organic material, such as dirt and mud, needs aggressive cleaning and monitoring for infection. It is reasonable to place a patient on prophylactic antibiotics in the setting of deeply contaminated wounds. Provided neurovascular integrity, these wounds should be irrigated copiously, cleansed, have antiseptic applied, and dressed as time allows and wound dictates. Dressing these wounds can be a challenge provided the time limitations of getting the athlete back into the race.

Wound dressings need to accommodate movement on perspiring skin for hours. Circumferential wrapped dressings, such as gauze, that wrap the extremity are

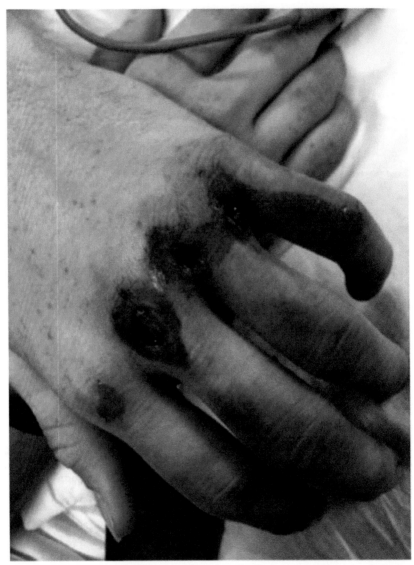

Fig. 17. It is important to assure that soft tissue injuries do not involve any deeper structures, such as bones, joint capsules, nerves, or blood vessels. Management of complicated wounds should not be deferred.

displaced distally with repetitive movement. For the lower extremities, this is particularly true; competitive cyclists ride at approximately 100 revolutions per minute. Wrapping dressings tighter to compensate is tolerated poorly and impedes performance. Adhesive tapes never should be circumferential and should be avoided when possible. For a majority of wounds on the extremities, dressings can be held into position by stocking gauze. There are several flexible and porous tapes that can accommodate movement much better than typical tapes.

Lacerations

Experienced clinicians may elect to use staples or loosely approximated sutures on sterilized wounds to gain hemostasis during competition. These wounds should have definitive repair at the end of the event. Skin staples offer the additional benefit of speed both for hemostasis and for getting an athlete back in competition. Definitive care should avoid use of nylon or other nonabsorbable suture material on lacerations that occur on abraded skin surfaces. These sutures often end up embedded in the wound and their removal can cause complications. Wounds generally should not be closed after 12 hours. Skin adhesives and glues are unlikely to be effective at the time of injury, given the nature of a bleeding and wet wound. They generally can be applied with success after the event. Skin glues and adhesives do not last as long during competition as out of competition but can be valuable tools (**Figs. 18–22**).

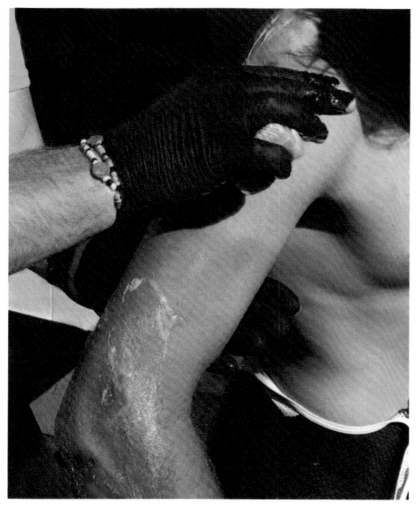

Fig. 18. Cleaning road rash. Area should be copiously irrigated with sterile solution and scrubbed clean of debris with an antiseptic solution.

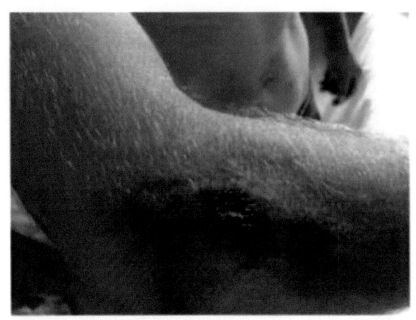

Fig. 19. Road rash after cleaning. Wound is inspected to assure that no deep structures are involved such as joint capsules.

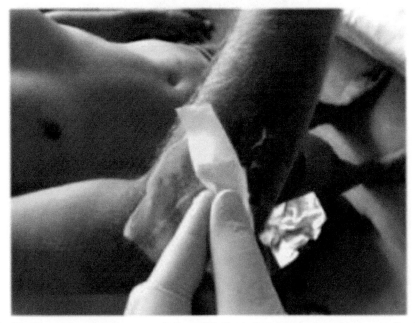

Fig. 20. Wound is covered generously in antibiotic ointment and covered in a nonadhesive dressing.

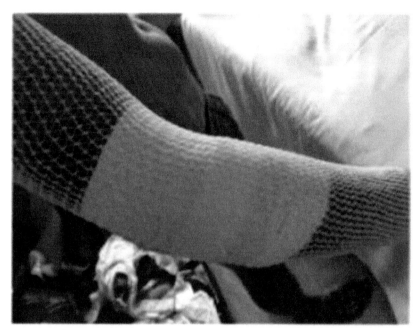

Fig. 21. Nonadhesive dressing is covered with gauze and area secured with stocking gauze. Leave generous margins to prevent slippage.

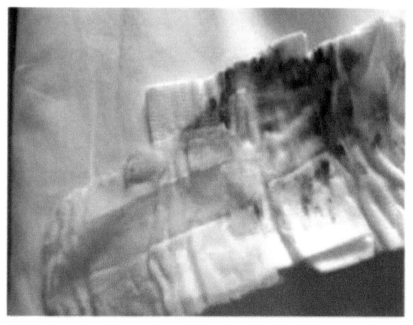

Fig. 22. Dressings after 12 hours. Gauze is fully saturated with dried serosanguinous fluid.

Depending on the depth and extent of injury, wounds typically require dressing changes twice a day for the first 24 hours to 48 hours after injury. They should be monitored closely for infection. Once a wound is dry, it can be left open to the air but should be covered during competition. Wounds can be cleaned gently during the healing process but should not be immersed.

Morel-Lavallée lesions are traumatic, closed degloving injuries that occur most frequently in the lower extremities, especially the upper thigh. Shearing effect on the capillaries occurring deep to subcutaneous plane may result in an effusion containing blood, lymph, and fat. These differ from normal hematomas in their composition, which often makes them difficult to heal without intervention. Externally they may appear the same as a large hematoma, but they fail to heal, become more edematous, and have high complication rates if not identified in the acute phase. MRI is the study of choice, but most can be identified by ultrasound imaging. These lesions often form a capsule, have high rates of infection, and require surgical débridement.[32]

SUMMARY

Physicians providing medical care to cyclists during competition should be prepared to manage a broad array of injuries and practice within ATLS guidelines. Serious injuries can occur and are more likely to involve the chest or brain. A vast majority are soft tissue injuries (road rash) and the riders can continue with competition. In competition, if riders are able to mount the bike after a crash, they generally are allowed to continue. This is not an appropriate screening tool for brain injury. Although the development of protocolized standards for the roadside assessment of concussed riders has been an important step, such steps are still in their infancy. Further developments in the science and technology of concussion diagnosis are likely to have a role in improved care but do not replace better awareness and access.

CLINICAL PEARLS

Bicycling has more in common with motor vehicle than other sports.
Know the ATLS.
Brain injury is the leading cause of death. Concussions are common.
Clavicles are the most fractured bone.
FOOSH mechanisms are common. Beware of the scaphoid.
Riders need to be able to bear weight on the lower extremities to get back on bike
Road rash is a burn. Treat it accordingly.

DISCLAIMER

The author has no conflicts of interest to report.

REFERENCES

1. Greve M, Baird J, Mello M. Health conditions and injury patterns in avid US cyclists : original research article. Int Sportmed J 2014;15:265–74.
2. Stigson, H., Åman, M., and Larsson, M. (2019). Incidence of acute injuries among licensed and non-licensed cyclists using insurance registry data. Conference: International conference on the biomechanics of injury. Florence, September 11-13, 2019.
3. Martinez JM. Medical coverage of cycling events. Curr Sports Med Rep 2006; 5(3):125–30.
4. Noakes TD. Fatal cycling injuries. Sports Med 1995;20(5):348–62.

5. Baldwin GT, Breiding MJ, Dawn Comstock R. Epidemiology of sports concussion in the United States. Handb Clin Neurol 2018;158:63–74.

6. Alfrey EJ, Tracy M, Alfrey JR, et al. Helmet Usage Reduces Serious Head Injury Without Decreasing Concussion After Bicycle Riders Crash. J Surg Res 2021; 257:593–6.

7. Haeberle HS, Navarro SM, Power EJ, et al. Prevalence and Epidemiology of Injuries Among Elite Cyclists in the Tour de France. Orthop J Sports Med 2018; 6(9):232.

8. Galvagno SM Jr, Nahmias JT, Young DA. Advanced Trauma Life Support® Update 2019: Management and Applications for Adults and Special Populations. Anesthesiol Clin 2019;37(1):13–32.

9. Elliott J, Anderson R, Collins S, et al. Sports-related concussion (SRC) assessment in road cycling: a systematic review and call to action. BMJ Open Sport Exerc Med 2019;5(1):525.

10. Heron N, Elliott J, Jones N, et al. Sports-related concussion (SRC) in road cycling: the RoadsIde heaD Injury assEssment (RIDE) for elite road cycling. Br J Sports Med 2020;54(3):127–8.

11. Greve MW, Zink BJ. Pathophysiology of traumatic brain injury. Mt Sinai J Med 2009;76(2):97–104.

12. Geeraerts T, Velly L, Abdennour L, et al. Management of severe traumatic brain injury (first 24hours). Anaesth Crit Care Pain Med 2018;37(2):171–86.

13. Jarrahi A, Braun M, Ahluwalia M, et al. Revisiting Traumatic Brain Injury: From Molecular Mechanisms to Therapeutic Interventions. Biomedicines 2020;8(10):389.

14. Stiell IG, Wells GA, Vandemheen K, et al. The Canadian CT Head Rule for patients with minor head injury. Lancet 2001;357(9266):1391–6.

15. Jackson WT, Starling AJ. Concussion Evaluation and Management. Med Clin North Am 2019;103(2):251–61.

16. Sanchez AR 2nd, Sugalski MT, LaPrade RF. Field-side and prehospital management of the spine-injured athlete. Curr Sports Med Rep 2005;4(1):50–5.

17. Bergaminelli C, Salvi R, Mattiacci DM, et al. Management of chest impalement injury. Int J Surg Case Rep 2019;61:123–6.

18. Winston FK, Shaw KN, Kreshak AA, et al. Hidden spears: handlebars as injury hazards to children. Pediatrics 1998;102(3 Pt 1):596–601.

19. Awad MA, Gaither TW, Murphy GP, et al. Cycling, and Male Sexual and Urinary Function: Results from a Large, Multinational, Cross-Sectional Study. J Urol 2018;199(3):798–804.

20. Gaither TW, Awad MA, Murphy GP, et al. Cycling and Female Sexual and Urinary Function: Results From a Large, Multinational, Cross-Sectional Study. J Sex Med 2018;15(4):510–8.

21. Bjurlin MA, Zhao LC, Goble SM, et al. Bicycle-related genitourinary injuries. Urology 2011;78(5):1187–90.

22. Alarhayem AQ, Cohn SM, Cantu-Nunez O, et al. Impact of time to repair on outcomes in patients with lower extremity arterial injuries. J Vasc Surg 2019;69(5): 1519–23.

23. Quinn RH, Macias DJ. The management of open fractures. Wilderness Environ Med 2006;17(1):41–8.

24. Ropars M, Thomazeau H, Huten D. Clavicle fractures. Orthop Traumatol Surg Res 2017;103(1S):S53–9.

25. Tagliapietra J, Belluzzi E, Biz C, et al. Midshaft Clavicle Fractures Treated Nonoperatively Using Figure-of-Eight Bandage: Are Fracture Type, Shortening, and

Displacement Radiographic Predictors of Failure? Diagnostics (Basel) 2020; 10(10):788.

26. Reichman EF. Sternoclavicular joint dislocation reduction. In: Reichman EF, editor. Emergency medicine procedures. 2nd edition. New York: McGraw Hill; 2013. p. 526–31.

27. Gaines RJ, Wilson A, Antevil J, et al. Parallel plating for a sternomanubrial dislocation. Orthopedics 2012;35(8):e1276–8.

28. LeBlanc KE, Muncie HL Jr, LeBlanc LL. Hip fracture: diagnosis, treatment, and secondary prevention. Am Fam Physician 2014;89(12):945–51.

29. Wood SP, Vrahas M, Wedel SK. Femur fracture immobilization with traction splints in multisystem trauma patients. Prehosp Emerg Care 2003;7(2):241–3.

30. Wedmore I, Young S, Franklin J. Emergency department evaluation and management of foot and ankle pain. Emerg Med Clin North Am 2015;33(2):363–96.

31. Yao K, Haque T. The Ottawa knee rules - a useful clinical decision tool. Aust Fam Physician 2012;41(4):223–4.

32. Porter D, Conley J, Ashurst J. Morel-Lavallée Lesion Following a Low-speed Injury: A Case Report. Clin Pract Cases Emerg Med 2020;4(4):642–4.

Nutrition in Cycling

Namrita Kumar Brooke, PhD, RD*, Ludmila Cosio-Lima, PhD

KEYWORDS

- Sports nutrition • Cycling • Personalized nutrition • Performance
- Periodized nutrition • Energy availability

KEY POINTS

- Athletes should match daily carbohydrate intake to energetic requirements of training and recovery.
- Male and female athletes should closely monitor energy availability throughout the season with the guidance of a qualified nutrition professional.
- Improving function of the gut microbiome through dietary strategies may be beneficial, particularly during periods of intense training and around competitions.
- Athletes should enlist the help of a qualified nutrition professional to establish risk versus reward of training modalities and nutrition interventions (eg, nutrient periodization, supplement usage, and body composition changes).
- Responses to nutrition interventions are highly individual and dependent on training history, training modality, training stress, event characteristics, and athlete goals.

BACKGROUND

The sport of cycling is diverse in nature with events ranging from less than 5 minutes to stage races taking place over several weeks. Overall, cycling, including both on-road and off-road disciplines, is considered an endurance-based sport in which utilization of fuel sources to provide energy and delay fatigue is primarily reliant on the availability of and delivery of oxygen to exercising muscle. There are many factors that can influence cycling power,[1] including athlete physiology, training, and nutrition strategies. When developing nutrition protocols to support cycling performance, the physiologic demands specific to the training or event, corresponding energy systems and fuel requirements, and individual characteristics should be considered. Fat oxidation is a primary contributor to long-duration steady-state cycling; however, most on- and off-road cycling disciplines involve periodic high-intensity bursts (breakaways, hill climbs, technical features, surges, and sprints). Thus, the ability to sustain higher-intensity

Department of Movement Sciences and Health, University of West Florida, 11000 University Parkway Building 782/220, Pensacola, FL 32514, USA
* Corresponding author.
E-mail address: nkumarbrooke@uwf.edu

Phys Med Rehabil Clin N Am 33 (2022) 159–172
https://doi.org/10.1016/j.pmr.2021.08.011
1047-9651/22/© 2021 Elsevier Inc. All rights reserved.

efforts throughout an event can be crucial to the outcome, emphasizing the importance of carbohydrate (CHO) availability for fuel oxidation.[2]

Training periodization involves phasic manipulation of volume, intensity, and training modalities for specific event preparation. To facilitate training adaptation, nutrition can also be periodized to support the physiologic requirements and relative energy demands[3–6] (**Table 1**). General preparation phases typically incorporate high-training volume and emphasize aerobic system development. As competition phase nears, training specificity increases for the goal event. Training intensity may increase to develop the anaerobic system, whereas volume may slightly decrease from the general preparation phase.[7] At a range of exercise intensities, CHO is a key substrate for both aerobic and anaerobic energy production. Thus, a primary goal of a nutrition strategy should be to ensure adequate CHO availability for performance and recovery.[8–11] Acute fueling strategies depend on factors, including the event type and duration, competition goals and relative pace of the athlete, demands of the course and terrain, the ability for an athlete to take in nutrition on the course, and specific environmental conditions. **Table 2** provides a summary of acute fueling strategies for optimizing CHO availability and performance.[8–10,12,13] The varying nature of on- and off-road cycling events poses numerous nutrition-related challenges for athletes (**Box 1**). This review focuses on existing literature that addresses some of these challenges and highlights recent advancements in the area of nutrition for cycling performance.

DISCUSSION
Periodized Nutrition to Optimize Carbohydrate Availability

Success in a competitive cycling event is determined by the ability to sustain the highest possible power output or velocity for the duration of the event. Lipids and CHOs must be readily available to resynthesize ATP to meet energy demands. In lieu of ingesting a chronically high-CHO diet, athletes may benefit from periodizing CHO availability corresponding to relative energy demands of the training cycle. During preparation phases, energy intake should be sufficient to maintain training load, facilitate recovery, and maintain general health (see **Table 1**). Nutrition strategies during the general preparation phase may facilitate body composition changes and fuel utilization adaptations or "metabolic flexibility."[7,14–16] Once specific preparation begins, nutrition interventions should support training and recovery to facilitate the desired responses. Athletes are also advised to incorporate trainings during which race-fueling strategies are practiced and to focus on "training the gut" to better tolerate high rates of CHO (eg, >60–90 g/h) during training and competition.[12,17]

Although nutrient periodization at a macro level parallels training periodization, nutrition can also be periodized at a micro level by optimizing CHO availability around training sessions (see **Table 2**).[8,13] Following exercise, glycogen restoration is a key consideration for recovery, particularly when performance during the subsequent session is important. If daily CHO intake is matched to energy requirements, there does not appear to be a critical "recovery window" in which an athlete should ingest postexercise nutrition.[18] Nevertheless, it is reasonable to advise ingesting postexercise nutrition as soon as is feasible based on convenience and preference.[8] Stage races and back-to-back events present the additional challenge of reduced available recovery time. In these scenarios, cyclists should refuel and rehydrate as promptly as possible following the event. Recommended is 1.0 to 1.2 g CHO/kg-hour for the first 4 hours before resuming normal daily intake.[8] When CHO availability is low, or during periods of energy restriction, there may be benefits to consuming protein with

Table 1
Periodization of training and nutrition

	General Preparation	Specific Preparation	Taper/Competition	Transition/Off-Season
Training focus	Aerobic system High volume Low intensity	Aerobic system Anaerobic system Lower volume Higher intensity Race-specific preparation Competitions begin	Low volume High intensity High specificity	Rest and recovery Cross-training Low volume Low intensity
Nutrition focus	Energy availability to support training, recovery, health, and desired body composition changes, targeted low-CHO availability	Energy availability to support training, recovery, higher intensity, race-specific fueling practice	Support high intensity but lower volume, recovery, race-specific preparation and fueling, nutrition for travel	Nutrition for health
Macronutrient recommendation	~6–12 g/kg-d CHO ~1.2–1.8 g/kg-d protein ~1–2 g/kg-d fat	~6–12 g/kg-d CHO ~1.2–1.8 g/kg-d protein ~1–1.5 g/kg-d fat	~6–12 g/kg-d CHO ~1.2–1.8 g/kg-d protein ~1 g/kg-d fat	~3–5 g/kg-d CHO ~1.2–1.8 g/kg-d protein ~1–1.5 g/kg-d fat

Data from Burke LM, Hawley JA, Wong SH, Jeukendrup AE. Carbohy-drates for training and competition. J Sports Sci. 2011;29 Suppl 1:S17-27; and Stellingwerff T, Maughan RJ, Burke LM. Nutrition for power sports: middle-distance running, track cycling, rowing, canoe-ing/kayaking, and swimming. J Sports Sci. 2011;29 Suppl 1:S79-89; and Mujika I, Halson S, Burke LM, Balague G, Farrow D. An Inte-grated, Multifactorial Approach to Periodization for Optimal Per-formance in Individual and Team Sports. Int J Sports Physiol Perform. 2018;13(5):538-561.

Table 2
Acute fueling strategies

	Purpose	Timing	CHO Intake	Other Considerations
Week of event	General fueling with high CHO foods that are familiar and tolerable for the gut, recovery from training sessions	5–7 d before event	7–12 g/kg-d	Moderate protein and low o moderate fat intake Low GI, complex CHO foods as tolerated
Preevent carbohydrate loading	Glycogen storage in preparation for events >90 min	36–48 h before event	10–12 g/kg per 24-h period	Moderate protein and low to moderate fat intake Low GI, complex CHO foods as tolerated
Preevent fueling	Ensure high CHO availability by topping off glycogen stores and maintaining blood glucose	1–4 h before event	1–4 g/kg	Moderate protein and low to moderate fat intake Low GI CHO foods as tolerated Familiar foods/drinks/supplements should be used to reduce risk of GI distress
During event (45–60 min)	Reduce sensation of fatigue via cental nervous system stimulation	As opportunities for intake are available	Small amounts, including CHO mouth rinse	Exogenous CHO generally not needed <60 min Ingesting small amounts of CHO and/or using CHO mouth rinse may have benefit
During event (1–2.5 h)	Ensure high CHO availability by maintaining blood glucose	As opportunities for intake are available	30–60 g/h	Familiar, tested sports supplements should be used Combination of liquid, gel, solid can be useful Intake depends on preevent fueling, duration and intensity of event, and timing of subsequent event
During event (>2.5 h)	Ensure high CHO availability by maintaining blood glucose	As opportunities for intake are available	30–90 g/h	Familiar, tested sports supplements and foods should be used Combination of liquid, gel, solid may be useful Multiple transportable carbohydrates should be used when CHO intake rates are high

Data from Burke LM, Hawley JA, Wong SH, Jeukendrup AE. Carbohy-drates for training and competition. J Sports Sci. 2011;29 Suppl 1:S17-27

> **Box 1**
> **Key nutrition challenges in cycling**
>
> Dehydration
>
> GI discomfort
>
> Steady-state and high-intensity efforts within a single event
>
> Power to weight
>
> Sprint capability after prolonged endurance effort
>
> Demands of terrain (eg, off-road)
>
> Environmental conditions
>
> Ability to take in nutrition on the course

postexercise CHO.[13,19] However, provided overall adequate energy availability (EA), daily protein intake of ~1.3 to 2.0 g/kg-day,[13,20] and adequate CHO intake,[8,21] there does not appear to be any specific benefit to consuming additional protein around or during training.[20]

Athletes may benefit from periodizing nutrition specific to training phases over the course of a cycling season such that energy and nutrient intake support the physiologic requirements and relative energy demands. CHO is a key substrate for both aerobic and anaerobic energy production and is important for cycling performance in most on- and off-road disciplines. Thus, in addition to overall energy intake, CHO availability should be a consideration for each athlete around and during training and competition.

Metabolic Flexibility

In theory, an athlete would benefit from optimizing use of all available muscular fuel stores for ATP resynthesis. The possibility of improving performance by enhancing fat oxidation at a higher percent of aerobic capacity[22] while maintaining the capability to oxidize CHO (eg, during a surge, breakaway, climb, or sprint) is a tempting prospect. With this in mind, cyclists use various training and nutrition strategies to attain a level of "metabolic flexibility."[14] Periodization of CHO and fat in the diet has been investigated as a strategy to optimize utilization of both substrates.[23–26] Studies have reported metabolic alterations and higher fat oxidation following ~5 days of a low-CHO high-fat (LCHF) protocol[24] before restoration of CHO availability. However, LCHF does not appear to improve performance when compared with a higher CHO diet.[14,27,28] Havemann and colleagues[27] reported impaired 100 km time trial (TT) time, reduced sprint power, and impaired glycogen oxidation, suggesting compromised CHO utilization after LCHF diet followed by restoration of CHO availability. Another study[29] examining long-term (>6 months) LCHF diet reported higher plasma glucose and delayed insulin response postoral glucose tolerance test, and decreased insulin receptor substrate IRS1 and glucose transporter protein GLUT4 in skeletal muscle, compared with cyclists following a mixed diet. It is unclear if these results suggest impaired glucose handling at rest or simply a temporary adaptation to an LCHF diet.

Enhancing fat oxidation at the expense of decreased CHO utilization carries the penalty of higher metabolic cost[24,30]; for an elite athlete, reduced economy and possible impairment of glycogen utilization would be counterproductive to optimal performance. Future research may uncover protocols effective in increasing utilization of exogenous CHO to compensate for impairments following LCHF diet.[14] However, outcomes of any such strategies are likely to be variable, highly individual, and dependent on training history, training modality, event characteristics, and athlete goals.[3,31] In a review of CHO periodization strategies, Stellingwerff and colleagues[5] emphasize that risk versus reward of such interventions should be evaluated for an individual athlete, and, that evidence to support metabolic adaptations translating to performance improvements remain equivocal.[5,26] In practice, certain training sessions that are less CHO-dependent (eg, steady-state training below lactate threshold) may be better suited for "train low CHO" modalities compared with implementing chronic (>3–5 days) LCHF,[5] which may add excessive strain to an athlete's training cycle.

Time-restricted eating (TRE) methods popularized by social media are increasingly common among athletes. However, evidence to support a benefit of TRE strategies on health or performance in athlete populations is lacking, and support in favor of TRE is overwhelmingly anecdotal. Metcalfe and colleagues[32] compared the effects of omitting breakfast on an evening 20 km TT; extension of the overnight fast until noon increased appetite and rating of perceived exertion, decreased power output (3%), and impaired time trial performance compared with ingesting a morning breakfast. Athletes who subscribe to forms of TRE may perceive benefits from alternative eating strategies and thus continue to abide by them despite a lack of current evidence supporting a performance benefit.

For cycling athletes whose primary goal is performance, the ability to use CHO is paramount for sustaining power and velocity. Currently, because there is insufficient evidence to suggest that LCHF and TRE strategies would improve cycling performance, it seems prudent to focus on adequate CHO availability to support workload and recovery during preparation and competition phases. Under guidance of a qualified nutrition professional and coach, athletes may carefully consider alternative dietary interventions during transition or general preparation phases, provided the interventions are specific to the overall goals of the athlete and the training plan.

Energy Availability

Athletes' energy needs fluctuate with changes in exercise volume and intensity. EA, the amount of energy available for the body to support normal physiologic functions after the cost of exercise is subtracted,[33] is related to optimal health and performance. EA is calculated as the difference between daily energy intake and exercise energy expenditure, relative to fat free mass (FFM). Chronic insufficient or low EA (LEA) may be associated with a variety of physiologic consequences; however, the threshold for LEA is not well defined, and impairments instead appear to occur over a continuum of reduced EA. It has been suggested that men may not experience impairments until lower values of EA compared with women,[34,35] but responses appear to be variable and highly individual. Female athletes reportedly have lower EA compared with men; athletes who intentionally restrict energy intake are at higher risk of long-term LEA complications.[36] Relative Energy Deficiency in Sport (RED-S) encompasses complications that may result in both male and female athletes as a result of chronic LEA. Adverse health outcomes in RED-S may occur in "menstrual function, bone health, endocrine, metabolic, hematological, growth and development, psychological, cardiovascular, gastrointestinal, and immunological systems."[13,37] Therefore, it is not surprising that performance would also be compromised, possibly manifesting as "decreased endurance, increased injury risk, decreased training response, impaired judgment, decreased coordination, decreased concentration, irritability, depression, decreased glycogen stores, or decreased muscle strength."[37]

At most levels in the sport of on- and off-road cycling, there is a common belief that leanness is a performance advantage. At the elite level, flat-terrain specialists generally focus on absolute power, whereas climbers aim to achieve a higher power-to-weight ratio (relative power), typically weigh less, and have leaner physiques.[38] Cyclists may intentionally restrict energy intake in an attempt to achieve a certain physique or body mass. It is also not unusual for athletes to undergo periods of very-high training stress and high-volume training blocks without a parallel increase in energy intake, resulting in unintentional LEA. Schofield and colleagues[34] highlighted the prevalence of LEA and markers of RED-S in male cyclists in periods of training and competition. LEA was associated with lower bone mineral density, decreased testosterone, decreased IGF-1, increased cortisol, and decreased resting metabolic rate (RMR), supporting that male athletes are also susceptible to metabolic and hormonal impairments in response to LEA. Stenqvist and colleagues[35] observed indications of RED-S in male cyclists after a 4-week training block. Participants improved performance markers (peak power output, VO_{2peak}, and functional threshold power), increased total testosterone, and did not change body weight, body composition, or energy intake while maintaining EA of 46 kcal/kg FFM-day. Despite these findings, the participants presented with decreased RMR, decreased T3, and increased cortisol levels. Thus, it is important for both male and female athletes and their coaches and nutritionists to closely monitor EA, particularly during periods of intensified training throughout the season. When left unaddressed, LEA may result in long-term consequences, but athletes who are able to increase EA with guided nutrition advice may restore levels of performance.[34,39]

During the competitive season, cyclists may be required to perform on back-to-back days or multiple times per week, possibly for several weeks at a time. In these scenarios, it can be challenging for cyclists to maintain EA, performance, and recovery throughout the season. Periodized nutrition guidelines (see **Tables 1** and **2**) provide a general framework for adjusting energy intake and macronutrient intake to "fuel for the work required."[26] However, in practice, cyclists may tend to intentionally or unintentionally undereat or overeat on a rest day, particularly when competitions are frequent. Heikura and colleagues[40] examined EA, CHO availability, and associated hormonal changes in professional male cyclists competing in the "Spring Classics," 4 single-day races over an 8-day period. Nutrition data were averaged over the 4 race days and 4 rest days and compared. Mean ($\pm$ standard deviation) EA for the athletes was 14 (8) kcal/kg FFM-day on race days compared with 57 (10) on rest days. Interestingly, alternating LEA with higher EA over 8 days was associated with a trend of decreased testosterone, decreased IGF-1, and decreased hemoglobin despite no change in body mass or body fat percentage. These findings suggest the physiologic perturbations resulting from short-term intermittent LEA may also be of consequence to otherwise healthy athletes performing at the highest level in the sport. The authors suggest that nutrition protocols for professional cyclists appear to be more aggressive during stage racing compared with the single-day races. In stage races, during-race intake is higher with the intention of supporting energy requirements of the current stage while also considering the subsequent stage.[40] In contrast, riders competing in frequent single-day races may be affected by intermittent LEA if they consume less energy and CHO during and following the race, knowing the subsequent day is not a race day.

Because it may be difficult to observe the effects of intentional or unintentional LEA before long-term consequences develop, athletes are advised to work with their dietitian and coach to monitor EA and related physiologic markers throughout the season. Because the threshold for LEA likely differs between individuals, body mass and body composition should be monitored in addition to measures related to sleep, mood, perceived effort, perceived energy and fatigue, and performance levels.

The Athlete's Gut

Although general endurance nutrition recommendations referred to in this review are accepted in the scientific literature and in practice, there are many individual factors[13,31,41] that necessitate a personalized approach to nutrition for training and performance. Individual factors influence energy intake, macronutrient ratios and micronutrient requirements, eating behavior, and efficacy of supplements.[31] Gut tolerance to sports nutrition products during exercise of varying duration and intensities also remains individual. CHO recommendations can be met with a variety of sources, including drinks, gels, and solid foods, and should be chosen according to personal preferences.[41] In order to maximize performance by increasing the absorptive capacity of the gut[17] and minimize chances of gastrointestinal (GI) distress during exercise, athletes should carefully test fueling strategies before an event.[12,41]

The gut microbiome may also influence food and supplement tolerance and related GI distress commonly experienced in endurance cycling. The gut microbiome affects nutrient uptake, vitamin synthesis, inflammation, and immune function[42]; thus, its function is fundamental to an athlete's overall health, exercise performance, and recovery. Weekly exercise time appears to be correlated with increased presence of gut bacteria associated with CHO and amino acid metabolism and a healthier metabolic profile.[42] Although chronic exercise appears to improve the diversity of the microbiome, it has also been suggested[43,44] that an acute bout of prolonged exercise can result in damage to enterocytes, ischemia, and possible cramping and diarrhea, particularly if the athlete is also dehydrated. An athlete's diet[45,46] also influences the microbiome.[42] The effect of protein intake on gut microbiota appears to depend on type of protein (animal vs plant), protein quality and digestibility, nutritional status, body composition of the athlete, and relative exercise intensity.[42] High-fiber CHO increases the diversity and richness of gut bacteria,[47] and in turn fermentation processes by bacteria yield byproducts that are beneficial to exercise recovery, performance, and body composition.[42] Despite health benefits of complex CHO, athletes often consume low-fiber CHO before and during exercise to reduce the likelihood of GI distress. Even when opportunities for consuming complex CHO in the regular diet are plenty, athletes may continue to self-select lower-fiber diets,[48,49] thereby compromising the microbiome and its effects on the immune system, metabolism, and performance.[42] Given that intense or prolonged exercise can have adverse effects on an athlete's gut, it is recommended that athletes take additional care to improve function of the gut microbiome through dietary strategies, particularly during periods of intense training and around competitions. In addition to prioritizing overall CHO intake, athletes should attempt to include a variety of complex, higher-fiber, nutrient-rich foods in their regular diet to meet their CHO needs. Further research can elucidate the specific dietary and supplement components that may be of benefit to athletes.

Hydration

Fluid consumption during prolonged cycling (>1 hours) decreases perceived exertion, reduces feelings of thirst, decreases thermal and cardiovascular strain, decreases glycogen utilization, and can improve performance when duration is greater than 1 hour. However, fluid intake during events less than 1 hour may decrease performance, likely because of feelings of bloating or other GI discomfort.[50,51] A meta-analysis[50] suggests a correlation between fluid intake of 0.15 to 0.27 mL/kg-min and increased power output during cycling greater than 1 hour in temperate to warm ambient conditions. Because athletes may not consume fluids reaching this range when ad libitum drinking "to thirst," drinking according to a planned rate may be a more effective hydration strategy[51] to avoid dehydration and improve performance during prolonged cycling.[50] Provided the athlete can establish euhydration before the event, preexercise hydration during a warmup period may also influence performance during the event in moderate ambient conditions. When developing and implementing a hydration strategy, environmental conditions, duration and intensity, and the athlete's perception of thirst, fullness, temperature, and energy should all be considered. Individual characteristics, such as age, body size, metabolic efficiency, heat acclimation status, and gender, also influence hydration considerations. Older athletes may have decreased thirst sensitivity when dehydrated; they may also be at greater risk of hyponatremia owing to blunted renal response to water and sodium.[51] Women typically have lower sweat rates and electrolyte losses compared with men[51] but may also have greater diuretic response to water load compared with men because of reduced arginine vasopressin (AVP) response.[52] However, estrogen increases AVP release, and both estrogen and progesterone increase water and electrolyte retention,[53] contributing to an increase in total body water.[54] Therefore, it has been suggested that women may be at higher risk of hyponatremia,[36] particularly during the luteal phase of the menstrual cycle when estrogen and progesterone are present in higher levels. Although it is acknowledged that the menstrual cycle, oral contraceptive use, and fluctuations in sex hormones may influence factors relating to hydration status (eg, internal body temperature, thirst, and other fluid regulatory functions),[36,55,56] the impacts on performance are less clear.[56] A systematic review and meta-analysis did not observe a strong or consistent relationship between menstrual cycle phase and performance; the authors emphasize the importance of furthering physiologic research in female athletes using more robust methodological procedures. Specifically, investigations should quantify hormone status with blood analysis, enabling physiologic and performance markers to be meaningfully compared between menstrual cycle phases.[57] Currently, there is insufficient evidence to make generalized recommendations to female athletes; thus, coaches and nutritionists should work with female athletes on an individual basis.

Nutrition support to prevent dehydration is an additional challenge for cyclists, particularly during long distance or back-to-back events, such as stage racing, and in hot and humid or high-altitude environments. However, athletes must balance avoidance of dehydration with avoidance of drinking in excess of sweat rate.[51] When athletes need to reestablish euhydration and electrolyte balance before an event such as a stage race, prehydration with 5 to 7 mL/kg fluid containing 20 to 50 mEq/L of sodium greater than 4 hours before the event may be beneficial.[51] At higher elevations (>4000 m), athletes may need to compensate for water losses from increased ventilation (1900 mL/d in men and 850 mL/d in women)[58] and urinary losses of ~500 mL/d.[59] When training or competing at altitude or in extreme environments, cyclists are recommended to monitor daily hydration and fluid balance using body mass measurement, and to increase fluid intake as needed to offset higher fluid losses.[60]

Hydration needs vary between individuals and fluctuate for each individual athlete according to heat acclimation status, season and environmental conditions, hormonal status, and duration and intensity of exercise. Athletes may implement general hydration recommendations in conjunction with measuring preexercise and postexercise body mass measurement and assessing perception of thirst to develop and adapt optimal hydration strategies throughout the cycling season.

Supplements

Use of ergogenic aids is prevalent in cycling, as athletes, particularly elite and older athletes,[13] are savvy to new technologies and products that may provide a competitive edge. Ergogenic aids used in cycling are generally categorized by their ability to reduce fatigue, reduce perceived effort, improve perceived energy, influence oxygen delivery and exercise economy, influence muscular properties and function, or provide buffering capabilities. Athletes seeking improvements in performance, recovery, and general health and well-being[61] may use supplements; however, a high proportion of athletes are not aware of the associated risks, including possible contamination, adverse effects and interactions, or simply the absence of active ingredients.[61–63] Many athletes use supplements without consulting with a sports nutrition professional, instead relying on self-guided research, social media, or other prominent spokespeople or sponsored athletes.[61,62] Relatively few supplements have ergogenic benefits that are supported by strong evidence.[13,18,63,64] Individual responses to supplements are variable; many studies have been conducted in narrow populations, making it difficult to translate results to others.[65,66] Although possibly improving performance, certain supplementation protocols may also inhibit desired training adaptations; thus, athletes considering supplement use are advised to consult with a sports nutrition professional[63] to complete a risk versus reward analysis before usage.[5,63]

SUMMARY

Cycling encompasses a variety of disciplines, each with a multitude of variables that influence physiologic demands and nutritional challenges. It is also common for athletes to participate in different types of cycling events over the course of a year. Combined with high interindividual variability within the sport, there exist endless combinations of potential training and nutrition interventions. Although general fueling recommendations referred to within this review can be applied for both amateur and professional cyclists, responses to training and nutrition interventions are individual. Thus, nutrition strategy should be approached on a personalized basis, continually adapting to the needs of the athlete. It is advantageous for athletes to work closely with a coach and a qualified nutrition professional when evaluating training modalities and nutrition interventions (eg, nutrient periodization protocols, supplement usage, and body composition changes). Finally, there continue to be many promising areas of research in nutrition for cycling, particularly relating to genomics, the gut microbiome, and in specific populations such as the female athlete.

CLINICS CARE POINTS

- Athletes should match daily carbohydrate intake to energetic requirements of training and recovery.
- Provided daily carbohydrate intake is adequate, athletes should ingest postexercise nutrition as soon as is feasible based on convenience and preference.
- Despite possible metabolic changes following LCHF diet, the effect on performance is equivocal when compared with a mixed diet.
- Training sessions that are less carbohydrate-dependent may be better suited for "train low" (carbohydrate) modalities.
- Improving function of the gut microbiome through dietary strategies may be beneficial during periods of intense training and competition.

- Fluid intake of 0.15 to 0.27 mL/kg-min may benefit performance in temperate to warm ambient conditions during cycling greater than 1-hour duration.
- Many athletes are not aware of associated risks with supplementation and should consult with a nutrition professional.
- Findings from research studies conducted in narrow populations may not translate to other groups within the diverse sport of cycling.

DISCLOSURE

The authors have nothing to disclose.

REFERENCES

1. Atkinson G, Davison R, Jeukendrup A, et al. Science and cycling: current knowledge and future directions for research. J Sports Sci 2003;21(9):767–87.
2. Romijn JA, Coyle EF, Sidossis LS, et al. Regulation of endogenous fat and carbohydrate metabolism in relation to exercise intensity and duration. Am J Physiol 1993;265(3 Pt 1):E380–91.
3. Burke LM, Castell LM, Casa DJ, et al. International Association of Athletics Federations consensus statement 2019: nutrition for athletics. Int J Sport Nutr Exerc Metab 2019;29(2):73–84.
4. Jeukendrup AE. Periodized nutrition for athletes. Sports Med 2017;47(Suppl 1): 51–63.
5. Stellingwerff T, Morton JP, Burke LM. A framework for periodized nutrition for athletics. Int J Sport Nutr Exerc Metab 2019;29(2):141–51.
6. Stellingwerff T, Maughan RJ, Burke LM. Nutrition for power sports: middle-distance running, track cycling, rowing, canoeing/kayaking, and swimming. J Sports Sci 2011;29(Suppl 1):S79–89.
7. Mujika I, Halson S, Burke LM, et al. An integrated, multifactorial approach to periodization for optimal performance in individual and team sports. Int J Sports Physiol Perform 2018;13(5):538–61.
8. Burke LM, Hawley JA, Wong SH, et al. Carbohydrates for training and competition. J Sports Sci 2011;29(Suppl 1):S17–27.
9. Cermak NM, van Loon LJ. The use of carbohydrates during exercise as an ergogenic aid. Sports Med 2013;43(11):1139–55.
10. Hargreaves M, Hawley JA, Jeukendrup A. Pre-exercise carbohydrate and fat ingestion: effects on metabolism and performance. J Sports Sci 2004;22(1):31–8.
11. Jeukendrup AE. Carbohydrate intake during exercise and performance. Nutrition 2004;20(7–8):669–77.
12. Jeukendrup AE. Nutrition for endurance sports: marathon, triathlon, and road cycling. J Sports Sci 2011;29(Suppl 1):S91–9.
13. Thomas DT, Erdman KA, Burke LM. American College of Sports Medicine Joint Position Statement. Nutrition and athletic performance. Med Sci Sports Exerc 2016;48(3):543–68.
14. Burke LM. Ketogenic low-CHO, high-fat diet: the future of elite endurance sport? J Physiol 2021;599(3):819–43.
15. Hulston CJ, Venables MC, Mann CH, et al. Training with low muscle glycogen enhances fat metabolism in well-trained cyclists. Med Sci Sports Exerc 2010;42(11): 2046–55.

16. Yeo WK, McGee SL, Carey AL, et al. Acute signalling responses to intense endurance training commenced with low or normal muscle glycogen. Exp Physiol 2010;95(2):351–8.

17. Cox GR, Clark SA, Cox AJ, et al. Daily training with high carbohydrate availability increases exogenous carbohydrate oxidation during endurance cycling. J Appl Physiol (1985) 2010;109(1):126–34.

18. Kerksick CM, Wilborn CD, Roberts MD, et al. ISSN exercise & sports nutrition review update: research & recommendations. J Int Soc Sports Nutr 2018;15(1):38.

19. Jentjens RL, van Loon LJ, Mann CH, et al. Addition of protein and amino acids to carbohydrates does not enhance postexercise muscle glycogen synthesis. J Appl Physiol (1985) 2001;91(2):839–46.

20. Phillips SM, Van Loon LJ. Dietary protein for athletes: from requirements to optimum adaptation. J Sports Sci 2011;29(Suppl 1):S29–38.

21. Alghannam AF, Gonzalez JT, Betts JA. Restoration of muscle glycogen and functional capacity: role of post-exercise carbohydrate and protein co-ingestion. Nutrients 2018;10(2):253.

22. Volek JS, Noakes T, Phinney SD. Rethinking fat as a fuel for endurance exercise. Eur J Sport Sci 2015;15(1):13–20.

23. Burke LM. Re-examining high-fat diets for sports performance: did we call the 'nail in the coffin' too soon? Sports Med 2015;45(Suppl 1):S33–49.

24. Burke LM, Hawley JA, Jeukendrup A, et al. Toward a common understanding of diet-exercise strategies to manipulate fuel availability for training and competition preparation in endurance sport. Int J Sport Nutr Exerc Metab 2018;28(5):451–63.

25. Burke LM, Whitfield J, Heikura IA, et al. Adaptation to a low carbohydrate high fat diet is rapid but impairs endurance exercise metabolism and performance despite enhanced glycogen availability. J Physiol 2021;599(3):771–90.

26. Impey SG, Hearris MA, Hammond KM, et al. Fuel for the work required: a theoretical framework for carbohydrate periodization and the glycogen threshold hypothesis. Sports Med 2018;48(5):1031–48.

27. Havemann L, West SJ, Goedecke JH, et al. Fat adaptation followed by carbohydrate loading compromises high-intensity sprint performance. J Appl Physiol (1985) 2006;100(1):194–202.

28. Burke LM, Angus DJ, Cox GR, et al. Effect of fat adaptation and carbohydrate restoration on metabolism and performance during prolonged cycling. J Appl Physiol (1985) 2000;89(6):2413–21.

29. Webster CC, van Boom KM, Armino N, et al. Reduced glucose tolerance and skeletal muscle GLUT4 and IRS1 content in cyclists habituated to a long-term low-carbohydrate, high-fat diet. Int J Sport Nutr Exerc Metab 2020;1–8.

30. Shaw DM, Merien F, Braakhuis A, et al. Effect of a ketogenic diet on submaximal exercise capacity and efficiency in runners. Med Sci Sports Exerc 2019;51(10):2135–46.

31. Guest NS, Horne J, Vanderhout SM, et al. Sport nutrigenomics: personalized nutrition for athletic performance. Front Nutr 2019;6:8.

32. Metcalfe RS, Thomas M, Lamb C, et al. Omission of a carbohydrate-rich breakfast impairs evening endurance exercise performance despite complete dietary compensation at lunch. Eur J Sport Sci 2020;21(7):1013–21.

33. Loucks AB, Stachenfeld NS, DiPietro L. The female athlete triad: do female athletes need to take special care to avoid low energy availability? Med Sci Sports Exerc 2006;38(10):1694–700.

34. Schofield KL, Thorpe H, Sims ST. Where are all the men? Low energy availability in male cyclists: a review. Eur J Sport Sci 2020;1–12.

35. Stenqvist TB, Torstveit MK, Faber J, et al. Impact of a 4-week intensified endurance training intervention on markers of relative energy deficiency in sport (RED-S) and performance among well-trained male cyclists. Front Endocrinol (Lausanne) 2020;11:512365.
36. Rossi KA. Nutritional aspects of the female athlete. Clin Sports Med 2017;36(4): 627–53.
37. Mountjoy M, Sundgot-Borgen J, Burke L, et al. The IOC consensus statement: beyond the female athlete triad–relative energy deficiency in sport (RED-S). Br J Sports Med 2014;48(7):491–7.
38. Mujika I, Padilla S. Physiological and performance characteristics of male professional road cyclists. Sports Med 2001;31(7):479–87.
39. Keay N, Francis G, Entwistle I, et al. Clinical evaluation of education relating to nutrition and skeletal loading in competitive male road cyclists at risk of relative energy deficiency in sports (RED-S): 6-month randomised controlled trial. BMJ Open Sport Exerc Med 2019;5(1):e000523.
40. Heikura IA, Quod M, Strobel N, et al. Alternate-day low energy availability during spring classics in professional cyclists. Int J Sports Physiol Perform 2019;1233–43.
41. Jeukendrup A. A step towards personalized sports nutrition: carbohydrate intake during exercise. Sports Med 2014;44(Suppl 1):S25–33.
42. Mohr AE, Jäger R, Carpenter KC, et al. The athletic gut microbiota. J Int Soc Sports Nutr 2020;17(1):24.
43. de Oliveira EP, Burini RC. The impact of physical exercise on the gastrointestinal tract. Curr Opin Clin Nutr Metab Care 2009;12(5):533–8.
44. Oktedalen O, Lunde OC, Opstad PK, et al. Changes in the gastrointestinal mucosa after long-distance running. Scand J Gastroenterol 1992;27(4):270–4.
45. Flint HJ, Duncan SH, Scott KP, et al. Links between diet, gut microbiota composition and gut metabolism. Proc Nutr Soc 2015;74(1):13–22.
46. Jang LG, Choi G, Kim SW, et al. The combination of sport and sport-specific diet is associated with characteristics of gut microbiota: an observational study. J Int Soc Sports Nutr 2019;16(1):21.
47. Tap J, Furet JP, Bensaada M, et al. Gut microbiota richness promotes its stability upon increased dietary fibre intake in healthy adults. Environ Microbiol 2015; 17(12):4954–64.
48. Clark A, Mach N. Exercise-induced stress behavior, gut-microbiota-brain axis and diet: a systematic review for athletes. J Int Soc Sports Nutr 2016;13:43.
49. Rehrer NJ, van Kemenade M, Meester W, et al. Gastrointestinal complaints in relation to dietary intake in triathletes. Int J Sport Nutr 1992;2(1):48–59.
50. Holland JJ, Skinner TL, Irwin CG, et al. The influence of drinking fluid on endurance cycling performance: a meta-analysis. Sports Med 2017;47(11):2269–84.
51. Sawka MN, Burke LM, Eichner ER, et al. American College of Sports Medicine position stand. Exercise and fluid replacement. Med Sci Sports Exerc 2007; 39(2):377–90.
52. Stachenfeld NS, Splenser AE, Calzone WL, et al. Sex differences in osmotic regulation of AVP and renal sodium handling. J Appl Physiol (1985) 2001;91(4): 1893–901.
53. Stachenfeld NS, Silva C, Keefe DL. Estrogen modifies the temperature effects of progesterone. J Appl Physiol (1985) 2000;88(5):1643–9.
54. Armstrong LE, Johnson EC, McKenzie AL, et al. Endurance cyclist fluid intake, hydration status, thirst, and thermal sensations: gender differences. Int J Sport Nutr Exerc Metab 2016;26(2):161–7.

55. Giersch GEW, Charkoudian N, Stearns RL, et al. Fluid balance and hydration considerations for women: review and future directions. Sports Med 2020;50(2): 253–61.

56. Giersch GEW, Morrissey MC, Katch RK, et al. Menstrual cycle and thermoregulation during exercise in the heat: a systematic review and meta-analysis. J Sci Med Sport 2020;23(12):1134–40.

57. McNulty KL, Elliott-Sale KJ, Dolan E, et al. The effects of menstrual cycle phase on exercise performance in eumenorrheic women: a systematic review and meta-analysis. Sports Med 2020;50(10):1813–27.

58. Mawson JT, Braun B, Rock PB, et al. Women at altitude: energy requirement at 4,300 m. J Appl Physiol (1985) 2000;88(1):272–81.

59. Butterfield GE. 19, Maintenance of body weight at altitude: In search of 500 kcal/day. In: Marriott BMCS, editor. Nutritional needs in Cold and high-altitude environments: applications for personnel in field operations. Washington, DC: National Academies Press (US); 1996.

60. Michalczyk M, Czuba M, Zydek G, et al. Dietary recommendations for cyclists during altitude training. Nutrients 2016;8(6):377.

61. Baltazar-Martins G, Brito de Souza D, Aguilar-Navarro M, et al. Prevalence and patterns of dietary supplement use in elite Spanish athletes. J Int Soc Sports Nutr 2019;16(1):30.

62. Gallardo EJ, Coggan AR. What's in your beet juice? Nitrate and nitrite content of beet juice products marketed to athletes. Int J Sport Nutr Exerc Metab 2019; 29(4):345–9.

63. Maughan RJ, Burke LM, Dvorak J, et al. IOC consensus statement: dietary supplements and the high-performance athlete. Br J Sports Med 2018;52(7):439–55.

64. Jeukendrup A, Tipton KD. Legal nutritional boosting for cycling. Curr Sports Med Rep 2009;8(4):186–91.

65. Senefeld JW, Wiggins CC, Regimbal RJ, et al. Ergogenic effect of nitrate supplementation: a systematic review and meta-analysis. Med Sci Sports Exerc 2020; 52(10):2250–61.

66. Wickham KA, Spriet LL. No longer beeting around the bush: a review of potential sex differences with dietary nitrate supplementation[1]. Appl Physiol Nutr Metab 2019;44(9):915–24.

A Coaching Perspective on Modern Training Metrics and Return from Injury and Illness

Kolie Moore, BS Biology

KEYWORDS

• Cycling • Injury • Illness • Training • Coaching • Recovery • Power • RPE

KEY POINTS

- Competitive and noncompetitive cyclists have metrics and models to quantify performance, including power, heart rate, and rating of perceived exertion
- Medical treatment providers can utilize training metrics to guide athletes' volume and intensity during return from illness and injury.
- Recovery from injury and illness can be energy intensive, and training too hard can delay the process, so ensuring common language via modern cycling metrics can lead to optimal outcomes.
- Power and rating of perceived exertion can be compared with monitor readiness to increase training intensity.
- Breaks in training required by the recovery process often is beneficial for cyclists and leads to improved fitness after a period of retraining.

INTRODUCTION

This article is a coaching perspective on returning to training and competition after illness or injury. Much of the following is opinion and should be taken as such, but, where physiologic mechanisms are known, they are referenced. My experience in coaching and consulting for athletes during return from injury and illness (RFII) includes noncompetitive cyclists, average cyclists, and elite regional cyclists as well as world class professionals.

In an ideal world, sporting injuries should be rare, but no activity is without risks. My experience coaching athletes during periods of stress or RFII almost always is done with some level of contact with a physician or physical therapist, although, in some populations without individual coaching feedback (discussed later), the treatment provider may be a cyclist's only point of contact, so more explicit guidance in training may be needed.

132 S Main Street, White River Junction, VT 05001, USA
E-mail address: empiricalcycling@gmail.com

Phys Med Rehabil Clin N Am 33 (2022) 173–186
https://doi.org/10.1016/j.pmr.2021.08.012
1047-9651/22/© 2021 Elsevier Inc. All rights reserved.

The purpose of this article is to introduce power-derived metrics to physicians and explore their utility in assisting cyclists in RFII. Training stress needs to be managed carefully for recreational, intermediate, and well-trained cyclists. This means understanding the benefits and drawbacks of modern cycling tools, including metrics, analytics, and estimations of significant physiologic thresholds in relation to everyday training and managing training stress during RFII.

The 3 different populations of recreational, semicoached, and coached cyclists are described in this article, based on the type of guidance and needs that a care provider may encounter. These populations were constructed for the purpose of describing and understanding different training loads and metrics, general amount of training stress, and potential complicating factors in guiding RFII.

MODERN CYCLING POWER METRICS

Cycling is one of several unique sports where nearly all work is performed through an external device. At many points in a bicycle drivetrain, between a foot and the driven wheel, it is possible to measure a person's work over time and thus power output. Cycling, therefore, is an easily quantifiable sport, although other sports, such as running and rowing, have developed similar methodologies.

Human performance on a bicycle can be quantified with a power meter (PM), although other methodologies can be utilized, such as rating of perceived effort (RPE) and heart rate (HR). It is power output as measured by a PM that forms the basis of the common modern training metrics. They are summarized with their most commonly used names.

The largest benefit of training with power is that it provides a consistent and objective measurement of effort level, both in absolute terms comparing cyclists with each other and tracking a cyclist's fitness or fatigue over time. A watt is defined as a work rate of 1 J per second. When combined with HR and RPE, a coach or athlete can assess the true state of fitness or fatigue more accurately. For example, if a regular workout prescribed by power is performed at a lower HR and RPE than usual, it might be inferred that an athlete is becoming more fit. On the other hand, if the same workout is performed with higher HR or RPE than usual, it can be interpreted as a sign of fatigue or detraining.

The most effective training typically does not use power, HR, or RPE in a vacuum; each provides important context for the others. Additional dimensionality occurs when putting HR and RPE in the context of other power-derived training metrics.

Familiarity with modern training metrics and the different cycling populations should aid in communicating with cyclists during treatment as well as ensuring that general terms like *rest*, *easy*, or *functional threshold of power* (*FTP*) have a common understanding. In this way, training guidelines or guidance during RFII can be prescribed in terms that cyclists generally use with each other.

Functional Threshold of Power

Some of the most commonly used metrics have a basis in physiology, and others are models that have benefits and drawbacks. FTP is the most popular, and is meant to represent work rate at maximal lactate steady state (MLSS).[1] Various methods exist to measure an athlete's FTP, but with modern power analysis programs, such as WKO5 (TrainingPeaks, Boulder, CO, USA), they generally are unnecessary. As shown in **Fig. 1**, FTP can be determined visually as an inflection point on a curve of aggregated mean maximal power (MMP), or highest average, data. Time ranges for finding the FTP inflection point is between 35 minutes and 75 minutes, although exceptions

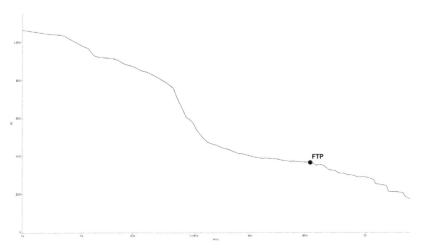

Fig. 1. MMP (W) plotted against logarithmic duration (in hours, minutes, and seconds) for an elite amateur athlete. The inflection point of FTP is noted and easily determined.

exist (personal observation). Normal values for trained adult men range from 200W to 400W and for adult women 100W to 300W. This value is related to Vo_{2max} (discussed later) and can fall with age or detraining.

FTP can be used to set training targets, based on a percentage below or above. This has a benefit in that as interval time at a particular power target is increased successfully, fitness is increasing. The drawback can be, however, that some methods to estimate FTP can overestimate it to enough that normal interval ranges are too fatiguing. Significant time training near or over MLSS without sufficient rest can lead to nonfunctional overreaching and overtraining. Underestimation of FTP occurs but seems to be a rare occurrence and does not lead to such outcomes.

There are many studies comparing the relationship between MLSS, FTP, critical power,[2] and exercise intensity domains,[3-7] which may find no significant differences between the metrics but on an individual level an athlete's anaerobic capacity can significantly raise their calculated FTP or critical power via use of tests over these thresholds.

Functional Reserve Capacity

Anaerobic capacity is another metric, most commonly called W', or functional reserve capacity (FRC). Calculation methods can vary but fall roughly onto the same value for an athlete's anaerobic capacity in kilojoules, which roughly represents the work capacity over a threshold.[8] This metric includes the phosphocreatine, glycolytic, and aerobic energy systems, because all contribute to power output over FTP.

Vo_{2max}

The Vo_{2max} cannot be measured directly with a cycling PM. The contribution of W' to workloads over FTP can affect estimation of this metric, although several models do exist. Typically, 5-minute MMP is used to estimate Vo_{2max}; although Vo_{2max} modeling software exists, it is not commonly available. Technically speaking, there is no such thing as Vo_{2max} power[9] due to the contribution of W' to all power outputs over FTP. An athlete's Vo_{2max} can be elicited in a variety of ways and at a variety of power outputs.[10]

Vo_{2max} sets an upper limit for aerobic energy contribution to power output. It has a relationship with FTP that can be measured accurately with gas exchange[11] and typically falls in the range of 60% to 80% of Vo_{2max}, although values outside that range are found.

Maximal Sprint Power

Maximal sprint power (Pmax) is an estimation of the maximum power an athlete can achieve in 1 complete pedal revolution. Typical rates of crank revolutions per minute (RPM) to achieve maximum power varies between approximately 90 RPM and 130 RPM (personal observation). Because the modern standard for power data recording is 1 Hz, a complete revolution is not recorded. Some hardware and software can either measure or interpolate a true 1-revolution Pmax, but this generally is unnecessary for most cyclists. A 1-second maximal power can be utilized except for erroneously high-power readings, so 5-second maximum power generally is a recognized field standard for Pmax.

Power Versus Other Metrics

Power metrics that relate to physiologic thresholds, such as FTP, do not change day to day, although with increasing or decreasing fitness and fatigue they may change, or appear to change, over weeks or months. In training, this is advantageous because it gives athletes and coaches a standard by which to compare training in the short term and long term. A metric, such as HR, can decouple or rise in relation to a steady power output, as seen in **Fig. 2**. Although environmental factors like heat can be a factor, during extensive endurance exercise, one of the largest contributors to decoupling is increasing motor unit recruitment.[10] This can occur during steady endurance pace exercise as well as during single or multiple intervals below, at, and above FTP. The fatigue presents via contractile dysfunction from initially recruited motor units. The body's response is to increase the enervating signal to recruit larger, often less efficient, motor units. This lower efficiency for the same power output requires a higher Vo_2, which is met by increased cardiac output, seen as increasing HR. This raises

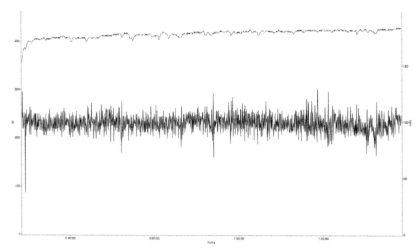

Fig. 2. This is an FTP test performed by a professional female cyclist. To illustrate HR decoupling, average HR in the third minute after stabilizing is 170 bpm, and the last minute average is 184 bpm.

doubts about whether it is possible to determine a threshold HR for most athletes when it decouples during an effort at FTP (see **Fig. 2**). During extensive intense exercise, athletes' ratings of perceived exertion (RPE) typically increase as well.

Although many modern cyclists overly focus on their power output as the only important metric, power is an external metric of stress, and using it alongside HR and RPE can add an internal focus on internal strain. This adds context to power output that can be used to guide training and RFII, discussed later.

There are important differences between power output, HR, and RPE. First, it must be recognized that myriad factors can affect HR and RPE on a daily basis, such as sleep, fatigue, or stress. Second, most athletes typically do not use or report with the Borg scale[12] and instead prefer a scale of 1 to 10, with 1 very easy and 10 a true all-out effort.

POPULATION CONSIDERATIONS

There is commonly received wisdom in endurance training: "the more you train, the more you can train." The statement implicitly acknowledges not only that the conditions that lead to aerobic adaptations are significant cellular stressors themselves but also that training leads to improved ability to handle these stressors, with a larger training "dose" being needed for further improvement. For instance, Place and colleagues[13] found that a bout of high-intensity interval training (HIIT) leads to flux of reactive oxygen species and site-specific fragmentation of muscular ryanodine receptors in recreationally active subjects but not in elite endurance athletes. Ryanodine receptor fragmentation leads directly to calcium leak out of the sarcoplasmic reticulum and into the sarcoplasm, which is one of many signals that can lead to up-regulation of aerobic adaptive pathways.[14] This suggests the need for different training strategies to improve elite athletes' fitness and easily can explain why many different training strategies are so effective on recreationally active or moderately trained subjects.

Understanding RFII requires understanding general athletic populations. Research, such as the Place and colleagues study, support the received wisdom that well-trained cyclists are able to absorb more training stress, although this does not necessarily imply HIIT, because even low-intensity and moderate-intensity training done for sufficient duration can provide needed training stress.[15] Perhaps the received wisdom should include the idea that the more well-trained a cyclist, the more significant training stress may be needed for further improvement. This principle is known as progressive overload. The takeaway is that training stress needs to be managed carefully for recreational, intermediate, and well-trained cyclists due to their training history. There is overlap between all populations, and important differences are emphasized but should not be taken as absolute; as always, consideration of each individual's history and needs is paramount.

When considering population differences and how much someone rides, consider that cyclists usually quantify riding volume by duration rather than distance. In part this is due to varying speeds encountered from terrain, wind, and the effects of drafting. Cycling also is a low-impact sport that has little, if any involvement of energy storage and release via eccentric contractions (some exceptions for mountain bike disciplines); there is little stress on joints and connective tissue. For this reason, a cyclist easily could double the duration or distance of their longest ride with relatively low injury risk compared with running. An exception to this is proper fitting on a bicycle, because improper fitting can lead to discomfort or pain. Thus, duration is the best indicator of a cyclist's training volume.

This discussion of different cycling populations exists only for the purposes of this discussion. Each population overlaps with the others, sometimes in large degrees; guidelines should be taken only as those, and assumptions should not be made hastily.

Recreational Cyclists

Recreational cyclists sometimes are called *weekend warriors*, although typically they do ride more often than just on weekends, in that they may commute or participate in social group rides during the week. Generally speaking, training volume and intensity are low. Total hours ridden per week for recreational cyclists, including work commutes, can be approximately 4 hours to 10 hours, depending on the length of the commute. The longest duration rides may not normally exceed 2 hours or 3 hours.

This population typically does not undertake structured training or may train for only a few months out of a year to participate in a longer noncompetitive or semicompetitive event. Due to a typical training history of low volume or low intensity, nearly any focused training plan can cause large and rapid improvements. Most cyclists in this population, however, may have only cursory to no knowledge of modern cycling metrics, so only generalized guidelines may be necessary.

During RFII, encouragement of enjoyment and low-intensity activity likely is well received. More serious interventions may not be necessary, although, if they are, the suggestions in the semicoached or coached populations should be referred to. Due to most recreational cyclists not being involved with a cycling coach or cycling-specific trainer (although many may have a personal trainer in a gym or at home for general strength and cardiovascular fitness), medical guidance likely is the only resource on RFII.

These cyclists may respond well to encouragement of new or additional sporting activities, if possible. If RFII precludes all sporting endeavors, then instruction on maintaining low volume or low intensity by pain score (eg, stop riding if the pain is more than 3 out of 10) may have high compliance. Because enjoyment typically is the primary motivator of recreational cyclists, permitting autoregulation of volume and intensity may work out well in most cases. In my coaching experience, long-term fatigue or signs of overtraining in this population is uncommon, because the motivation for cycling enjoyment typically seems to outweigh any desire to become the fastest a cyclist can become, so breaks and rest often are self-determined to rest or focus on other activities.

Semicoached Cyclists

The population of semicoached cyclists exists only for the purpose of RFII practices and should be used in other contexts with caution. There exist a variety of athlete types in this group that share many similar characteristics. The term, *semi-coached*, is an attempt to describe competitive and noncompetitive cyclists who write their own training plans, use algorithm-based training programs or prewritten training plans from coaches (with limited coach contact, if any), or have a coach with low amounts of contact; for example, some cycling coaches only check in with their athletes once a week or month or less. This contact may be a call but also can be a cursory check of power files and an e-mail.

Training volume with these athletes can be 6 hours to 18 hours per week, with some exceptions for rest weeks (easy weeks interspersed in a training schedule) or more intense periods of training like camps with friends or cycling club teammates. Intensity can be varied, because some athletes perform a large number of intervals per week (sometimes 2 days to 6 days per week) at intensities usually based on their FTP. This has benefits and drawbacks, discussed later.

There are many common threads among these athletes, but two are pertinent for RFII advice. The first is that the contact infrequency with a trusted and knowledgeable coach is supplemented with scouring the Internet (which can include inquiring on forums) for information on training, which can be oversimplified, incorrect, or misleading. The second is that these cyclists typically are driven by performance metrics, which can be race results or power-derived metrics like FTP or Pmax, or also can be self-improvement in terms of the desire to see increasing power or decreasing time on a local hill or course. Additionally, because training plans at this level usually are not customized or an athlete has low confidence in proper plan modification, training plans often are seen as rigid, rather than the flexible plans usually adopted by fully coached cyclists.

A seemingly common characteristic with semicoached athletes is that they are afraid to rest. The importance of rest commonly is undersold in articles, books, and forums, in favor of training methods that appear to shortcut normal training, rest, and adaptation timelines. Where a fully coached athlete often has a season structure defined by an experienced coach that includes periods of dedicated training, racing, and rest, semicoached athletes frequently determine the structure of their own seasons and may train through injury and illness out of the fear that resting results in fitness loss. In treating these athletes during RFII, the importance of rest must be impressed on them, and my coaching and athletic experience suggest that the additional stress of hard training uses energy that would be used for recovery and prolongs the process.

Given that cycling is a sport where low body weight is at a premium, another potential pitfall during RFII with semicoached cyclists is weight loss. Because semicoached cyclists may choose their training guidance or coaching based on budget, professional nutrition guidance often is too expensive for most semicoached cyclists, so it can be difficult to adjust a diet to meet the energetic demand of training while simultaneously achieving a sustainable weight loss rate and amount during a training season. Therefore, a period of low training stress can seem an ideal time to lose weight because there are no additional energetic demands associated with training. Additionally, cyclists may be afraid of weight gain during periods of inactivity or tapering. These two factors can lead to energy deficit and prolonged healing. A well-known example from 2020 is Remco Evenepoel, a professional cyclist who crashed in August 2020 and suffered a pelvis fracture, whose recovery timeline was delayed by energy deficit due to his dieting to lose "puppy fat." This example indicates that RFII should not include weight loss.

For semicoached cyclists, the role of health care providers during RFII is similar to a coach because the point of care likely is the best and most reliable resource this population has access to and usually is taken the most seriously. Fears of fitness loss and weight gain must be assuaged to ensure full healing before returning to intense training. In the long term, it may be impressed upon patients that delaying RFII results in a delay in proper training and, therefore, delays return to fitness. Details of detraining and retraining are discussed later in terms of modern cycling metrics and should be discussed with patients.

Coached Cyclists

The largest difference between the two populations is that a coached cyclist has regular communication with a coach, who writes a custom training plan or adjusts a pre-written plan that is adaptable to the needs of the cyclist. A continuum does exist between recreational, coached, and semicoached athletes because some coaches offer different levels of contact, for example, daily, weekly, or monthly, and take athlete feedback to varying degrees. These athletes also have a good understanding of modern training metrics.

Coached athletes have the widest range of training duration, intensity, and goals. This can include recreational cyclists at 6 hours to 8 hours per week, training for general fitness, or 1 or several noncompetitive or semicompetitive events per year. Coached athletes also can include average amateur competitive cyclists training more intensely for 6 hours to 18 hours per week, or professional cyclists training 15 hours to 25 hours per week or more, mostly at low intensity but including periods of very high intensity.

Communication between athlete and coach allows a cyclist many opportunities to discuss training plans, details of stress or injury, and myriad things that allow a coach to adjust a training plan to best suit someone's needs. This means that the nominal role of the medical provider is to assign guidelines to be followed by the coach and athlete.

Discussion between the medical provider, coach, and athlete is ideal, because coaches can ask questions directly pertaining to the limitations of movement, training intensity, and other pertinent information, such as when outdoor rides or off-road rides can be resumed. The medical provider also would benefit from asking a cyclist if their coach has any questions or concerns about training limitations or guidance for programming training during RFII. This gives coaches — in particular, strength coaches, should the athlete have one — the opportunity to review different training modalities that are to be explicitly avoided or to get medical approval for a training progression to complement an athlete's RFII, including especially rehabilitation exercise.

UTILIZING METRICS TO GUIDE RETURN FROM INJURY AND ILLNESS

The following section of this article is meant to provide care providers with tools to communicate with cyclists under the guidelines of the previous section in order to address their concerns. In addition are suggestions for utilizing training metrics, including power, HR, and RPE, to provide intensity suggestions and guide athletes to properly autoregulate training progression during RFII.

Expected Detraining Effects and Resting Benefits

In the course of several weeks off the bike, the most volatile component of fitness is plasma volume,[16,17] which can affect stroke volume and cardiac output directly. This also is one of the first things to be retrained[18] and primarily affects Vo_{2max}, which in turn affects FTP. Re-expansion of plasma volume during retraining brings Vo_{2max} back to near fully trained values by increasing heart stroke volume and cardiac output.[18,19] Because FTP is the simplest metric to measure (discussed later), lowered FTP from detraining (or fatigue) can affect athletes' perception of their fitness and can motivate them to begin intense training before they are ready.

It may seem counterintuitive that RFII-required rest, or low intensity and low volume, may allow for an adaptive process to occur, but in my experience that is exactly what happens. Chronic training stress without time for rest does not allow the body to recover from the training stress itself. A cogent analogy is strength training. If performing 3 sets of 5 heavy squats to near failure, a repeat of this is impossible until an athlete is recovered and supercompensation occurs. The exact mechanism of chronic fatigue and subsequent adaptation in endurance training is unknown, but there are some clues that implicate oxidative stress[20,21] or potentially any adaptive signal that creates a greater than normally experienced perturbation of cellular homeostasis.

An example of this from my coaching career is an athlete who sustained a clavicle fracture in a crash. This athlete spent 2 weeks completely off the bike, then did several weeks of easy riding with slowly increasing volume, and then increased intensity gradually in a logical manner. Shortly thereafter, he was ready for a hard training block. Before the crash and RFII, his FTP was 330W. After recovering from the hard training block, his FTP was 365W. This amount of progression is rare in athletes, when a 5W to 10W improvement in FTP is typical. The time off and dissipation of the previous 6 months of chronic training stress, however, allowed him to train harder than he could while carrying chronic fatigue, and reach new levels of fitness.

Even a short break for a minor cold can leave cyclists feeling fresh. Two days or 3 days off the bike followed by 2 days or 3 days of increasing intensity gradually often is a good example of how a minor period of RFII can increase performance greatly. An example of this for 2 days off the bike is a 1-hour recovery ride the first day back, 1 hour to 2 hours of 3/10 RPE to 4/10 RPE endurance riding on the second day, and 20 minutes to 50 minutes of 6/10 RPE tempo on day 3. Cyclists usually call a progression like this "openers," which generally are done in the days before a competition, after a period of rest or taper. The physiologic mechanism of openers is unknown, but I speculate it is related to autonomic function and sympathetic hormone signaling.

Functional Threshold of Power Testing

It is my opinion that assessment of an athlete's FTP can and should be done within 5W, rounded down to err on the conservative side due to the potential drawbacks of fatigue. Ensuring that FTP is set accurately can aid a cyclist's RFII greatly. In utilizing FTP as a main marker of fitness, particularly with coached and semicoached athletes, the method used to perform FTP testing is important, because some methods often can overestimate values, especially for cyclists with a high W'. Methods of estimating FTP include 95% of 20-minute MMP, or 90% of the average MMP of 2 maximal 8-minute intervals with a 10-minute rest interval between. Athletes with large anaerobic capacity (the amount of work that can be done over FTP [**Fig. 3**]) can increase the results of these tests greatly. As an example, an individual with a 1500W Pmax and 27-kJ W'

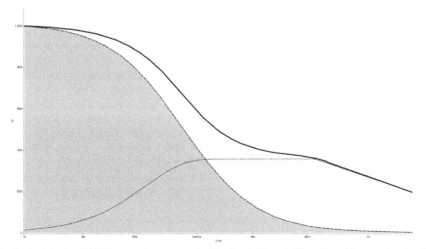

Fig. 3. An idealized MMP curve is represented by the thick solid line. Aerobic contribution is represented with the thin solid line and reaches its maximum at FTP. W' is represented by the integral of the shaded area.

can do a 20-minute time trial effort at 300W. According to this test, their FTP is 285W, when in fact it is 270W. Particularly when performing intervals intended to be at 100% FTP, the additional fatigue caused by the overestimation is large and can lead to nonfunctional overtraining.

Two other common testing methods that typically cause overestimation are the ramp test, either with or without blood lactate measurements, and the 8-minute FTP test. Ramp tests typically assign FTP between 70% and 75% of the maximum power value achieved in the test, but as Adami and colleagues[9] found, this value is affected by W' and the rate of workload increase. In laboratory or field settings, this can provide a place to begin searching for MLSS or FTP, but it should not be strictly assigned. The 8-minute FTP test is a protocol utilizing two 8-minute maximal efforts with a 10-minute rest interval in-between. The average power outputs from the two 8-minute bouts are averaged again, and 90% of the average is taken to be FTP. This testing method suffers from the same problems as the 20-minute and ramp tests.

Proper FTP testing requires either blood lactate testing to determine MLSS or a field test of a 35-minute to 60-minute time trial in order to infer an inflection point, as seen in **Fig. 1**. A qualitative description of this time trial is that the athlete ride just under the intensity at which they feel like they would fatigue quickly, because FTP is the border of faster or slower fatigue rates, over MLSS and under MLSS, respectively. This is the functional part of FTP.

Training Black Holes

In my experience, FTP overestimation is the single largest detriment to effective training, and can delay RFII. During times of rest, recovery, or RFII, FTP overestimation and cumulative workload at this overestimated intensity can be particularly detrimental to both the healing and training processes. Discussion of the metabolic process involved is beyond the scope of this article and seems not to be described in the current body of literature. Regardless, it sometimes is popularly referred to as a black hole of intensity. The pattern is such that workouts at the same overestimated FTP become progressively more difficult, until failure becomes imminent and without proper rest might be consistently recurring on a weekly or even daily basis. The fatigue associated accumulates so fast that a normal recovery timeline is longer than athletes expect and may be ignored as HR and RPE decouple from power, as described later.

This black hole might be described as a situation where the actual recovery needed is incompatible with the athlete's expected training frequency. For example, an average trained cyclist could be expected to perform an FTP workout with three 15-minute intervals at an intensity equal to 100% FTP, with 5-minute rest periods between intervals. This normally could be done 3 times per week, which indicates the recovery from this workout is approximately 24 hours to 48 hours. The total workout RPE would be 7 or 8 out of 10. If FTP is overestimated by as little as 10W to 20W, however, full recovery from the same workout may take 3 days to 5 days or longer. In this instance, the accumulated fatigue eventually leads to failure in 1 of 2 ways, which are the inability to achieve the expected power targets for the full interval durations or the failure to achieve the expected power target for significantly less than the full workout duration. This is accompanied by an RPE of 10 out of 10, rather than the expected 7 or 8.

How Easy Is Easy?

For the purposes of allowing energy to aid the healing process rather than recovery, assigning active recovery or endurance training to the modern cyclist may not be a simple task. There is day-to-day variation in the upper limit for easy cycling, often described as the first lactate threshold (LT1), sometimes known as aerobic threshold, because the power output associated with LT1 can vary widely as a percentage of FTP and can be reduced with fatigue (personal observation). This makes it nearly impossible to assign a single power target that is consistent every day. Thus, in my coaching practice, active recovery or endurance rides are assigned by RPE only, because they are intended to be below LT1. The RPE associated with being above LT1 or below LT1 also seems to shift in tandem, allowing cyclists to maintain adequately nonfatiguing effort that still allows for training adaptations to occur. It, therefore, is useful during normal training to assign easy rides by RPE, but, particularly during RFII, RPE tends to be a much more useful tool than power or even HR.

Easy rides by RPE usually are given as 1/10 RPE to 2/10 RPE for the purpose of active recovery, and 3/10 RPE to 4/10 RPE as endurance pace below LT1. In more experienced athletes, a 5/10 RPE also can be below LT1. Regardless, additional descriptors are useful. Cyclists who are riding at these intensities should be able to have full conversations not interrupted by catching their breath; this does not necessarily equate to metabolic or ventilatory thresholds, because they may decouple in well-trained athletes,[22] but it is a useful guideline nonetheless.

Practitioners may find it better to describe easy or endurance pace rides by the resultant expected fatigue. A description of an active recovery ride may be "put little to no pressure on the pedals, and feel better when you finish the ride than when you started." Qualitative description of an endurance ride could be "the pace should feel like you're not accumulating too much fatigue, and you're not empty when you finish."

Due to cycling being a low-impact sport and that increasing volume is relatively accomplishable, an easy ride still may accumulate a significant fatigue if it is longer than a cyclist is accustomed to. Therefore, logical progression of a cyclist's longest ride can help control training load and fatigue. Where runners typically use a 10% rule for increasing volume, the low-impact nature of cycling means a 30-minute rule likely is sufficient. For instance, if a cyclist's longest ride is 120 minutes, the 10% rule would add only 12 minutes, where a 30-minute rule would add 30 minutes. If an athlete's longest ride is done only once or twice per week, this rule may be sufficient until they reach their maximum training time allowed by their schedule. Vigilance for typical signs of overtraining still should be done, particularly when energetic demands of RFII are high.

Another potential black hole of endurance training is when the low-intensity rides (active recovery or endurance), discussed previously, are done too hard, which can be seen in all populations. This can occur when training intensities like FTP or endurance pace are overestimated. For instance, a typical range for an athlete's "endurance pace" may be assigned as 55% to 75% of FTP. When endurance intensity is assigned with this method, it implies that 75% FTP is the upper limit for a sustainable, nonfatiguing pace or perhaps even represents LT1, which is not necessarily the case. There is a similar implication with active recovery, typically assigned as less than 55% FTP. It is the tendency of many cyclists—of all populations—to ride at the upper limit of their training zone, regardless of the amount of fatigue they experience. No common power training (and often HR training) prescriptions properly individualize a target or range that works for all individuals because there is not yet any power prescription tool or algorithm that can determine quickly and accurately a cyclist's easy training intensities better than an athlete's own RPE.

Easy intensity rides done too hard can lead to fatigue accumulation, often indicated by unusual amounts of decoupling of HR and RPE from power, frequent failure of previously achievable workouts, or even decreased Pmax. Further indicators of this training black hole also can be when athletes are unable to train at volumes greater than approximately 8 hours to 12 hours per week, along with normal signs of overtraining.

Integrating Training Metrics with Return from Injury and Illness

Utilizing training metrics to guide RFII should begin with guidelines of volume and intensity in terms of FTP or RPE. There should be differentiation between intensities, such as active recovery, endurance pace, threshold training between LT1 and FTP (typically intensities called tempo, sweet spot, and threshold or FTP), or any training above FTP, which includes Vo_{2max}, anaerobic capacity, and sprints. Increasing training intensity comes with increased energy demands and recovery time.

Determining an optimal timeline for RFII intensity may be as simple as "for 6 weeks ride below 4/10 RPE, with no endurance ride longer than 3 hours, and a maximum 10 hours per week total," followed by reevaluation. The necessary duration of low training load, by intensity, volume, or both, can be up to the treatment provider. Athletes and coaches usually defer to medical advice in order to avoid exacerbating illness or injury or delaying recovery time. The prescription also may be as simple as "stop riding for any pain over a 3/10," and the cyclist or coach can regulate training load via volume and intensity based on that guideline. In cases of chronic fatigue and overtraining, re-evaluation of anchor training intensities, such as FTP or aerobic threshold, always should be suggested

Should any overtraining symptoms present in addition to any other clinical findings, re-evaluation of anchor training intensities may be necessary to add into the treatment. Consultation with an outside cycling coach may be necessary to ensure appropriate evaluation.

As a cyclist begins to build back up to preinjury or preillness training loads, it should be made clear that expected recovery times may be longer than when at peak fitness. Because of additional energy demands during RFII that reduce recovery time, guidance also may be needed to help with recovery time from harder workouts. For example, if an athlete performing three 15-minute intervals at 100% FTP and a 7/10 RPE or 8/10 RPE cannot do so again the next day, then easier intervals, active recovery, or rest must be done until the power and RPE come back into alignment. This allows for a degree of autoregulation by athletes during RFII.

When in doubt, RFII guidelines should be made by RPE and cyclists encouraged to ignore power and HR metrics and data until fully recovered and ready to resume normal training. Particularly when a medical provider is a cyclist's only point of contact for training advice, a conservative approach should lead to the best outcomes in RFII.

SUMMARY

For anyone involved with RFII guidance with cyclists, open communication between personnel, coaches, and cyclista is invaluable. This should take into consideration a training timeline, fatigue or intensity management, and realistic expectations with regard to fitness levels or bodyweight. Highly internally motivated cyclists may wish for shorter RFII timelines, but communication with language and metrics they are familiar with may ease fears and increase compliance.

CLINICS CARE POINTS

- Modern power-derived training metrics can be used to communicate with cyclists and guide the recovery process.
- Training guidelines during recovery should include volume and intensity components.
- Cyclists should ride to perceived exertion when returning from illness and injury.

- If a cyclist has one or several coaches, particularly for strength or technique coaching, they can be included in communication to learn and inquire about medically advised limitations.
- Cyclists should be monitored for signs of overtraining. Reassessment of power-derived training metrics may be advised.

CONFLICT OF INTEREST

The author has no conflict of interest to report.

REFERENCES

1. Billat VL, Sirvent P, Py G, et al. The concept of maximal lactate steady state: a bridge between biochemistry, physiology and sport science. Sports Med 2003; 33(6):407–26.
2. Monod H, Scherrer J. The work capacity of a synergic muscular group. Ergonomics 1965;3:329–38.
3. Jamnick NA, Pettitt RW, Granata C, et al. An examination and critique of current methods to determine exercise intensity. Sports Med 2020;50(10):1729–56.
4. Jones AM, Burnley M, Black MI, et al. The maximal metabolic steady state: redefining the 'gold standard. Physiol Rep 2019;7(10):e14098.
5. Mattioni Maturana F, Keir DA, McLay KM, et al. Can measures of critical power precisely estimate the maximal metabolic steady-state? Appl Physiol Nutr Metab 2016;41(11):1197–203.
6. Dekerle J, Pelayo P, Clipet B, et al. Critical swimming speed does not represent the speed at maximal lactate steady state. Int J Sports Med 2005;26(7):524–30.
7. Pringle JS, Jones AM. Maximal lactate steady state, critical power and EMG during cycling. Eur J Appl Physiol 2002;88(3):214–26.
8. Poole DC, Burnley M, Vanhatalo A, et al. Critical power: an important fatigue threshold in exercise physiology. Med Sci Sports Exerc 2016;48(11):2320–34.
9. Adami A, Sivieri A, Moia C, et al. Effects of step duration in incremental ramp protocols on peak power and maximal oxygen consumption. Eur J Appl Physiol 2013;113(10):2647–53.
10. Vanhatalo A, Poole DC, DiMenna FJ, et al. Muscle fiber recruitment and the slow component of O2 uptake: constant work rate vs. all-out sprint exercise. Am J Physiol Regul Integr Comp Physiol 2011;300(3):R700–7.
11. Coyle EF, Coggan AR, Hopper MK, et al. Determinants of endurance in well-trained cyclists. J Appl Physiol (1985) 1988;64(6):2622–30.
12. Borg GA. Psychophysical bases of perceived exertion. Med Sci Sports Exerc 1982;14(5):377–81.
13. Place N, Ivarsson N, Venckunas T, et al. Ryanodine receptor fragmentation and sarcoplasmic reticulum Ca2+ leak after one session of high-intensity interval exercise. Proc Natl Acad Sci U S A 2015;112(50):15492–7.
14. Kang C, Li Ji L. Role of PGC-1α signaling in skeletal muscle health and disease. Ann N Y Acad Sci 2012;1271(1):110–7.
15. Jones TE, Baar K, Ojuka E, et al. Exercise induces an increase in muscle UCP3 as a component of the increase in mitochondrial biogenesis. Am J Physiol Endocrinol Metab 2003;284(1):E96–101.
16. Mujika I, Padilla S. Muscular characteristics of detraining in humans. Med Sci Sports Exerc 2001;33(8):1297–303.

17. Mujika I, Padilla S. Cardiorespiratory and metabolic characteristics of detraining in humans. Med Sci Sports Exerc 2001;33(3):413–21.

18. Montero D, Cathomen A, Jacobs RA, et al. Haematological rather than skeletal muscle adaptations contribute to the increase in peak oxygen uptake induced by moderate endurance training. J Physiol 2015;593(20):4677–88.

19. Coyle EF, Hemmert MK, Coggan AR. Effects of detraining on cardiovascular responses to exercise: role of blood volume. J Appl Physiol (1985) 1986; 60(1):95–9.

20. Aon MA, Cortassa S, O'Rourke B. Redox-optimized ROS balance: a unifying hypothesis. Biochim Biophys Acta 2010;1797(6–7):865–77.

21. Nikolaidis MG, Margaritelis NV, Matsakas A. Quantitative redox biology of exercise. Int J Sports Med 2020;41(10):633–45.

22. Wang L, Yoshikawa T, Hara T, et al. Which common NIRS variable reflects muscle estimated lactate threshold most closely? Appl Physiol Nutr Metab 2006;31(5): 612–20.

Cervical Spine, Upper Extremity Neuropathies, and Overuse Injuries in Cyclists

Andrea Cyr, DO

KEYWORDS

- Carpal tunnel syndrome • Ulnar neuropathy • Guyon's canal • Neck pain
- Biker's elbow

KEY POINTS

- Ulnar neuropathy and carpal tunnel are 2 upper extremity neuropathies common among cyclists.
- Biker's elbow is a tendinopathy of the common flexor or extensor tendon and the most common overuse injury in cycling.
- A bicycle fit assessment is recommended as part of the conservative management for upper extremity neuropathies or overuse injuries worsened from cycling.
- Neck pain is a common complaint among cyclists, and prolonged hyperextension of the cervical spine may contribute to symptoms.

INTRODUCTION

Neck pain, upper extremity neuropathies such as ulnar neuropathy and carpal tunnel syndrome, and overuse injuries of the upper extremity are common injuries in cyclists. Physician and medical professionals can aid in prevention, recognition, and treatment of these injuries. This often involves addressing bicycle fit, evaluation for improper equipment, and assessing individual factors.

UPPER EXTREMITY NEUROPATHIES

Upper extremity neuropathies are common in both competitive and recreational cyclists.[1,2] Ulnar neuropathy sometimes called *handlebar palsy* or *cyclist's palsy* and carpal tunnel syndrome presents as numbness or tingling in the hands and is a common complaint in cyclists. These are 2 well-defined upper extremity neuropathies found in the general population, but the prevalence among cyclists is unknown. Peripheral

Department of Family Medicine, University of Illinois – College of Medicine, UIC Sports Medicine Center, Flames Athletic Center, 839 Roosevelt Road. Suite 102, Chicago, IL 60608, USA
E-mail address: Acyr3@uic.edu
Twitter: @AndreaCyrDO (A.C.)

Phys Med Rehabil Clin N Am 33 (2022) 187–199
https://doi.org/10.1016/j.pmr.2021.08.013
1047-9651/22/© 2021 Elsevier Inc. All rights reserved.
pmr.theclinics.com

nerve lesions that occur with these conditions can be classified based on the degree of injury. The Seddon classification of nerve lesions is divided into 3 stages, neuro-praxia, axonotmesis, and neurotmesis.[3,4] Sunderland further classifies nerve lesions into grades 1 to 5 depending on severity. These classifications aid in assessing the de-gree of nerve injury and provide prognostic information for recovery. Regarding chronic neuropathies of the upper extremity in cycling, it can be expected that most nerve lesions will be neuropraxia or grade 1, injuries caused by a temporary mechanical compression (**Table 1**).

ULNAR NEUROPATHY

In cyclists, ulnar nerve compression typically occurs near or within Guyon's canal distally in the wrist. Compression of the distal ulnar nerve at the wrist can affect the superficial or deep branches of the ulnar nerve leading to motor deficits, sensory changes, or both.[2] Distal ulnar neuropathy can be localized as proximal, within or distal to Guyon's canal. Guyon's canal is an area of the wrist formed by a fibro-osseous tunnel bordered by the hook of hamate at the radial-sided boundary and the pisiform along its ulnar-sided boundary. The volar carpal and transverse carpal lig-aments create the "roof" and "floor" of the Guyon's canal, respectively[3] (**Fig. 1**). Ulnar nerve is divided into the deep motor branch, which provides motor innervation to all ulnar-innervated hand muscles, and the superficial branch, which provides sensory fi-bers only to the ulnar side of the hand.[4,5] Four locations of ulnar nerve compression related to Guyon's canal have been defined as follows:

- Type 1
  - Location: Proximal lesion that affects both deep motor and superficial branches of ulnar nerve.
  - Clinical findings: Sensory loss and weakness of all ulnar intrinsic hand muscles.
- Type 2
  - Location: Lesion to deep motor branch only.
  - Clinical findings: Weakness of all ulnar intrinsic muscles and no sensory loss.
- Type 3
  - Location: Lesion to deep motor branch, more distal than type 2.
  - Clinical findings: Isolated weakness to ulnar-innervated intrinsic muscles except hypothenar muscles (abductor digiti minimi muscle is unaffected). No sensory loss.
- Type 4
  - Location: Distal lesion to superficial branch only.
  - Clinical findings: Sensory loss only, no weakness.

Physical Examination Signs that May be Seen in Ulnar Neuropathy

- Tinel sign: Percussion over the ulnar side of the wrist causes pain or paresthesias in the index or pinky finger.[3]
- Froment sign: The patient tries to hold a piece of paper between their thumb and index finger. In cases of ulnar neuropathy with weakness, the patient will compensate with flexion of the thumb's interphalangeal joint instead of their ulnar-innervated adductor pollicis muscle; this causes the thumb's interphalan-geal joint to be in a flexed position.
- Wartenberg sign: The pinky finger remains in abduction due to weakness of ulnar-innervated intrinsic muscles.

Table 1				

Seddon and Sunderland classifications of nerve injuries and prognosis				
Seddon	Sunderland	Injury		Prognosis
Neuropraxia	Grade I	Temporary mechanical compression, local ischemia, or traction injury		Full recovery usually possible
Axonotmesis	Grade II	Lesion to axon. Schwann cell remains intact		Complete, recovery weeks to months
Axonotmesis	Grade III	Lesion to axon. Schwann cell remains intact		Incomplete and variable, recovery months
Axonotmesis	Grade IV	Lesion to axon. Schwann cell remains intact		Incomplete and variable, recovery months to years
Neurotmesis	Grade V	Serious injury, defined as complete axon and Schwann cell disruption		Incomplete, recovery is guarded

Studies show that prolonged biking and repetitive compression, as occurs in road cycling, can cause an ulnar nerve injury.[6] Nerve compression secondary to poor hand positioning on handlebars and vibration from ground terrain are well-known risk factors for developing ulnar neuropathy at the wrist. Hand positioning on the bicycle handlebars can lead to ulnar deviation and nerve compression in various locations of Guyon's canal. In addition, during long descents on a bicycle, more body weight is supported by the upper extremities, leading to a high load and pressure on the wrists and hands.[5]

An ulnar nerve lesion in this population typically occurs with recurrence of temporary, mechanical compression of the nerve; however, there has been evidence of a single prolonged event eliciting symptoms consistent with an ulnar neuropathy. One case has been described of a cyclist participating in a single downhill mountain bike trip, with prolonged downhill riding, who presented with paresthesias and hand weakness. Therefore, this condition should be considered in any individual with any amount of previous cycling events in their history and clinical signs of ulnar nerve injury.[5]

Proximal Ulnar Neuropathy

Proximal ulnar nerve lesions are less common among cyclists but should be considered. At the elbow, the ulnar nerve travels through the cubital tunnel. A snapping triceps phenomenon may cause ulnar nerve symptoms that are exacerbated by forcefully gripping the handlebars. In this syndrome, there is dislocation of the medial head of the triceps in combination with ulnar nerve dislocation. This syndrome would lead to discomfort on the medial side of the elbow with or without ulnar neuropathy[7]; this has not been studied in cyclists but is postulated as a possible cause of elbow pain and ulnar neuropathy in this population.

CARPAL TUNNEL SYNDROME

Long-distance cycling may exacerbate symptoms of carpal tunnel syndrome.[8] Carpal tunnel syndrome is a mononeuropathy of the median nerve at the wrist and is the most common entrapment neuropathy of the upper extremity, affecting approximately 3% of the general population.[9] The carpal tunnel is bordered superiorly by the transverse carpal ligament and is bordered inferiorly by the carpal bones. Structures that pass

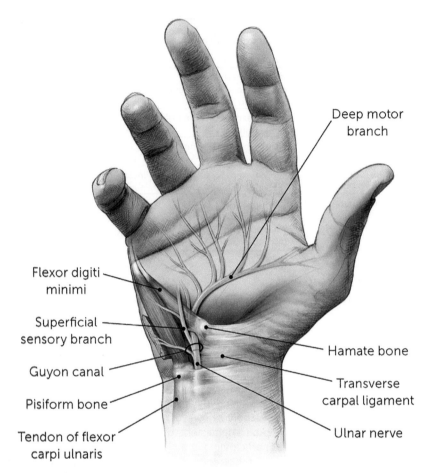

Fig. 1. Guyon's canal. Ulnar nerve entrapment can occur at the wrist as it passes through Guyon's canal, which contains the ulnar nerve with its superficial sensory and deep motor branches. Two carpal bones are important in relation to the ulnar nerve in the wrist: the pisiform and hamate. (*From* ©Christy Krames 2013 ckrames@swbell.net.)

through the carpal tunnel include 9 flexor tendons and the median nerve, which is susceptible to compression with any increased pressure of this space (**Fig. 2**). Symptoms of carpal tunnel include paresthesias in the distribution of the median nerve, which involves the palmar thumb, index and middle fingers, and radial half of the ring finger.[10]

Physical examination findings in carpal tunnel syndrome include a flick sign, Tinel sign causing pain and paresthesias in the hand with percussion over the volar wrist, or symptoms with Phalen maneuver or median nerve compression test. Mild or moderate symptoms of carpal tunnel syndrome may not show any physical examination findings, so a degree of suspicion is required based on history.

THORACIC OUTLET SYNDROME

Thoracic outlet syndrome in cyclists can present as a condition on its own or a confounding issue and should remain on the differential of hand paresthesias.[11]

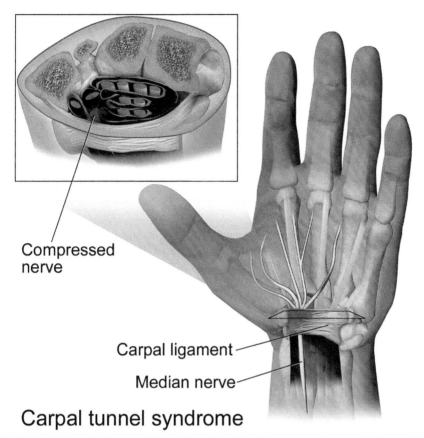

Compressed nerve

Carpal ligament

Median nerve

Carpal tunnel syndrome

Fig. 2. Carpal tunnel. The carpal tunnel is a site of median nerve entrapment. The median nerve traverses underneath the superficial flexor retinaculum through the carpal tunnel with the 4 tendons of the flexor digitorum profundus, the 4 tendons of the flexor digitorum superficialis, and the flexor pollicis longus tendon. (*From* Blausen.com staff (2014). "Medical gallery of Blausen Medical 2014." WikiJournal of Medicine 1 (2). https://doi.org/10.15347/ wjm/2014.010. ISSN 2002-4436; by (CC BY 4.0).)

Symptoms of an ulnar neuropathy and thoracic outlet syndrome in cyclists may present similarly given the overlap of sensation with the dermatomal pattern of a lower trunk brachial plexus injury and a peripheral ulnar nerve lesion. It may not be possible to distinguish an ulnar neuropathy from thoracic outlet syndrome from clinical examination only. Thoracic outlet syndrome in cyclists typically effects the lower trunk (C8-T1 nerve roots) of the brachial plexus as it traverses over the first rib toward the upper extremity. Anterior or middle scalene dysfunction can affect the first rib and cause symptoms, such as paresthesias in the hand, if the brachial plexus is involved.[6,11]

EVALUATION OF UPPER EXTREMITY NEUROPATHIES

Many compressive neuropathies in cyclists will resolve on their own with rest from activity and conservative management. Evaluation includes a thorough history with attention to timing and exacerbation of symptoms and any history of previous injuries.

Weakness on clinical examination warrants further workup as that suggests a progression of the nerve injury or an underlying condition.

Electrodiagnostic Studies

In diagnosis of upper extremity neuropathies, nerve conduction studies and electromyography are the gold standard that can assess for axon damage, grade severity of the nerve lesion, and provide information regarding prognosis. Even in cases of axonal damage, which is seen in more severe cases, spontaneous recovery can be possible over weeks to months. Electrodiagnostic studies can exclude other conditions as well, such as polyneuropathy, and evaluate for a radiculopathy. Electrodiagnostic studies may also differentiate symptoms due to an ulnar neuropathy versus thoracic outlet syndrome.[12]

Ultrasonography

In addition to nerve conduction studies, ultrasonography can also be useful to confirm a nerve lesion diagnosis as well as localization.[10] Ultrasonography can be useful to assess for any structural lesions such as a ganglion cyst, or in the case of an ulnar nerve lesion, assessment can include a hook of the hamate fracture or nonunion that may compromise nerve function. In cases that are unclear, an MRI should be considered.

MANAGEMENT OF UPPER EXTREMITY NEUROPATHIES
Conservative Treatment

Goals of management for mild- or moderate-grade ulnar neuropathy or carpal tunnel syndrome include reducing ongoing compression and conservative management; this can be achieved by activity rest with or without splinting, therapy with strengthening and nerve glide exercises, yoga, therapeutic ultrasonography, or local administration of corticosteroids for cases of carpal tunnel syndrome.[10]

Activity Modification

In severe cases, cyclists should reduce or alter their biking activities to prevent further nerve damage and allow for nerve regeneration to occur.[5] Upon resumption of biking activities, bicycle fit with special attention to handlebar positioning is recommended.

Splinting

Management of compressive nerve lesions includes use of neutral wrist splints for carpal tunnel syndrome or ulnar neuropathy, or nighttime elbow extension splint to minimize traction forces across the nerves of the wrist or elbow. Bracing allows for avoidance of prolonged nerve compression.[8,10]

Riding Modifications

Prevention and management of compressive upper extremity neuropathies in cycling includes avoiding excessive or prolonged weight-bearing through the hands and alternating hand and upper extremity positioning during long rides. Padded bicycle gloves lessen hand vibrations from the ground terrain. Riding with lower tire pressure also reduces terrain vibration. A study found that hand position and padded gloves reduced the magnitude and duration of loading patterns at the wrist, which mitigated the risk of ulnar neuropathy during longer rides.[13] Padded gloves provide a significant decrease of pressure over the hypothenar region (**Fig. 3**). Compliant foam padding of 3 mm provided the greatest pressure reduction, and thicker padding did not lessen hypothenar pressure any further.[13]

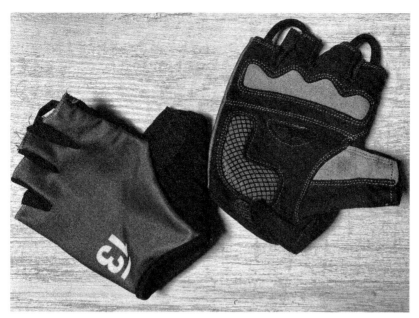

Fig. 3. Padded cycling gloves. The padded palm area of cycling gloves can provide protection, reducing pressure on the ulnar and median nerves of the hands and reducing the impact of vibrations through the handlebars.

Bicycle Fit

Proper bicycle fit assessment to determine the best saddle and handlebar type/shape and positioning is recommended including assessment of appropriate stem height and use of stem extensions if needed. A competitive cyclist may choose a lower handlebar height, several centimeters below the height of the saddle, for a more aerodynamic position. A recreational cyclist should aim for handlebars nearly equal to the saddle height to distribute weight evenly across the bike. Handlebar width should be roughly the width of the shoulders.

Surgical Treatment

Surgical nerve decompression for upper extremity compressive neuropathies is an option for the most severe cases. Severe carpal tunnel syndrome or ulnar neuropathy without improvement with conservative management after 4 to 6 months should be evaluated for surgical decompression.[10]

NECK PAIN AND THE CERVICAL SPINE

Neck pain is a common complaint of cyclists particularly when in an aerodynamic position as seen during racing or triathlons. Neck pain was reported in nearly 50% of recreational cyclists in one questionnaire, with reported neck and shoulder issues being 1.5 to 2.2 times more common in female cyclists than males, possibly related to less upper body strength.[14] Majority (91.3%) of these individuals reported neck and shoulder symptoms as mild.[14] Symptoms of chronic neck pain without traumatic injury may be described as "dull" or an "ache" specifically at the base of the skull and trapezius muscles. There may be associated headaches and referred pain down the periscapular region. A complete history and examination should always be done with any complaint of neck pain with a wide differential to include discogenic neck pain, facet arthropathy, cervical spine stenosis, radiculopathy, and spondylotic myelopathy. Any history of concussion or whiplash injury should also warrant further evaluation of cervical spine pain.

In cases of suspected radiculopathy, cervical nerve root lesions may cause motor or sensory changes of the upper extremity such as pain, numbness, tingling, or weakness. When a cervical nerve root compression occurs in conjunction with a peripheral nerve lesion, this phenomenon is known as "double crush syndrome," which has been described in a cyclist in one study.[15]

In a cycling position, the cervical spine can be forced into extension with shoulder protraction, and poor muscular endurance can fatigue the cervical paraspinals and trapezius muscles over time[16] (Fig. 4). Poor bike posture can be the root cause of chronic neck pain with cycling in the absence of serious neurologic findings. Issues with bicycle fit includes handlebar reach as too far or too low, saddle tilted forward increasing weight-bearing through upper extremities, or factors that lead to increased cervical spine extension such as a rounded thoracic spine, too aggressive aerodynamic positioning, or poorly fitting helmet and/or eyeglasses causing hyperextension of the cervical spine.[17]

Bike position for indoor cycling should also be considered. With increasing popularity of indoor cycling classes and at-home workout equipment, more individuals are using stationary bicycles where they may hyperextend their neck to maintain forward gaze as occurs with watching a class leader or video screen. Neck pain may also result from upper extremity positioning on the bike if elbows are in a locked extended position, which leads to shoulder elevation. This poor bike posture causes prolonged muscle tension around the upper shoulders and cervical spine, and consequently pain and discomfort associated with cycling. Adjustments to bike positioning should be made to decrease cervical extension.[16,18]

OVERUSE INJURIES OF THE UPPER EXTREMITY

Overuse injuries in cycling more commonly involves the lower extremities. Less literature explains susceptibility to overuse injuries of the upper extremity in cycling. One condition, termed *biker's elbow* can result in elbow and forearm pain, which has the same pathophysiology of lateral or medial epicondylosis, otherwise more commonly known as *tennis and golfer's elbow*. Pain at the lateral elbow can result from overuse injury to the common extensor tendon that leads to tendinopathy, or lateral epicondylosis.[19] Conversely, pain over the medial aspect of the elbow leads to medial epicondylosis, or a stress injury to the common flexor tendon.[20] Overuse injuries of the upper extremity are less frequent overall, but certain cycling disciplines carry greater risk. The risk of upper extremity overuse injury is present in an off-road discipline of cycling called *cyclocross*, in which riders must dismount their bicycle to traverse obstacles such as barriers on the ground, requiring the rider to repeatedly lift their bicycle to waist or shoulder height, which can lead to injuries of the wrist, elbow, or shoulder. These injuries may include tendinopathies of the wrist or elbow, as well as rotator cuff injury or injury to the acromioclavicular joint.

Mountain biking may predispose to chronic elbow pain due to frequent steering, increased vibratory forces, and tension in the forearm from navigating through rough terrain. Conservative management includes a bicycle fit assessment, strengthening exercises, counterforce bracing, nonsteroidal anti-inflammatory medications, and then injections or surgery if needed.[19] Bicycle fit in mountain bikers should address the saddle height in relation to handlebars. Proper handlebars and positioning are

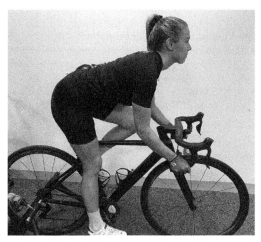

Fig. 4. Cervical spine and positioning. Poor bicycle fit or various posturing can alter the spinal mechanics by causing hyperextension of the cervical spine and is a cause for neck discomfort with cycling. Cyclists should alter their hand positions on the handlebars frequently to prevent prolonged neck extension. The cyclist in this photograph is extending her cervical spine to gaze forward.

paramount for a mountain bike fit, with attention to handlebar (1) width, (2) rise, and (3) sweep. Handlebar width is measured end to end and determines elbow and shoulder positioning while cycling. Handlebar rise is the vertical angulation from the center of the bar. Sweep refers to how much the bar bends back toward the rider as measured in degrees.[21] A bar with little to no sweep or otherwise a straight bar results in the wrist being slightly radially deviated and the elbow flexed outward. Positioning of the wrists, elbow, and shoulders can be improved with an increased sweep of the handlebars that will adjust the rider to a more relaxed position. Using handlebars of proper width, increased sweep, and rise adjustment can help chronic overuse injuries of the wrist, elbow, and shoulder in mountain biking.

Road cycling can also lead to chronic overuse injuries of the upper extremity, because this discipline involves longer hours of bike riding, sometimes 4 to 5 hours at once. Overuse injuries in these cases is caused by a position on the bike that creates stress on the wrist, elbows, shoulders, and spine by increased weight distribution over the upper extremities. Similarly, overuse injuries involve wrist tendinopathies or medial or lateral epicondylosis at the elbow. Combined shoulder elevation, locked elbow extension, and ulnar deviation may worsen symptoms, which can be adjusted by handlebar height and changes to hood positioning to achieve a more relaxed position of the upper extremity and improved cycling posture.[21] In addition, attention to saddle height positioning in relation to handlebars and degree of saddle tilt will influence the amount of forward weight distribution onto the handlebars. A saddle that is too high or tilted forward will cause increased weight and stress onto the upper extremities and can result in pain. Similar to the management of upper extremity neuropathies, stem height is an important consideration for proper bike fit for management of overuse injury. The stem may be a couple of inches below the height of the saddle, but there is variability depending on the skill and goals of the cyclist. A lower stem results in more aerodynamic positioning and is more advantageous for racing. A common rule of thumb with stem height is that the top of the handlebars should obscure the axle of the front wheel when the rider is looking down.[18]

DISCUSSION

Chronic and repetitive trauma from increased pressure due to road vibration, as occurs with cycling, can cause neuropathies of the upper extremities. One prospective study found that 70% of long-distance cyclists reported motor and/or sensory symptoms during the course of a 4-day ride.[2] Prolonged biking has been well defined as cause of ulnar neuropathy at the wrist.[5,6]

Handlebar shape is an important consideration in any upper extremity symptom in cycling. In cyclists, upper extremity neuropathies are commonly caused by poor bicycle fit and improper handlebar positioning causing nerve compression due to wrist or elbow strain. Road bikes typically have 3 components to their handlebars: drops, tops, and hoods (**Fig. 5**). Typical road bike handlebars have drops, which are the downward, curved parts of the handlebars. Drop handlebars increase the likelihood of an ulnar-deviated wrist and can redistribute more weight through the upper extremities. Although a less stable position for novice riders, hands on the tops, or the flat part of the handlebars, is an alternative hand position. This is a common hand position during climbing; however, it places the hands further away from the shifting gears and brakes. It is recommended that cyclists frequently change the riding positions of their hands throughout a ride to reduce prolonged compression and strain. Upper extremity overuse injury or pain is often a result of poor compensation patterns due to muscle strain and fatigue of a repetitive action such as cycling over time. Although there are different pathophysiological causes, there is overlap to the management of upper extremity conditions whether caused by an ulnar or median neuropathy or an overuse injury.

Recommendations for Hand Paresthesias or Upper Extremity Pain

- Reduce milage and readapt slowly[18]
- Reposition hands frequently
- Riders should be mindful of not tensing up their arms while riding
- Wear padded gloves
- Recommend wider tires
- Reduce tire pressure while riding

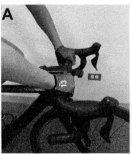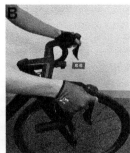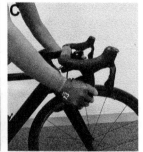

Fig. 5. Various hand positions on handlebars. Hands on different parts of the bike handlebars including on the tops (*A*) or hands in the hoods position (*B*). Riding on the tops provides less stability especially for novice cyclists. Hands on the drops is typically the most comfortable position with easy access to the gears and brakes. (*C*) Hands on the drops, which leads to a more aerodynamic position on the bike but is most likely to compress the ulnar nerve in Guyon's canal with increased pressure through the hands and possible ulnar deviation of the wrist.

- Use thicker, gel- or foam-based handlebar tape
- Alter the stem height
- Avoid tilting the saddle down
- Adjust the seat positioning; likely move backward

Handlebar height has an effect on cervical and thoracic spine postures.[22] Elevating the height of bicycle handlebars is recommended in cyclists who experience cervical spine discomfort during riding. High handlebars reduce the load on the lower cervical spine and decrease the risk of a hyperextended cervical spine.[22]

Stationary, indoor cycling has gained recent popularity. Indoor cycling produces less impact and vibratory forces; however, factors related to poor bike fit, such as overgripping of the handlebars and excessive wrist extension, can lead to similar issues as described earlier.[21]

SUMMARY

The most common upper extremity nerve injuries in cyclists are distal ulnar neuropathy in the wrist and carpal tunnel syndrome. Neck pain can also be a problem for cyclists caused by poor positioning on the bike or deconditioned cervical musculature. Overuse injuries of the upper extremities in cycling are less common but can present in the wrist, elbow, and shoulder. Treatment of these conditions varies from conservative management to surgical options. Regardless of the treatment approach, a bicycle fit assessment should be a key component for the management of these conditions. The prevalence of upper extremity neuropathies in the cycling population is unknown and could be an area of future studies. It would be advantageous to determine if there is a correlation between upper extremity neuropathies and overuse injuries, including neck pain with increased duration of riding, or if specific cycling disciplines have a greater prevalence of these conditions, such as mountain biking versus long-distance road cycling. Understanding the role of proper bicycle fit as it pertains to the individual is key to prevention and management of common cervical spine and upper extremity injuries.

CLINICS CARE POINTS

- Ulnar neuropathy at the wrist, also known as *cyclist palsy* or *handlebar palsy* is a common diagnosis for hand numbness and tingling in cyclists.

- Carpal tunnel syndrome may cause hand paresthesias and weakness; however, the literature is not as well defined in cyclists as it is in the general population.

- The cervical spine can be in a prolonged hyperextended position leading to cervical spine discomfort while cycling.

- Electromyography and nerve conduction tests are the gold standard in diagnosis of upper extremity neuropathies or cervical radiculopathies.

- MRI and diagnostic ultrasonography can also be used to assess for the degree and localization of nerve injury or compression.

- Prevention of compressive upper extremity neuropathies in cycling includes avoiding excessive or prolonged weight bearing through the hands, alternating hand and upper extremity positioning frequently during rides, and the use of padded cycling gloves.

- The most common overuse injury in the upper extremity in cycling is biker's elbow that presents as an insidious, chronic tendinopathy to the medial or lateral elbow.

- Conservative management of upper extremity conditions including neuropathies and overuse conditions related to cycling should always include a bicycle fit assessment with a focus on saddle and handlebar positioning.
- Medications; physical therapy, including strengthening or nerve glide exercises; proper bracing; and various injections can be helpful.
- Surgical nerve decompression should be considered for upper extremity compressive neuropathies for the most severe cases.

DISCLOSURE

The author has nothing to disclose.

ACKNOWLEDGMENTS

Lane Lagatutta, DO.

REFERENCES

1. Mellion MB. Common cycling injuries. Management and prevention. Sports Med 1991;11(1):52–70.
2. Patterson JM, Jaggars MM, Boyer MI. Ulnar and median nerve palsy in long-distance cyclists. A prospective study. Am J Sports Med 2003;31(4):585–9.
3. Depukat P, Mróz I, Tomaszewski K, et al. Syndrome of canal of Guyon — definition, diagnosis, treatment and complication. Folia Med Cracov 2015;55(1):17–23.
4. Andreisek G, Crook DW, Burg D, et al. Peripheral neuropathies of the median, radial, and ulnar nerves: MR imaging features. Radiographics 2006;26(5): 1267–87.
5. Capitani D, Beer S. Handlebar palsy–a compression syndrome of the deep terminal (motor) branch of the ulnar nerve in biking. J Neurol 2002;249(10):1441–5.
6. Brubacher JW, Leversedge FJ. Ulnar Neuropathy in Cyclists. Hand Clin 2017; 33(1):199–205.
7. Spinner RJ, Goldner RD. Snapping of the medial head of the triceps and recurrent dislocation of the ulnar nerve. Anatomical and dynamic factors. J Bone Joint Surg Am 1998;80(2):239–47.
8. Akuthota V, Plastaras C, Lindberg K, et al. The effect of long-distance bicycling on ulnar and median nerves: an electrophysiologic evaluation of cyclist palsy. Am J Sports Med 2005;33(8):1224–30.
9. Atroshi I, Gummesson C, Johnsson R, et al. Prevalence of Carpal Tunnel Syndrome in a General Population. JAMA 1999;282(2):153–8.
10. Wipperman J, Goerl K. Carpal Tunnel Syndrome: Diagnosis and Management. Am Fam Physician 2016;94(12):993–9.
11. Smith TM, Sawyer SF, Sizer PS, et al. The double crush syndrome: a common occurrence in cyclists with ulnar nerve neuropathy-a case-control study. Clin J Sport Med 2008;18(1):55–61.
12. Fitzpatrick KF. Cyclists - ulnar nerve and double crush. Clin J Sport Med 2010; 20(1):69–70 [author reply: 70–1].
13. Slane J, Timmerman M, Ploeg HL, et al. The influence of glove and hand position on pressure over the ulnar nerve during cycling. Clin Biomech (Bristol, Avon) 2011;26(6):642–8.
14. Wilber CA, Holland GJ, Madison RE, et al. An epidemiological analysis of overuse injuries among recreational cyclists. Int J Sports Med 1995;16(3):201–6.

15. Briggs MS, Rethman KK, Lopez MT. Clinical decision making and differential diagnosis in a cyclist with upper quarter pain, numbness, and weakness: a case report. Int J Sports Phys Ther 2018;13(2):255–68.
16. Kotler DH, Babu AN, Robidoux G. Prevention, Evaluation, and Rehabilitation of Cycling-Related Injury. Curr Sports Med Rep 2016;15(3):199–206.
17. Asplund C, Webb C, Barkdull T. Neck and back pain in bicycling. Curr Sports Med Rep 2005;4(5):271–4.
18. Arnie Baker M. Bicycling medicine. New York: Fireside; 1998.
19. Tosti R, Jennings J, Sewards JM. Lateral epicondylitis of the elbow. Am J Med 2013;126(4):357.e1-6.
20. Amin NH, Kumar NS, Schickendantz MS. Medial epicondylitis: evaluation and management. J Am Acad Orthop Surg 2015;23(6):348–55.
21. Willette A. Why cycling + mountain biking causes golfer's or tennis elbow and how to treat it. 2019. Available at: https://tenniselbowclassroom.com/sports-injuries/bikers-elbow/.
22. Kolehmainen I, Harms-Ringdahl K, Lanshammart H. Cervical spine positions and load moments during bicycling with different handlebar positions. Clin Biomech 1989;4(2):105–10.

Lumbar Spine and Lower Extremity Overuse Injuries

Tracey Isidro, MD, Elaine Gregory, MD, Laura Lachman, MD, Stacey Isidro, MD, Angela N. Cortez, MD*

KEYWORDS

- Cycling • Low back pain • Lower extremity pain • Overuse injury

KEY POINTS

- Lower extremity pain is a common source of overuse injury for cyclists.
- Knee pain is the most commonly affected area for overuse injuries in the lower extremities.
- Low back pain is a common source of overuse injury for cyclists.
- Understanding the relationship between the athlete and the bicycle can be an important component of treating both lower extremity pain and low back pain.

INTRODUCTION

Both lower extremities and the lower back are common sources of injury for cyclists.[1,2] In order for providers to optimize care within this specialized area of sports medicine, they need to understand the most common sources of injury in this population. To achieve this, cycling presents a unique challenge: treating both the athlete and the complex relationship between rider and bicycle. Physicians, however knowledgeable, should not replace the role of a professional bike fitter and should view these individuals as integral members of the team to alleviate current and prevent future injury. This article explores the most common lower extremity and lumbar back overuse injuries in cyclists and their medical management.

CYCLING-RELATED LOWER EXTREMITY PAIN

Cyclists can experience chronic overuse injuries in multiple parts of the body from repetitive movements.[1] Various studies report that the knee is the second most affected area for overuse injuries overall and the most commonly affected in the lower limb.[3,4]

H. Ben Taub Department of Physical Medicine and Rehabilitation, Baylor College of Medicine; 7200 Cambridge Street, Houston, TX 77030, USA
* Corresponding author. Baylor Medicine at McNair Campus, A10.264, Houston, TX 77030.
E-mail address: angela.cortez@bcm.edu

Phys Med Rehabil Clin N Am 33 (2022) 201–214
https://doi.org/10.1016/j.pmr.2021.08.014
1047-9651/22/© 2021 Elsevier Inc. All rights reserved.

According to the 2020 SAFER XIII cross-sectional study of more than 21,000 cyclists, the prevalence of injuries in the lower limb is 43.4%.[4] The incidence of injuries in the knee ranges from 14.2% to 62% compared with a 7% to 31% incidence in the rest of the lower extremity.[2–10] This wide range is attributed to level and intensity of training as well as different forces of the leg due to bike fit and alignment.[5,7,11–15] These musculoskeletal injuries of the lower extremity can cause pain and impede performance in the cyclist. With the goal of helping cyclists achieve improved function, cyclists and medical professionals can become familiar in chronic overuse injuries, management, and injury prevention Common causes of lower extremity pain in cyclists are explored.

Anterior Knee Pain——Patellofemoral Pain Syndrome, Patellar Tendinosis, and Quadriceps Tendinosis

Clinical presentation

Anterior knee pain can be a common complaint in cyclists. Differential diagnoses include patellofemoral pain (PFP) syndrome, patellar tendinosis, and quadriceps tendinosis. Of these 3, PFP is the most common cause of chronic overuse injury in the lower extremity.[1,16–18] PFP syndrome has multiple contributing factors. Anatomic factors include patellofemoral malalignment and maltracking, where the patella is not situated properly over the intercondylar notch, varus or valgus abnormalities at the knee or ankle, and muscular conditions from weak quadriceps or tight hamstrings.[1,16–18] Some external factors that contribute to PFP syndrome include low seat height and anterior seat position,[1,19] causing further knee flexion and anterior forces on the knees. Training issues related to excessive use of high gears or uphill climbing with a slow cadence also can lead to or exacerbate PFP syndrome.[1,16–18,20–22] In patellar tendinosis, cyclists may have pain directly over the patellar tendon on the downstroke during knee extension.[1] Repetitive knee flexion and extension, in combination with genu valgum, tibial internal rotation, and foot hyperpronation[1] may cause microtears or disruption of patellar tendon architecture. In quadriceps tendinosis, cyclists typically present with anterolateral knee pain.[1] Other factors contributing to quadriceps tendonitis include genu valgum and suboptimal seat positioning, including a low saddle height.[1]

Physical examination findings

Physical examination should include range of motion (ROM) of the hip, knee, and ankle, and strength of the hip flexors, extensors, abductors, and adductors. The knee joint should be assessed for patellar mobility as well as tenderness over the patellar facets, quadriceps, or patellar tendons. The key findings on examination for patellar and quadriceps tendinosis are pain with palpation or swelling over the patellar or quadriceps tendon, respectively.[1] In a cycling-specific clinic setup, physician may collaborate with a physical therapist or a bike fitter to identify potential causes of the cyclist's knee pain. Alternatively, a slow-motion video recorded in the frontal plane is helpful in evaluating knee deviations. The foot and ankle along with cleat position may also be examined to determine if there are uneven forces from foot hyperpronation, resulting in upstream anterior knee pain.

Treatment/management

There are multiple ways to treat anterior knee pain. For pain management, rest, ice, heat, over-the-counter oral medications like acetaminophen or ibuprofen, or topical anti-inflammatories, such as diclofenac gel, may be helpful. In the acute setting, cyclists may avoid exercises that cause increased stress on the quadriceps tendon like squats but may restart strengthening exercises once pain improves.[1] Modifications to cycling technique and habit,s including use of gears that allow a higher cadence of at least 80 rpm to 90 rpm, and reducing hill-climbing in the short term may be helpful.[1,16–18,20,21] Ensuring there is an efficient alignment of the hip, knee, and ankle during pedaling to reduce forces on the patellofemoral joint may be accomplished by improved hip abductor strength and proper foot support. A cyclist may engage in stretches, massage, foam rolling, therapeutic tape, and strength training. Because the vastus medialis oblique is responsible for patellar stabilization and tracking, focusing on this quadricep muscle in addition to the hamstrings, iliotibial band (ITB), and core stabilization may be beneficial.[1,16–18,20,21,23] Supportive inserts, wedges in cycling shoes, adjustments to the cleat angle or position, and exercises to strengthen arch support may correct foot hyperpronation for better alignment but should be done by a trained bike fitter as a part of a comprehensive bike fit.[1,19]

Iliotibial Band Friction Syndrome

Clinical presentation
Lateral knee pain is most commonly caused by ITB friction syndrome.[16] The ITB originates from the iliac crest and courses over the lateral femoral epicondyle before attaching to the anterolateral tibia.[1,16] Cyclists present with lateral knee pain worse at the ITB impingement angle, which is 30° of knee flexion. This is due to repetitive knee flexion and extension while cycling and may be exacerbated with a taller seat height or fast cadence.[1,16,18]

Physical examination findings
When evaluating for ITB friction syndrome, a physician may appreciate tenderness and/or swelling over the lateral femoral condyle.[1,16] A positive Ober test may be indicative of ITB tightness.[1] The physician also may note genu varus or similar findings from other chronic knee overuse injuries, such as tibial internal rotation and foot hyperpronation.[1]

Treatment/management
One way to treat ITB friction syndrome is to lower the seat height or adjust the seat position anteriorly and decrease cadence.[17,18] Another is to adjust stance width, which is the distance between the center of each pedal, typically through a cleat adjustment, addition of pedal washers, or use of pedal spindle extenders. Other options include adjusting cleats, using wedges, and stretching and strengthening hip abductors, all of which may decrease rotational strain over the ITB.[1,18,23]

Pes Anserine Bursitis

Clinical presentation
The pes anserine bursa is located distal to the medial tibial tubercle and is the site of insertion of the tendons of the sartorius, gracilis, and semitendinosus. Similar to the ITB friction syndrome, pes anserine bursitis also presents after repetitive friction of these 3 tendons over the bursa.[1] Risk factors include excessive valgus knee angulation, resulting in excessive traction forces on the medial knee and knee osteoarthritis. Although further research is needed, cleat wedges and shoe inserts that affect knee angulation may be factors.[24]

Physical examination findings
A cyclist presents with medial knee pain with palpation over the pes anserine bursa or pain with resisted internal rotation and resisted flexion of the knee. The clinician also may notice hamstring tightness or genu valgum on examination.[1]

Treatment/management

In addition to conservative treatment options, discussed previously, stretching the hamstrings and hip adductors may relieve medial knee pain.[23] Other possible treatment options include ultrasound and corticosteroid injections to the pes anserine bursa.[1,25]

Achilles Tendinopathy or Tendonitis

Clinical presentation

Cyclists, especially multisport athletes, such as triathletes, who experience posterior distal leg or heel pain, may have Achilles tendinopathy or tendonitis, particularly from running activities. Prevalence ranges from 6.4% to 15% and may be caused by a multitude of factors similar to other overuse leg injuries.[3,26,27] These include suboptimal pedaling like standing during uphill and excessive dorsiflexion, low cadence, low seat height, hyperpronation, tight and weak plantarflexors, poor recovery time, and osteophytes.[1,14,28,29]

Physical examination findings

There may be swelling, thickening, and pain on palpation over the Achilles tendon midportion or at its insertion on the calcaneus. There also may be restricted passive dorsiflexion, gastrocnemius weakness or myofascial trigger points, and/or pain with active plantarflexion exercises, including single-leg heel raises.

Treatment/management

Suggestions include ice, heat, pain medications, stretching, and strengthening of the gastrocnemius and soleus.[23,30] Sufficient rest along with these conservative measures have been found to be helpful. If the etiology for a cyclist's Achilles tendinopathy or tendonitis is due to improper bike fit, then seat height may be raised in order to increase plantarflexion while cycling. If it is due to foot misplacement or malalignment, the center of the foot may be placed over the center of the pedal in a neutral position, which helps decrease the excessive angle of dorsiflexion and provides symptomatic relief.[1,28,29]

Plantar Fasciitis

Clinical presentation

A common cause of heel pain is plantar fasciitis, a condition that affects the fibrous band of tissue at the bottom of the foot from the heel to the toes. Typically, symptoms are worse in the morning, with weight bearing, and usually after multisport activities like triathlons. Structural issues like pes planus or a weak tibialis posterior and external factors like improper footwear, low cadence with high resistance, and a low seat height may predispose cyclists to plantar fasciitis.[1,18]

Physical examination findings

There may be pain with palpation over the medial calcaneal tubercle and weakness in plantarflexors. Because the plantar fascia also helps with arch support, there may be decreased arch height on the affected side. If ultrasound is available, a thickened plantar fascia may be appreciated.

Treatment/management

Nonsurgical treatment options include orthotics for arch support. Physical therapy with stretching and night splints may be beneficial in addition to strengthening muscles involved in supporting the arch, including the intrinsic foot muscles, posterior tibialis, flexor digitorum longus, and flexor hallucis longus. Regenerative interventions, including shockwave therapy, prolotherapy, and orthobiologics, are options for treatment. Steroid injections also may be performed, although there is a risk of fat atrophy and tendon rupture with repeated steroid injections.[1] Training with a lower resistance and slightly increasing the seat height to relieve pressure on the plantar fascia may be useful as well.[1]

Metatarsalgia

Clinical presentation
Cycling shoes are rigid to allow efficient power transfer to the pedals. Pain at the ball of the foot over the metatarsal bones, or metatarsalgia, may result from training issues like high resistance or low cadence and equipment issues like poorly fit shoes,[1] causing pain with pedaling. Another cause that increases pressure over the forefoot is abnormal foot alignment.

Physical examination findings
There can be pain with palpation to the plantar surface of the foot along the metatarsal heads. Evaluating the cyclist's shoes and pedaling technique may provide useful information as to the etiology of pain.

Treatment/management
Similar to other conditions that cause foot pain, metatarsalgia may be managed by using well-fitting shoes with good arch and metatarsal support, checking cleats, and decreasing resistance with a faster cadence.[1]

External Iliac Artery Endofibrosis

Clinical presentation
External iliac artery endofibrosis is an underappreciated condition that often is misdiagnosed, leading to delays in proper management. Leg symptoms of cramping, swelling, and numbness or pain of the calf, thigh, or buttock during near-maximal exercise that resolves within 5 minutes of rest is a sign of potential external iliac artery endofibrosis.[31] It is thought to be due to arterial injury caused by some combination of high blood flow stresses and mechanical kinking from hip hyperflexion. One study suggested that as many as 10% to 20% of professional road cyclists may experience blood-flow restrictions due to either intravascular endofibrosis or functional kinking of iliac arteries.[32] Cycling greater than 14,500 km/y may be a risk factor.[33,34]

Physical examination findings
Femoral bruit with the hip in flexion is a diagnostic sign of iliac endofibrosis. Examination of the hip and back to rule out nonvascular causes is essential. Diagnostic confirmation is through measurement of pre-exercise and postexercise ankle pressures (ankle-brachial index) and duplex ultrasound while supine and with the hips and knees in 90° flexion. Computed tomography angiography or magnetic resonance angiography also may be used to support the diagnosis.[32]

Treatment/management
Conservative management consists of avoiding maximal hip-flexion by adjusting saddle and handlebar height, decreasing psoas hypertrophy by refraining from pulling up in clipless pedals, and folate supplementation.[32] Because the disease is progressive, surgical options often are pursued, such as endofibroscectomy and arterial shortening, allowing athletes to return to sport within a few months of intervention with good results.[32,34]

Pudendal Neuralgia

Clinical presentation
Genital pain, numbness, and tingling while cycling can be a sign of pudendal nerve injury. Mechanisms of injury are incompletely understood but may be due to mechanical compression, stretching of the nerve, friction, or ischemia from vascular compression

during pedaling.[35,36] Symptoms may be found in up to 9% to 34% of professional cyclists, with increased risk in those older than 50 years, with greater body weight, with more than 10-year cycling history, and from high-intensity training.[35,37]

Physical examination findings
Nantes criteria are recommended, which include (1) pain in the anatomic region of the pudendal nerve, (2) pain aggravated by sitting, (3) absence of nocturnal pain, (4) no sensory loss on clinical examination, and (5) resolution of symptoms with anesthetic block of the pudendal nerve.[17,38]

Treatment/management
Choosing a wider saddle or alternate shape in order to distribute weight over a wider area of the buttocks and ischial tuberosities may prevent direct compression of the pudendal nerve and perineal soft tissues.[35,37] Additionally, intermittent periods of standing for pressure relief and avoidance of prolonged aero position may reduce nerve irritation.[36]

CYCLING-RELATED LOW BACK PAIN

Low back pain (LBP) is a frequent complaint of cyclists, with an incidence of 15% to 60%, and may become a source of frustration for both the cyclists and treating physicians, particularly if there are recurrent injuries/issues.[3,6,39] There are multiple hypotheses theorizing the pathomechanics of cycling-induced LBP, including the flexion-relaxation hypothesis, the muscle fatigue hypothesis, the over-activation of spinal extensors hypothesis, the mechanical creep hypothesis, and the disc ischemia hypothesis. The evidence supporting any of these theories, however, is lacking.[39] The common thread among all these hypotheses is that LBP stems from the prolonged, flexed lumbar posture assumed while riding, in combination with poor bike fit or due to spinal extensor muscle fatigue. These hypotheses all focus on the direct or indirect impact that the riding position has on the extensor/flexor spinal musculature, posterior spinal elements, intervertebral discs and how the interaction of these factors can lead to LBP. LBP can originate at any level, including the spinal musculature (due to muscular fatigue), soft tissues (musculotendinous strains or ligamentous sprains), intervertebral discs, and facet joints (due to prolonged traction on the joint capsule).[15–17,38,40–42]

Most of the current literature is based on retrospective data collection and lacks a specific etiology of the LBP; specific diagnoses and their frequencies, therefore, are lacking. Patients often are diagnosed with nonspecific chronic LBP.[38] Although many of these complaints resolve with conservative interventions, LBP often recurs and may be progressive if the causative factors are not addressed. This can result in missed training, loss of income for professional cyclists, and potential withdrawal from cycling all together. Clinicians should focus on the identification and mitigation of modifiable factors contributing to LBP. To prepare the clinician in this effort, elements reviewed in this section include the components of a comprehensive cyclist history; the risk factors for developing LBP, important components of bike fit, and specific diagnoses that should be considered.

Important Factors to Consider

Comprehensive cyclist history
In addition to the standard history of present illness, including prior injuries/trauma, the presence of symptoms on and off the bike is essential. A comprehensive cycling history, including the type of cycling, training/racing schedule, cross-training activities, duration of climbing hills/sprinting/riding long distances, typical cadence, and recent changes in equipment, is vital to determining potential interventions.[43]

Risk factors for the development of back pain

Risk factors are divided into 2 groups: intrinsic risk factors related to the cyclist and extrinsic factors related to the bicycle or environment. Intrinsic risk factors for LBP are related to muscle dysfunction, flexibility limitations, body asymmetry, and degenerative change. Some examples include asymmetric spinal muscle firing patterns, imbalance of flexor and extensor trunk muscles, weak or tight hip flexors/abductors, and leg length differences (LLDs). Extrinsic factors include bike position and fit and training/racing factors including training volume, ride duration, intensity, and low-cadence high-resistance cycling.[39,44]

Cyclist physical examination

Examination includes

- Inspection for lumbar paraspinal and iliac asymmetry, palpation to assess reproducibility of pain and trigger points
- ROM assessment to determine limitations and directional preference of flexion or extension
- Special maneuvers, including the slump test and straight leg raise to assess dural tension and facet loading
- Neurologic testing, including manual muscle testing, reflexes, and sensation
- Single-leg squats to test for weakness or decreased recruitment of hip abductors and poor knee tracking
- Evaluation of asymmetry, including LLDs.[45]
- Assessment of lumbosacral, hamstring, and quadricep flexibility and hip ROM to determine how much forward flexion patients can tolerate and their pelvic positioning. Flexibility of the hamstrings can be assessed by evaluating the popliteal angle while flexibility of the quadriceps can be assessed with the Ely test. Evaluation of these is important because inflexibility of the quadriceps favors anterior pelvic tilt whereas tight hamstrings favor posterior pelvic tilt.[35,43]

Critical Aspect of Bike Fit

A comprehensive evaluation of cycling-related LBP includes an evaluation of bicycle fit and the cyclist's biomechanics on the bicycle. Familiarity with the main considerations of bike fit is helpful because it can be integral to the development of LBP as well as an area for potential intervention. Physicians, however, should not attempt to replace the role of a professional bike fitter because they are specially trained to ensure proper frame size, saddle height/position, cleat placement, and handlebar reach distance/height.

Frame size

Appropriate frame size is the most important condition to achieve a proper fit and varies depending on the type of bike selection (mountain, commuter/hybrid, or road) and manufacturer. A competent bike fitter should be collaborated with to ensure proper alignment/fit.

Reach distance

Top tube length, saddle height and angle, and stem and handlebar reach are factors that have an impact on reach distance and are important considerations in the development of cycling-related LBP. A too short reach forces an individual to sit more upright, causing the sacral spine to flex and increasing the pressure on the intervertebral discs. When the reach is too long, it extends the cyclists lumbar posture and can result in increased pressure on the posterior spinal elements and the intervertebral discs. A short reach distance favors an increased amount of lumbar flexion and a posterior pelvic tilt, although a longer reach distance decreases lumbar flexion, favoring an anterior pelvic tilt.[39] This relation between reach distance and top tube length can be adjusted by varying the length of the seat stem. Using a stem shorter than 40 mm or longer than 140 mm, however, affects the stability of the bike.[36] Poor fit can result in constant isometric contraction of supporting muscles of the back resulting in pain from muscle fatigue.[36] It is important to differentiate maladaptive lower lumbar kinematics from issues that can be minimized through proper bike fit.[46]

Handlebar height, grip placement, and saddle angle

The lumbar spine changes from a lordotic curvature to a kyphotic curvature when positioned on the bike.[47] This results in increased lumbar flexion and changes the lumbosacral angle, predisposing the cyclist to LBP (**Fig. 1**).[48] Investigations have established that handlebar grip, height/distance from the saddle, and saddle fit (angle, shape, height, and comfort) can be adjusted to minimize these changes.[36,41,47,48] These studies indicate that higher handlebar height and grip can decrease the degree of lumbar flexion. Changes in saddle also can decrease the degree of lumbar flexion. Increasing the anterior saddle tilt may increase the lumbosacral angle; therefore, decreasing the tensile forces across the anterior lumbar spine and subsequent loading of the posterior spinal elements. Other factors that can increase the degree of lumbar flexion include handlebar hand positions that are farther away and lower than the saddle of the bicycle.[36,41] Studies also have demonstrated that anterior pelvic tilt can mitigate the forces across the lumbar spine whereas posterior pelvic tilt exacerbates them.[36,41,48] Alterations in saddle angle, handlebar height, and grip placement to relieve LBP also should be evaluated for unintended consequences, such as painful hands (handlebars lower than saddle) or groin pain (saddle position).

Levels of low back pain in cyclists

It is useful to conceptualize LBP in cyclists on a continuum ranging from muscular fatigue or muscular strains to injury to the posterior spinal components. Diagnoses considered in this section include (1) lumbar strains and sprains, (2) discogenic pain/disc herniation, (3) facet joint syndrome, and (4) radiculopathy. The clinical

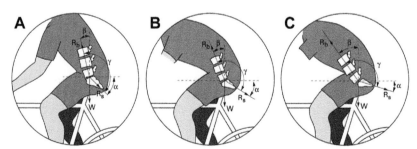

Fig. 1. Lateral pelvic/spine schema drawn from radiographs taken while the subject was sitting on various bicycles with various body positions, showing the related force vectors at the promontorium. W, weight; R_b, lumbar vector; R_s, pelvic vector; α, angle between ground and R_s vector; β, angle between weight axis and R_b vector; γ, lumbosacral/pelvic angle. (A) Town bike; (B) mountain bike; (C) racing bike. (*From* Salai M, Brosh T, Blankstein A, Oran A, Chechik A. Effect of changing the saddle angle on the incidence of low back pain in recreational bicyclists. Br J Sports Med. 1999 Dec;33(6):398-400. https://doi.org/10.1136/bjsm.33.6.398. PMID: 10597848; PMCID: PMC1756210.)

presentation and presumed pathophysiology, physical examination findings, and treatment recommendations are discussed for each. Because these injuries represent a spectrum of causes, treatment recommendations may be applied to multiple diagnoses and should be considered unless expressly contraindicated.

Lumbar Strains and Sprains

Clinical presentation
Strains result from disruption of the muscle fibers within the muscle belly or in the musculotendinous junction and can be categorized as acute, chronic, or recurrent. A patient's presentation may vary based on the location, severity, and chronicity of the muscle strain. In general, acute strains present with intense pain for the first 24 hours to 48 hours after injury and often are associated with spasms. Days later, the pain may be localized to a trigger point. Chronic strains are characterized by continued pain in the muscle due to injury whereas recurrent strains are denoted by frequent flares with short asymptomatic periods.[37,40]

Ligamentous sprains occur by stretching of the spinal ligaments, which remain intact because only some of the fibers are involved. Although not well defined, the proposed pain generator with ligament sprains is thought to be via nociceptive innervation of the spinal ligament, which has been characterized on anatomic and histologic studies.[49] The interspinous process ligament has been proposed as the most affected by sprains.[37,40]

Physical examination findings
Findings usually include paraspinal muscle tenderness with or without associated muscle spasm, and without localized bruising or radicular symptoms. Trigger points likely are present in patients with acute, chronic, or recurrent muscular strain. Muscular sprains and ligamentous strains are not discernible based on physical examination.

Treatment of strains and sprains
Initial treatment begins with a period of rest and cryotherapy. Nonsteroidal anti-inflammatory drugs (NSAIDS) are particularly useful in acute injuries. Gentle and progressive stretching, follows ideally under the guidance of a trainer or physical therapist. LLDs of 3 mm to 6 mm can be addressed by moving the cleat backward on the long leg or forward on the short leg. LLDs greater than 6 mm should be addressed with a shim or combination of shim and adjustment of cleats.[45] Patients should resume their normal activities only when they are pain-free and without functional limitations. If all the intrinsic and extrinsic factors, such as cycling activities, duration, frequency, issues with bike fit, and technical riding errors, are not addressed, patients are at risk of recurrence of their symptoms once they completely resume their cycling activities.

Intervertebral Discogenic Pain

Clinical presentation
Following soft tissue injuries, discogenic pain is theorized to be the next most common etiology of LBP in cyclists and its onset may be gradual or acute. Discogenic pain potentially is associated with disc ischemia, increased discal forces related to the seated lumbar flexed position, and disc erniation.[18,50] The literature suggests that disc ischemia, increased discal forces, or combination of these results in microtears in the posterior annulus, resulting in discogenic type pain. During an active flare, flexion activities, including cycling, may exacerbate the pain. Disc herniation results from focal protrusions of the nucleus pulposus through the annulus fibrosis; patients

report increased pain associated with hills and rough terrain.[40,45] An acute onset of discogenic pain with or without radiation suggests a tiny annular fissure or an acute herniation. Signs and symptoms reported vary widely. Pain can present unilaterally or bilaterally with or without radiation to the buttock or lower extremity.

Physical examination findings
Physical examination reveals pain with forward flexion or load lifting and pain with dural tension maneuvers, such as straight leg raise. As with strains and sprains, the neurologic examination usually is normal. Assessment of a patient's posture off the bike as well as observing the patient on the bike for technical saddle errors, such as sitting behind the ischial tuberosity, is helpful in identifying contributing factors.[43] Although plain films frequently are pursued, they do not prove a causative relationship. Multilevel disc disease on plain film likely is required to produce symptoms. Depending on the acuity, severity, or persistence of the patient's symptoms, however, plain films or more advanced imaging may be considered.

Treatment
When pain is flexion-based, McKenzie back extension exercises are the mainstay treatment of disc disease and have been found especially useful in cyclists (**Fig. 2**).[37,40] Similar to strains and sprains, these injuries are treated in a progressive manner, including a brief rest period and NSAIDs. When pain is controlled, efforts to enhance spinal stability by improving abdominal muscles and lumbar extensor muscle control should be pursued. Progressive strengthening of the lumbar muscles to improve neuromuscular firing then is recommended. The goal is restoration of the balance between the spinal extensors and flexors. Studies have shown that increased trunk flexor training or decreased trunk extensor to flexor ratios are more frequently associated with complaints of LBP.[15,51,52] Returning to sport activities usually requires the patient to have painless ROM, return of muscle strength/endurance, less lumbar flexion, and improved pelvic stability.[37] Upon resuming cycling activities, the cyclist is advised to dismount the bike intermittently to perform the McKenzie back extension exercises. This can progress to performing hyperextension exercises while upright on the bike during competitions and training.[40]

Lumbar Facet Syndrome

Clinical presentation
Lumbar facet syndrome usually affects athletes by repeated forceful hyperextension of the lumbar spine and, therefore, does not tend to limit cyclists from their ability to ride. Symptoms result from direct irritation of the facet joint or indirectly by irritation of the intervertebral discs. Symptomatology ranges from localized signs to radiating symptoms.[40]

Physical examination findings
Physical examination usually reveals pain on lumbar extension and facet loading maneuver (extension and rotation). There may be paraspinal tenderness. Neurologic examination typically is normal.[40] Patients who do not have pain with extension may have pain when rising from forward flexed to upright positions.

Treatment
Similar to sprains/strains and discogenic pain, treatment begins with a short period of rest and maintenance of a pain-free position. Physical therapy for these patients has a similar objective of gradually improving spinal stability. As with prior diagnoses, imaging is not confirmatory but may show facet arthropathy, effusions, spondylolisthesis,

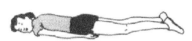
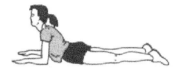

1. Prone lying. Lie on your stomach with arms along your sides and head turned to one side. Maintain this position for 5 to 10 minutes.

2. Prone lying on elbows. Lie on your stomach with your weight on elbows and forearms and your hips touching the floor or mat. Relax your low back. Remain in this position 5 to 10 minutes. If this causes pain, repeat exercise 1, then try again.

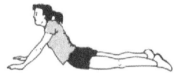
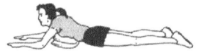

3. Prone press-ups. Lie on your stomach with palms near your shoulders, as if to do a standard push-up. Slowly push your shoulders up, keeping your hips on the surface and letting your back and stomach sag. Slowly lower your shoulders. Repeat 10 times.

4. Progressive extension with pillows. Lie on your stomach and place a pillow under your chest. After several minutes, add a second pillow. If this does not hurt, add a third pillow after a few more minutes. Stay in this position up to 10 minutes. Remove pillows one at a time over several minutes.

Fig. 2. Examples of McKenzie extension exercises.[40] (*From* Harvey J, Tanner S. (1991). Low Back Pain in Young Atheletes A Practical Approach. Sports Medicine, 12(6), 394-406.)

or facet synovial cysts, which may cause nerve root impingement. Based on the acuity or persistence of a patient's symptoms, interventions, such as medial branch blocks, can be performed for diagnostic purposes with subsequent radiofrequency ablation for treatment.

Radiculopathy/Radicular Pain

Clinical presentation
Radicular pain may be caused by irritation or mechanical compression of the nerve roots in the spinal canal or neural foramen, either by disc, bone, or other space-occupying mass. Annular tears may cause an acute radiculitis, which may cause pain and altered sensation, whereas mechanical compression can result in objective neurologic findings, including sensory loss or motor weakness in a lumbosacral radiculopathy. In cases of disc herniation, exacerbating factors are similar to those discussed in discogenic pain, often flexion-based. In cases of spinal or foraminal stenosis with radiculopathy or claudication, pain often is alleviated in a flexed-posture, and cycling may be well tolerated.[43]

Physical examination findings
Physical examination findings are similar to those of lumbar facet syndrome. Radicular symptoms may be reproducible with dural tension tests. A detailed neurologic examination identifies sensory or motor deficits as well as asymmetry in reflexes.[40]

Treatment
Because these radicular symptoms are often associated with inflammation near the nerve root or disc herniation, treatment of the underlying cause results in centralization

of pain and resolution of radicular symptoms. Any radiculopathy that is progressive or fails to centralize with conservative therapies or is associated with sensory or strength impairments warrants further evaluation, including advanced imaging.[40]

SUMMARY

Lower extremity and lower back issues are common injuries faced by competitive and recreational cyclists alike. When treating such injuries, it is important to understand the most common sources of pain and to account for the complex relationship between the athlete and the bicycle. This article presents the most common sources of these injuries and how best to treat them. As to future directions, in order to improve treatment and care, the authors suggest additional focus be placed on understanding how the complex relationship between athlete and bicycle can have an impact on these injuries.

DISCLOSURE

The authors have nothing to disclose.

REFERENCES

1. Wanich T, Hodgkins C, Columbier JA, et al. Cycling injuries of the lower extremity. J Am Acad Orthop Surg 2007;15:748–56.
2. Johnston TE, Baskins TA, Koppel RV, et al. The influence of extrinsic factors on knee biomechanics during cycling: a systematic review of the literature. Int J Sports Phys Ther 2017;12(7):1023.
3. Clarsen B, Krosshaug T, Bahr R. Overuse Injuries in Professional Road Cyclists. Am J Sports Med 2010;38:2494–501.
4. Du Toit F, Schwellnus M, Wood P, et al. Epidemiology, clinical characteristics and severity of gradual onset injuries in recreational road cyclists: A cross-sectional study in 21,824 cyclists - SAFER XIII. Phys Ther Sport 2020;46:113e119.
5. Bini R, Hume PA, Croft JL. Effects of bicycle saddle height on knee injury risk and cycling performance. Sports Med 2011;41:463–76.
6. Dannenberg AL, Needle S, Mullady D, et al. Predictors of injury among 1638 riders in a recreational long-distance bicycle tour: cycle across Maryland. Am J Sports Med 1996;24(6):747–53.
7. Wilber CA, Holland GJ, Madison RE, et al. An epidemiological analysis of overuse injuries among recreational cyclists. Int J Sports Med 1995;16:201–6.
8. Vleck VE, Garbutt G. Injury and training characteristics of male elite, development squad, and club triathletes. Int J Sports Med 1998;19:38–42.
9. Kulund DN, Brubaker CE. Injuries in the bikecentennial tour. Phys Sportsmed 1978;6:74–8.
10. Borgers A, Claes S, Vanbeek N, et al. Etiology of knee pain in elite cyclists: A 14-month consecutive case series. Acta Orthop Belg 2020;86(2):262–71.
11. Weiss BD. Nontraumatic injuries in amateur long distance bicyclists. Am J Sports Med 1985;13(3):187–92.
12. Zwingenberger S, Valladares RD, Walther A, et al. An epidemiological investigation of training and injury patterns in triathletes. J Sports Sci 2014;32:583–90.
13. Berkovich Y, Nierenberg G, Falah M, et al. Knee injury in cyclers. Harefuah 2010; 149:726–8, 748.
14. Silberman MR. Bicycling injuries. Curr Sports Med Rep 2013;12:337–45.

15. Deakon RT. Chronic musculoskeletal conditions associated with the cycling segment of the triathlon; prevention and treatment with an emphasis on proper bicycle fitting. Sports Med Arthrosc Rev 2012;20:200–5.

16. Schwellnus MP, Derman EW. Common injuries in cycling: Prevention, diagnosis and management. South Afr Fam Pract 2005;47(7):14–9.

17. Campbell ML, Lebec MT. Etiology and Intervention for Common Overuse Syndromes Associated with Mountain Biking. Ann Sports Med Res 2015;2(3):1022.

18. Dettori N, Norvell D. Non-traumatic bicycle injuries: A review of the literature. Sports Med 2006;36(1):7–18.

19. Wang Y, Liang L, Wang D, et al. Cycling with Low Saddle Height is Related to Increased Knee Adduction Moments in Healthy Recreational Cyclists. Eur J Sport Sci 2020;20(4):461–7.

20. Holmes JC, Pruitt AL, Whalen NJ. Lower extremity overuse in bicycling. Clin Sports Med 1994;13:187–205.

21. Sabeti-Aschraf M, Serek M, Geisler M, et al. Overuse injuries correlated to the mountain bike's adjustment: a prospective field study. Open Sports Sci J 2010; 3:1–6.

22. Shen G, Zhang S, Bennett HJ, et al. Effects of Knee Alignments and Toe Clip on Frontal Plane Knee Biomechanics in Cycling. J Sports Sci Med 2018;17(2): 312–21.

23. Piotrowska SE, Majchrzycki M, Rogala P, et al. Lower extremity and spine pain in cyclists. Ann Agric Environ Med 2017;24(4):654–8.

24. Alvarez-Nenemegyei J. Risk factors for pes anserinus tendinitis/bursitis syndrome: a case control study. J Clin Rheumatol 2007;13(2):63–5.

25. Helfenstein M Jr, Kuromoto J. Anserine syndrome. Rev Bras Reumatol 2010; 50(3):313–27.

26. Barrios C, Bernardo ND, Vera P, et al. Changes in sports injuries incidence over time in world-class road cyclists. Int J Sports Med 2015;36:241–8.

27. De Bernardo N, Barrios C, Vera P, et al. Incidence and risk for traumatic and overuse injuries in top-level road cyclists. J Sports Sci 2012;30:1047–53.

28. Althunyan AK, Darwish MA, Sabra AA, et al. Factors associated with Achilles tendon pain in cyclists in eastern province of Saudi Arabia. J Fam Community Med 2021;28(1):35–41.

29. Chisari E, Rehak L, Khan WS, et al. Tendon healing in presence of chronic low-level inflammation: A systematic review. Br Med Bull 2019;132:97–116.

30. Gregor RJ, Komi PV, Järvinen M. Achilles tendon forces during cycling. Int J Sports Med 1987;8(Suppl 1):9–14.

31. Peach G, Schep G, Palfreeman R, et al. Endofibrosis and kinking of the iliac arteries in athletes: a systematic review. Eur J Vasc Endovasc Surg 2012;43(2): 208–17.

32. Gähwiler R, Hirschmüller A, Grumann T, et al. Exercise induced leg pain due to endofibrosis of external iliac artery. Vasa 2021;50(2):92–100.

33. Schep G, Bender MH, van de Tempel G, et al. Detection and treatment of claudication due to functional iliac obstruction in top endurance athletes: a prospective study. Lancet 2002;359(9305):466–73.

34. Khan A, Al-Dawoud M, Salaman R, et al. Management of Endurance Athletes with Flow Limitation in the Iliac Arteries: A Case Series. EJVES Short Rep 2018; 40:7–11.

35. Ansari MN. Mountain Biking Injuries. Curr Sports Med Rep 2017;16(6):404–12.

36. Asplund C WC. Neck and Back Pain in Bicycling. Curr Sports Med Rep 2005;4: 271–4.

37. Bono CM. Current Concepts Review Low-Back Pain in Atheletes. J Bone Joint Surg 2004;86-A(2):382–96.
38. Burnett AF, Cornelius MW, Dankaerts W, Peter B O'sullivan. Spinal Kinematics and trunk muscle activity in cyclists: a comparision between healthy controls and non-specific chronic low back pain subjects. Man Ther 2004;9:211–9.
39. Marsden MS. Lower back pain in cyclists: A review of epidemiology, pathomechanics and risk factors. Int SportMed J 2010;11(1):216–25. Available at: http://www.ismj.com.
40. Harvey J, Tanner S. Low Back Pain in Young Atheletes A Practical Approach. Sports Med 1991;12(6):394–406.
41. Muyor J. The influence of handlebar-hand position on spinal posture in professional cyclists. J Back Musculoskeletl Rehabil 2015;28:167–72.
42. Pardal-Fernandez G-M, Godes-Medrano B, Jerez-García P. Bilateral sacral radiculopathy in a cyclist. Electromyogr Clin Neurophys 2005;45:155–60.
43. Kotler DB. Preventon, Evaluation and Rehabilitation of Cycling-Related Injury. Curr Sports Med Rep 2016;15(3):199–206.
44. Lebec MT, Cook K, Baumgartel D. Overuse Injuries Assocated with Mountain Biking: Is Single-Speed Riding a Predisopsing Factor. Sports 2014;2:1–13, 10:3390/sports2010001.
45. Madden CC, P. M. Netter's sports medicine. (S. Edition, Ed.) Philadelphia: Saunders/Elsevier; 2018. p. 713-731.
46. Van Hoof W, Volkaerts K, O'Sullivan K, et al. Low back pain in cycling: does it matter how you sit? Br J Sports Med 2014;48(7):609.
47. Muyor JM, López-Miñarro PA, Alacid F. Spinal posture of thoracic and lumbar spine and pelvic tilt in highly trained cyclists. J Sports Sci Med 2011;10:355–61.
48. Salai M, Brosh T, Blankstein A, et al. Effect of changing the saddle angle on the incidence of low back pain in recereational bicyclists. Br J Sports Med 1999;33:398–400.
49. Konttinen YT, Grönblad M, Antti-Poika I, S Seitsalo. Neuroimmunohistochemical Analysis of Peridiscal Nociceptive Neural Elements. Spine 1990;15(5):383–6.
50. Nachemson A. Towards a better understanding of low-back pain: a review of the mechanics of the lumbar disc. Rheumatol Rehabil 1975;14(3):129–43.
51. Seppo OM, Kallinen M. Low back pain and other overuse injuries in a group of Japanese triathletes. Br J Sports Med 1996;30:134–9.
52. Silberman M. Bicycling Injuries. Sport Specif Illness Inj 2013;12(5):337–45.

Moving?

Make sure your subscription moves with you!

To notify us of your new address, find your **Clinics Account Number** (located on your mailing label above your name), and contact customer service at:

Email: journalscustomerservice-usa@elsevier.com

800-654-2452 (subscribers in the U.S. & Canada)
314-447-8871 (subscribers outside of the U.S. & Canada)

Fax number: 314-447-8029

Elsevier Health Sciences Division
Subscription Customer Service
3251 Riverport Lane
Maryland Heights, MO 63043

*To ensure uninterrupted delivery of your subscription, please notify us at least 4 weeks in advance of move.

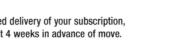

Printed and bound by CPI Group (UK) Ltd, Croydon, CR0 4YY

03/10/2024

01040473-0001